Managing Human Resources in Health Care Organizations

Leiyu Shi, DrPH, MBA, MPA

Co-Director
Primary Care Policy Center for Underserved Populations
Johns Hopkins Bloomberg School of Public Health
Department of Health Policy and Management

JONES AND BARTLETT PUBLISHERS
Sudbury, Massachusetts
BOSTON   TORONTO   LONDON   SINGAPORE

World Headquarters
Jones and Bartlett Publishers
40 Tall Pine Drive
Sudbury, MA 01776
978-443-5000
info@jbpub.com
www.jbpub.com

Jones and Bartlett Publishers
Canada
6339 Ormindale Way
Mississauga, Ontario L5V 1J2
CANADA

Jones and Bartlett Publishers
International
Barb House, Barb Mews
London W6 7PA
UK

Jones and Bartlett's books and products are available through most bookstores and online book-sellers. To contact Jones and Bartlett Publishers directly, call 800-832-0034, fax 978-443-8000, or visit our website www.jbpub.com.

Substantial discounts on bulk quantities of Jones and Bartlett's publications are available to corporations, professional associations, and other qualified organizations. For details and specific discount information, contact the special sales department at Jones and Bartlett via the above contact information or send an email to specialsales@jbpub.com.

Library of Congress Cataloging-in-Publication Data

Managing human resources in health care organizations / [edited by] Leiyu Shi.
    p. ; cm.
    Includes bibliographical references and index.
    ISBN-13: 978-0-7637-2997-4 (pbk.)
    ISBN-10: 0-7637-2997-3
    1. Health facilities—United States—Personnel management. I. Shi, Leiyu.
    [DNLM: 1. Personnel Management. 2. Health Facilities—organization & administration.
WX 159 M266 2006]
    RA971.35.M268 2006
    362.1068'3—dc22

                                        2006010088
6048

Production Credits
Publisher: Michael Brown
Associate Editor: Kylah Goodfellow McNeill
Production Director: Amy Rose
Production Editor: Renée Sekerak
Marketing Manager: Sophie Fleck
Manufacturing Buyer: Amy Bacus
Composition: ATLIS Graphics
Cover Design: Kristin E. Ohlin
Printing and Binding: Malloy, Inc.
Cover Printing: Malloy, Inc.

Printed in the United States of America
10 09 08 07 06   10 9 8 7 6 5 4 3 2 1

Contents

About the Editor

Dr. Leiyu Shi is an Associate Professor in the Department of Health Policy and Management at Johns Hopkins School of Public Health, and Co-Director of Johns Hopkins Primary Care Policy Center for the Underserved Populations. Dr. Shi's research focuses on primary care, health disparities, and vulnerable populations. He has conducted extensive studies about the association between primary care and health outcomes, particularly on the role of primary care in mediating the adverse impact of income inequality on health outcomes. Dr. Shi is also well-known for his extensive research on the nation's vulnerable populations, in particular community health centers that serve vulnerable populations, including their sustainability, provider recruitment and retention experiences, financial performance, experience under managed care, and quality of care. Dr. Shi is the author of six textbooks and over 100 journal articles.

Contributors

Steven D. Berkshire, EdD, MHA, SPHR, CHE
Associate Academic Dean
Regis University
Denver, Colorado

Karen S. Burnett, MA, SPHR
Regional Director, Human Resources
Urban North Region
Intermountain Healthcare
Salt Lake City, Utah

Mark Burns, PhD
Associate Professor
Auburn University
Auburn, Alabama

Daniel F. Fahey, PhD, MPH, FACHE
Associate Professor
Department of Health Science
California State University
San Bernardino, California

Kanak Gautam, MBA, PhD
Associate Professor
St. Louis University School of Public Health
St. Louis, Missouri

Donna L. Gellatly, MBA, FHFMA, CPA
University Professor
Health Administration Program
Governors State University
University Park, Illinois

Gretchen Gemeinhardt, PhD
Assistant Professor
Department of Healthcare Administration
Texas Woman's University
Houston, Texas

Lloyd Greene, EdD
Associate Professor
Texas State University
San Marcos, Texas

Harold Ray Griffin, MBA, PhD
Dean
DeVry University
Houston Galleria Center
Houston, Texas

Anne M. Hewitt, PhD, CHES
Assistant Professor
Graduate Department of Public
    and Healthcare Administration
Director
Seton Center for Community
    Health
Seton Hall University
South Orange, New Jersey

Marie L. Kotter, PhD
Professor and Department Chair
Health Sciences Department
Weber State University
Ogden, Utah

**Sarah Lindstrom, PhD
    Candidate**
Johns Hopkins Bloomberg School
    of Public Health
Johns Hopkins University
Baltimore, Maryland

Leiyu Shi, DrPH, MBA, MPA
Co-Director
Johns Hopkins Primary Care
    Policy Center for Underserved
    Populations
Johns Hopkins University
Baltimore, Maryland

Susan Sportsman, RN, PhD
Dean
College of Health Sciences and
    Human Services
Midwestern State University
Wichita Falls, Texas

**Charles F. Wainright III, MHA,
    PhD, FACHE**
Associate Professor and Program
    Director
Department of Public Health
Western Kentucky University
Bowling Green, Kentucky

Preface

PURPOSE

The purpose of this book is to explore how human resources management is applied in different healthcare settings. Each chapter explains both the current state of human resources management as well as suggests possible ways that human resources management could be altered in order to address a chronic challenge or adapt to a changing situation. Each of the chapters focuses on the major elements of human resources management, as well as discusses ways in which human resources can be used in the strategic planning of the organization. While the chapters individually could be used as a human resources how-to guide for a particular sector of the healthcare system, taken in its entirety the book offers a glimpse into the myriad of ways human resources management is applied in the healthcare setting and emphasizes its importance.

SCOPE

This book encompasses the human resource needs for the continuum of health care. Public health organizations are the first stage of this continuum as they attempt to prevent disease and disability. They do this through efforts at the population level (Chapters 4 and 5) as well as through efforts at the individual level (Chapter 10, 11, and 12). Managed Care Organizations also provide many prevention services as well as serving as a gateway into the healthcare system (Chapter 7). As a diagnosis becomes more serious or involves more intensive treatment or specialty care, healthcare may begin to take place in Hospitals (Chapter 8). And then as individuals' age and/or a disease or co-morbidities become chronic, care may start to take place in Long-Term Care Settings (Chapter 9). This book also acknowledges the different human resources needs of an Integrated Delivery System (Chapter 6) with its attempts to coordinate the continuum of care.

TARGETS

This book is aimed to be useful to both students and instructors in a variety of educational settings such as business colleges, nursing schools, public health schools, medical schools, allied health institutes, and healthcare administration programs, and current human resource managers. Students and instructors may find the book useful in its entirety in understanding the nuances of the applications of human resources in various healthcare settings. Students and instructors in practice and not management related fields may also find only specific chapters relate to their interests. This also may be true for current human resource managers or physicians operating in private practices or medical groups.

The book is written assuming little or no previous experience with human resources management. Chapter 3 is dedicated to a simple, but thorough explanation of the common features of human resources management. Technical terms both relating to human resources management and the healthcare setting are explained in a way that even a novice to both fields would understand.

ORGANIZATION

The first three chapters of the book offer an overview of the healthcare sector and its employees and the importance and significance in studying human resources. They also explain the essential components of human resources management and highlight important issues in human resources management in healthcare. The next eight chapters each deal with the human resources practices and issues of a specific healthcare setting. These eight chapters focus on recruitment, contract/agreement, training/ education/support, retention, performance evaluation, compensation, legal/regulatory issues, and strategic planning. Each of these chapters begins with a vignette that emphasizes the daily problems faced by human resources in that setting. The final chapter of the book addresses the key human resources challenges that have been identified in the eight setting specific chapters and offers an outlook for the future of human resources in the healthcare settings.

The organization of this book by healthcare setting and not by human resource function is what sets it apart from other books discussing healthcare human resources. Most healthcare human resource textbooks or guides are grouped according to human resource functions, for example, with chapters devoted to recruitment and compensation. By organizing this book by healthcare sector, a more in-depth analysis of the particulars of human resource management in the setting can be undertaken. It also then becomes more readily useful for human resources practitioners in each of the settings.

Leiyu Shi
Johns Hopkins University

Acknowledgments

The Editor would like to acknowledge the contributors of the chapters: Steven Berkshire, Mark Burns, Harold R. Griffin, Lloyd Greene, Kanak Gautam, Marie Kotter, Karen Burnett, Susan Sportsman, Donna L. Gellatly, Gretchen Gemeinhardt, Daniel F. Fahey, Anne Hewitt, and Charles F. Wainright III.

The Editor also gratefully acknowledges Sarah Lindstrom (Research Assistant) and Normalie Barton (Administrative Assistant), from Johns Hopkins University, for their work in putting this book together.

The assistance of the reviewers and editors from Jones and Bartlett is also greatly appreciated.

CHAPTER 1

Human Resources in the Healthcare Sector

Leiyu Shi and Sarah Lindstrom

The healthcare industry is the largest employer in the United States and by far the most labor-intensive. In 2002, the healthcare industry consisted of 518,000 organizations that employed 12.9 million individuals.[1] The healthcare sector accounts for 10.7% of all employment in the United States, with 41% of the healthcare workforce being employed in hospitals.[1] Besides being the largest employer, the healthcare industry is one of the fastest-growing industries in the United States. Ten out of 20 of the fastest-growing jobs are in health care, with 16% of all new job growth occurring in the healthcare industry.[1]

This sector's growth, size, and power are driven by an economy that spends $1 out of every $6 on health care, or more than $3,000 per person per year—$1,000 more than any other country.[2] The healthcare industry is second only to the manufacturing sector in terms of its dollar volume.[3] Healthcare costs exceed $1.3 trillion and consume almost 13% of the U.S. gross domestic product (GDP).[3] The amount spent on the U.S. healthcare system would make it the world's eighth largest economy,[3] and this amount seems to be rising, with projections that the health share of GDP will reach 17.7% in 2012.[4] Private healthcare expenditure growth in the mid-1990s was about 3–4%, but climbed to 8.4% in 2004.[4] This growth rate is troubling, as overall economic growth has not kept pace: The GDP growth rate was only 5.6% in 2004.[4]

The continuing growth of the healthcare industry is primarily due to two factors: increased use of technology and the continued aging of the baby boomer population.

Prompted by a specialist orientation in medical care and assisted by much more lucrative reimbursement streams that favor technology and specialization, the last few decades have seen significant developments in medical technology and its increased availability and use. This advancement in medical technology is most evident in the treatment of heart and circulatory ailments.[5] While it has proven effective at extending the lives of the sick (many with terminal illnesses), the new technology is invariably costly, and investment in it typically comes at the expense of preventive services, even though the latter might be more critical for improving the health of the general population.[3] Evidence-based outcome research on new technology is being advocated to identify beneficial technology that is not worth the cost.[5] Suggested evaluative questions include the following:

How does the new technology benefit the patient?

Is it worth the cost?

Are the new methods better than previous methods, and can they replace them?

Is treatment planning enhanced?

Is the outcome from disease better, or is the mortality rate improved?[3] (p. 22)

The second reason for the continuing growth of the healthcare industry is the aging of the baby boomer generation. This cohort will begin to reach retirement age in 2011. As the elderly are traditionally strong advocates of health care, the political importance of this group will begin to affect the healthcare sector.[6] As they age, the baby boomers may also place increased demands on the healthcare system. However, the extent of this increased demand is not known for certain. Advances in medicine and public health have created a generation of older people who are healthier and less disabled than their counterparts in the past.[7] Of course, these same advances have created a generation of elderly who expect to be physically active.[6] Additionally, medical technology advances promise to prolong the lives of chronically ill or severely injured patients.[1] While the baby boomer generation may be a burden in terms of services utilized, the medical technology improvements have resulted in a group of people who will be less of a labor drain on the healthcare system. Given that the elderly now expect to be productive later in life, potential changes in Social Security could increase the age of retirement and drop the earnings limit between the ages of 65 and 69. These changes will allow older employees to work later in life.[8]

Due to the increasing size of the healthcare system and the costs associated with it, reforms are being instituted that will change the healthcare industry from one dominated by providers' decisions, with no checks on costs or quality of care and no regard for consumer satisfaction, to a market-based system.[2] The market-based system encourages consolidation and coordination of care to reduce costs and improve services.[2] Coordination of care will make medical group practices and integrated health systems a more prominent feature of the healthcare industry. These trends have already resulted in most healthcare markets being dominated by a relatively few insurance providers. With market control comes the ability to compete for the business of large employers that are looking for ways to decrease their insurance costs.[2] In this way, healthcare systems create a cheaper product for both employees and employers, even as they improve the quality of services offered. Along with changing the healthcare market, integrated systems and medical group practices will increase the need for office and administrative support workers.[1]

These changes are not directed by a central entity, and the pace of change has differed among various areas, depending on the type of services offered and the system's organizing body. The healthcare system is massive, not only in terms of the number of organizations and the size of the workforce, but also in terms of the multiplicity of entities providing care. Figure 1-1 illustrates the potential providers of care, depending on the nature of the disease.

Against this backdrop of growth and change, the healthcare industry faces unprecedented challenges. Industry leaders and policymakers have to figure out the answer to the fundamental question of how to maintain and even enhance services to a growing population with increasingly more chronic health problems, and to do so while dealing with increasing financial constraints. In this chapter (and the rest of this book), we provide a human resources perspective while addressing this question. Although other perspectives (including other managerial components and policy, system, and culture) have to be considered, a clear understanding of the human resources issues in the healthcare sector is a prerequisite for instituting effective changes. Specifically, this chapter provides an overview of the human resources issues in the healthcare sector, and the remaining chapters focus on these issues in major public and private

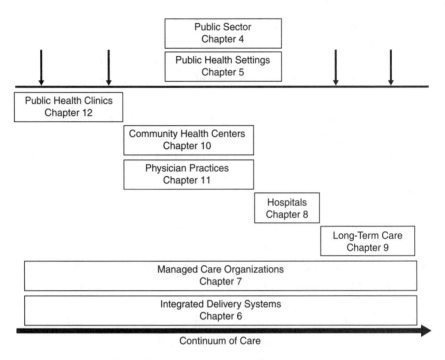

FIGURE 1-1   Providers Along the Continuum of Care

healthcare settings. We first identify the major human resources within the healthcare sector. Next we summarize the managerial functions related to human resources. We then discuss the challenges facing human resources professionals in the health sector and the legal environment in which they function. Human resources issues related to specific healthcare settings are highlighted as well. Finally, we identify future trends that will affect human resources development within the healthcare sector.

HEALTHCARE HUMAN RESOURCES

The healthcare industry is labor-intensive. The primary expenses for healthcare organizations are their salary-related costs. Large numbers of individuals are necessary to provide, record, and bill for the services provided to the patients. Contrary to common perception, the majority of jobs in the healthcare industry require fewer than four years of college.[1] More than half of all workers in nursing and residential care and one-fourth of those employed in hospitals have a high school diploma or less.[1]

While these jobs represent the majority of jobs, the healthcare industry also employs some of the workforce's most educated individuals as diagnostic and treatment practitioners.[1] Because of the high level of training required for these professionals, healthcare industry employees tend to be older than workers in other industries. The healthcare industry also has a sizable number of employees (16%) who work part-time.[1]

The occupations encompassed by the healthcare industry can be divided into professional and service occupations. This distinction would cover three-fourths of all jobs in the industry, with the remainder of the jobs belonging in office and administrative support and management, business, and financial operations.[1] Professional occupations include physicians, surgeons, dentists, nurses, social workers, and allied health workers. Service occupations include nursing aides, home health aides, building cleaning workers, dental assistants, medical assistants, and personal and home care aides. While it is impossible to discuss all of the jobs in the healthcare industry, this book will address a great many, albeit focusing more on the professional occupations than the service occupations.

Physicians

Physicians traditionally have been the focus of the healthcare industry. They are the people who primarily evaluate and diagnose patients' conditions and prescribe treatment. As health care has advanced and become more medically and technologically complex, more individuals are becoming involved in the evaluation, diagnosis, and treatment of health-related problems. Eventually demand for physician services may decrease due to this reliance on other providers.[1] Nevertheless, physicians still play key roles in health care and are the symbolic icons of the industry.

Not all physicians practice medicine; some are involved in research to find better methods to evaluate, diagnose, treat, and deliver health care. Those who do practice must be licensed in the state where they practice. A license requires graduation from an accredited school of medicine or osteopathic medicine (MD or DO degree). Following graduation, would-be physicians have to pass a licensing examination and complete a supervised internship/residency program.[9] Internship/residency is a form of paid on-the-job training that usually occurs in a hospital. Because of the need to fulfill these qualifications, it takes a long time to train a physician, and this long lead time determines how rapidly a response can be made to a physician shortage.

Currently, there are 126 accredited schools of medicine and 20 schools of osteopathic medicine in the United States. The differences between the schools' curricula and the types of doctors they produce deal less with accepted methods of treatment and more with philosophy. Osteopathic medicine, which is practiced by DOs, recognizes the "interrelationship between the body's nerves, muscles, bones, and organs" and "applies the philosophy of treating the whole person to the prevention, diagnosis, and treatment of illness, disease, and injury."[10] MDs are trained in and practice allopathic medicine—a type of medicine that involves an active intervention to alter a diseased state, in which the intervention might produce its own effects (known as side effects).

Because of their holistic approach to medicine, most DOs are considered generalists. Most MDs are specialists, with those practicing in family practice, internal medicine, or pediatrics being considered generalists or, more commonly, primary care physicians. Primary care physicians are usually the first to see a patient. They treat the person as a whole and therefore are more aware of the interrelations between conditions. In contrast, specialists are concerned usually with a specific organ or situation. With the advent of managed care, the gap between primary care physicians and specialists has grown, as primary care physicians are used as a "gatekeeping" mechanism. As a consequence, primary care physicians typically must first evaluate a patient before the patient receives a referral to a specialist.

Physicians work in a variety of settings. New physicians today are much less likely to enter into a single physician practice and more likely to take jobs in a managed care setting, an integrated system, or a group physician practice. This book discusses physicians in the context of federal, state, and local governments; integrated delivery systems; hospitals; long-term care; physician practices, community health centers; managed care; and public health clinics.

Dentists

Dentists provide care for teeth and mouth tissue. A dentist's duties might include filling cavities, performing corrective surgery on gums, replacing missing teeth with dentures, and providing preventive information on diet, brushing, and flossing. Like physicians, dentists must be licensed to practice. Licensure requirements include graduation from an accredited school of dentistry with a Doctor of Dental Surgery (DDS) or Doctor of

Dental Medicine (DMD) degree and completion of written and practical exams. Specialty dentists may be required to obtain a specialty license in certain states to practice.[9] Eight dental specialties are recognized by the American Dental Association: orthodontics, oral and maxillofacial surgery, pediatric dentistry, periodontics, prosthodontics, endodontics, public health dentistry, and oral pathology.[11]

Most dentists work in solo practices. As a consequence, they must oversee many administrative tasks, such as bookkeeping, buying equipment, and hiring staff such as dental hygienists and dental assistants to provide preventive dental care (i.e., cleanings). The solo nature of most dental practices reflects the fact that dentistry has been traditionally left out of the healthcare industry's cost and management structure decisions and, therefore, has remained a cottage industry. In actuality, dentistry services represent 7% of all healthcare expenditures.[2] The field of dentistry is expected to grow more slowly than the average for all occupations through 2012.[1] The baby boomer generation's retirement, however, may provide more opportunities for dentists, as older patients typically need more complicated dental services. Dental offices may also find more of their work centering on prevention efforts, which means greater demand for dental hygienists and dental assistants. Another area of growth may lie in providing dental services to underserved populations who do not have dental coverage.[3]

Pharmacists

Pharmacists traditionally dispense medications prescribed by physicians and nonphysician providers and provide information about usage to patients. Recently, pharmacists have begun to play a role in comprehensive drug therapy management, which is a collaborative process of selecting drug therapies, educating patients, monitoring patients, and continually assessing outcomes of therapy. A license is required to practice pharmacy in all 50 states; it is granted to graduates of one of the 85 accredited schools of pharmacy (PharmD). Additionally, pharmacists must pass the North American Pharmacist Licensure Exam (NAPLEX) and the Multistate Pharmacy Jurisprudence Exam (MPJE) or, in California, the California Pharmacy Jurisprudence Exam.

A pharmacist shortage was recognized in the 1980s.[12] This shortage was attributed to a rapid increase in the demand for pharmacists and an inability to increase the supply of pharmacists due to limited slots for pharmacist education.[12] Additionally, a downturn in pharmacy school applications occurred during the 1990s.[1, 12] This shortage of workers resulted in sharp increases in salaries for pharmacists, especially in community pharmacies, which have particular difficulty filling positions.[12] New developments in genome research and medication distribution and greater coverage of prescription drugs by more health insurance plans and by Medicare could result in an increase in prescription drug usage, which could make the shortage of pharmacists even worse in the future.

Allied Health Workers

There are more than 200 allied health occupations; workers in these occupations represent 60% of the U.S. healthcare workforce.[3] These workers assist physicians, dentists, and other health professionals in the evaluation, diagnosis, and treatment of patients' conditions. They are also employed in health education, disease prevention, and environmental health control. Allied health professionals can be classified into four (and sometimes more) categories: laboratory technologists and technicians, therapeutic science practitioners, behavioral sciences, and support services.[3] Laboratory technologists and technicians are involved in the application of highly technical procedures that aid in the diagnosis and treatment of disease or in the monitoring of the effectiveness of treatment. This category includes radiologic technologists, nuclear medicine technologists, medical technologists, and cytotechnologists, among others. Therapeutic science practitioners are involved in the treatment of patients. This category includes physical therapists, occupational therapists, speech pathologists, radiation therapists, respiratory therapists, dietitians, dental hygienists, and nonphysician practitioners. Behavioral scientists are involved in health education and disease prevention activities. Behavioral science professions include social workers, rehabilitation counselors, and health educators. The support services category includes jobs created to cope with the complexity of the healthcare system. These personnel usually work behind the scenes and include health information administrators, dental laboratory technologists, electroencephalagraphic technologists, food service administrators, and surgical technologists, among others.

Training for allied health professionals depends on the type of job being performed. Laboratory technologists/technicians and support services personnel usually require fewer than two years of secondary education, with most skills being learned on the job. Jobs in the therapeutic science practitioners and behavioral sciences fields usually require a bachelor's or master's degree and accreditation by the field's professional body.

Nonphysician Practitioners

Nonphysician practitioners (NPPs) provide healthcare services in areas similar to those of physicians, but do not have an MD or DO degree. They include physician assistants (PAs), who provide care under the direction of a physician; nurse practitioners (NPs), who provide mostly primary care; and certified nurse midwives (CNMs), who are involved in gynecological and obstetric care. In 2001, 103,600 NPs and PAs practiced medicine, as well as 8,000 CNMs.[13]

PAs are trained to perform diagnostic, preventive, and therapeutic services, as delegated by a physician. In 47 states and the District of Columbia, they can prescribe medication. While PAs must work under the supervision of a physician, the level of supervision may differ depending on the setting. For example, in rural or inner-city areas, the physician may be present only one or two days or by phone consultation. Most PAs work in primary care settings and provide evaluation, monitoring, diagnostics, therapeutics, counseling, and referral services.[14] Others specialize in general or thoracic surgery, emergency medicine, orthopedics, and geriatrics.[1] Most PA programs take two years to complete and require two previous years of college and some healthcare experience.

NPs are the largest group of nonphysician practitioners, although their new enrollments are gradually declining.[15] These registered nurses (RNs) have completed some additional training (either a certificate program or a master's degree), allowing them to practice in an expanded capacity. Most NPs must also complete clinical training in direct patient care to be certified. NPs are primarily interested in patient education and spend extra time with patients to help them understand their role in their treatment. Their specialties include pediatric, family, adult, psychiatric, and geriatric medicine.

Certified nurse midwives are RNs with additional training from a nurse midwifery program. They are certified by the American College of Nurse-Midwives (ACNM). CNMs provide care for normal expectant mothers, and refer abnormal or high-risk pregnancies to physicians or jointly manage their care. CNMs are less likely to continuously and electronically monitor a birth, induce labor, or use epidural anethesia.

Nurses

Nurses provide primary care to patients in both hospital and clinic settings. Duties for nurses differ, depending on the type of setting in which they work. Nurses work in hospitals, nursing homes, private practice, ambulatory care centers, community and migrant health centers, emergency medical centers, managed care organizations, worksites, government and private agencies, clinics, schools, retirement communities, and rehabilitation centers. Because of the trends toward discharging patients from hospitals faster and performing many procedures in outpatient settings, nurses are increasingly being employed by outpatient centers and home healthcare organizations.

Nurses must be licensed to practice. Licensure is achieved by graduating from an accredited nursing school and completing a national exam. Two levels of practice are distinguished among nurses. Registered nurses (RNs) complete an associate degree, a diploma program, or a baccalaureate degree; these programs take between two and five years to complete. Licensed practical nurses (LPNs) complete a state-approved program that lasts about one year.

HUMAN RESOURCES: FUNCTIONS

Like other service industries, the healthcare industry aims to provide services to people. Unlike in most service industries, however, the work provided is actually on the person who seeks assistance. This level of trust mandates an intimate relationship, one whose intimacy has recently been protected by legislation (the Health Insurance Portability and Accountability Act). People skills, it can be argued, are not just important for employees of the healthcare industry, but imperative.

The human resources department of any healthcare entity is responsible for the people side of the business. Not only must the human resources department protect and encourage the quality of the patient's relationship with the healthcare entity, but it also must protect and encourage the quality of the employee's relationship with the healthcare entity. For employees of the healthcare industry to provide compassionate and considerate care, their job satisfaction is important. In this section, we summarize the major managerial functions surrounding human resources.

Strategic Planning

Strategic planning is a process of matching the human resources of an organization with its goals and objectives. It implies an active process of determining key personnel and skills needed for the attainment of organizational progress. When this determination is made, gaps in personnel and skills can be discovered and can guide recruitment or training programs. In strategic human resources planning, the human resources department is an important member of the executive committee.

Recruitment and Selection

Effective recruitment and selection allow hiring of the best candidate with the needed skills. Recruitment efforts should be tailored to attract the desired candidates and should use recruiting avenues that have the greatest possibility to attracting these individuals. When recruiting for new positions, it is important to recruit internally as well as externally, because a member of the current staff may be appropriate for the position or may know someone who is qualified for the position. One advantage of internal recruiting is that the staff member already knows and presumably fits into the organizational culture. Organizational culture consists of the external environment, which shapes the economic situation of the organization; the organization's values or philosophy; the current staffing situation; the rites and rituals of the organization, which are manifested in its daily routine; and the organization's network of communication.

Retention

Recruiting and selecting the "right" people will help greatly with retention of staff. While it is important to ensure that new recruits will fit into the organizational culture, it is also critical to assess the organizational culture to ensure that it is not a source of retention problems. For example, doctors' lack of respect for nurses in some organizations, as well as system-wide, has created a retention problem for nurses. The process of recruitment, selection, and training is intensive and expensive, in both actual costs and opportunity costs, and should be avoided if at all possible.

Compensation and Benefits

One factor that will enhance retention of workers is high compensation and—perhaps even more important than compensation—good benefits. Compensation is usually based on the education and skills needed to perform the job. However, in this age of professional shortages and competition for certain types of healthcare providers, compensation for certain classes of professionals has been elevated as a recruitment strategy, and many organizations are also offering hiring bonuses. Likewise, organizations now recognize the importance of nonmonetary incentives and rewards and are structuring their benefits packages to include not only health care, but also childcare services and gym memberships.

Performance Evaluation

Performance evaluation is a way to define the level of competence of an employee as measured against a certain standard level of skills and knowledge. In the busy environment of health care, performance evaluation is reported to be difficult, in terms of both finding the time to assess an employee's performance and actually attaining a meaningful evaluation. To encourage the practice of performance evaluation, many healthcare organizations—especially integrated healthcare systems—are implementing, "pay for performance" compensation plans. Pay raises in these systems and perhaps even base pay are linked to quantifiable skills and/or results. Pay for performance can be based on individual, team, or organizational goals.

Training and Education

Due to the highly regulated environment in which health care operates, training and education are not merely important for organizational efficiency, but mandated in many cases by the Joint Council on Accreditation of Healthcare Organizations (JCAHO). Many healthcare providers are required to pass yearly competency examinations to prove they possess certain skills. Besides satisfying such legal obligations, training and education are important to stay abreast of new technological developments. Given the rapid pace of healthcare information growth, keeping staff up-to-date on new developments in diagnostic and treatment information and technology is challenging. It is the human resources department's duty to ensure that the organization has this knowledge.

Legal and Regulatory Issues

In addition to training and education mandates, healthcare organizations must be cognizant of the legal and regulatory issues related to human resources in general, especially safety of the workplace and union regulations. Because of the potential for exposure to blood-borne pathogens and radiological substances, healthcare organizations must have appropriate safety measures in place to protect against any injury, as well as appropriate training to facilitate the use of these safety measures. These measures also protect the organization from unionization. Specific legal issues affecting the human resources practice in healthcare organizations will be discussed later in this chapter.

Figure 1-2 highlights the interconnectedness of human resources functions. It shows that human resources management does not occur in a vacuum, but rather in an environment governed strictly by laws and regulations coming either from the federal or state government or from within the organization itself. In this environment, the human resources functions are fluid, with the success of and need for one component being dependent on another component. For example, who is recruited and selected is determined by the staffing needs identified via strategic planning. Whether the desired individual actually accepts the offered position is determined by the compensation and benefits package. If the individual

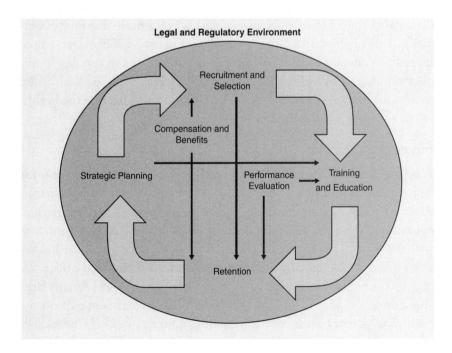

FIGURE 1-2 Integrated Human Resources Functions

accepts the position, his or her training and education needs will be determined by strategic planning indicators and the individual's current skill set. Successful recruitment and selection and training will, in turn, improve retention.

HUMAN RESOURCES: CHALLENGES

Health care is essential, so much so that care at certain levels is mandated by the government, and the elderly and poor populations, who are least likely to receive health insurance through an employer, are covered by government-sponsored insurance programs. Increasing awareness of the importance of preventive health care and the cost savings associated with such care is furthering discussions about how to change the healthcare system to be more proactive toward health. However, while the system realizes the importance of preventive efforts, new technological advances are simultaneously pushing the system toward treatment and curative focuses.

The United States has the most expensive healthcare system in the world. Because it is primarily a market-based system, cost is an important driver of change. However, change is difficult to achieve due to the complex nature of the healthcare system and its myriad stakeholders, whose interests frequently conflict. As most of the cost of health care lies in human resources, the study of the human resources issues of health care takes on an urgent nature. Some of the critical issues affecting the healthcare labor force are discussed in this section.

Increasing Demand

Demand for health care is determined by the amount of services for which patients will pay. This demand is influenced by insurance status, access to health care, health status, advice from providers, age, gender, and education. Given the changing demographics of the U.S. population, as well as the changing nature of disease, it is not surprising that the healthcare system is experiencing increasing demand. As mentioned earlier, the baby boomer generation will be at retirement age in 2011. As this large segment of the population ages, they will place greater demands on the healthcare system because of the increasing number of elderly individuals with chronic diseases. In 1999, more than 15% of Medicare beneficiaries reported having in excess of five chronic conditions.[16] Chronic conditions require more care. A 65-year-old with one chronic condition spends $1,000–$2,000 more on health care than a similar adult without a chronic condition.[17] Additionally, as care for chronic diseases improves and individuals with chronic disease live longer, these patients will consume a greater proportion of care given through the healthcare system.

Outdated System

The increased demands have made evident the fact that the U.S. healthcare system was designed for the treatment of acute diseases and, in its current state, cannot handle the continuous and coordinated care needed for chronic diseases.[18, 19] A system designed for acute care focuses on diagnosing the immediate problem and offers a treatment that will "fix" the problem in a short amount of time. It is not designed to encourage self-management skills or patient tracking.[18] System shortcomings have resulted in poor-quality health care, with fewer than half of all asthma, hypertension, diabetes, and depression patients receiving appropriate care.[18]

The system is also technology oriented, which, for the diagnosis and treatment of chronic diseases, has resulted in skyrocketing costs. These extreme costs have hindered healthcare access for patients with insurance (high copayments) and made it especially difficult for patients without insurance to obtain care. More than 45.8 million Americans currently lack health insurance.[20] These individuals have difficulty finding health care, especially preventive care, and are forced to seek the majority of their care from more expensive providers, such as hospital emergency rooms, which further escalates the overall cost of health care.

Medical reimbursement favors specialty care and treatment of patients with comorbidities. Preventive care, that delays onset of diseases or reduces symptoms, does not pay off to the practitioners.

Erosion in Caring and Personal Touch

Today there is a growing concern about the lack of human involvement— the doctor's touch—in the healthcare system. New technologies have altered almost every aspect of care and have replaced services that once were administered by the doctor. While these technologies may be as effective as the doctor's care, they do not offer the same level of personal attention. This depersonalization, along with the increasing regulation of care by insurance companies, has furthered the notion that the healthcare system is a business, all about science and the bottom line, and one that is abandoning the art of caring. There are also increasing concerns that many of the new technologies are not cost-effective and that their benefits to society do not outweigh their costs, especially when opportunity costs are considered.[21]

Increasing Dissatisfaction

In addition to the public concerns about the healthcare system, there is a growing dissatisfaction with the healthcare system within the healthcare sector. Physician satisfaction has been shown to consist of five domains: income, relationships, autonomy, practice, and broader market environment.[22] Managed care has greatly affected physician autonomy, by limiting which services are covered or requiring extensive preauthorization, as well as physician income, through prepaid capitation and other price-controlling mechanisms. High malpractice premiums have also diminished physician satisfaction, by changing the nature of the relationship between the patient and the provider, and by decreasing physicians' income.[22] By contrast, unhappiness with the healthcare system due to the long and hard work hours has been associated more with nurses than with physicians.[23] This dissatisfaction is partly contributing to the difficulty in recruiting nurses, which is also explained by their low and variable levels of compensation and the stressful environments in which they work.[23]

Shortages and Surpluses

In the professional occupations, some concern has been voiced about either an over- or under-supply of certain types of personnel. Because these professions require a tremendous amount of training, it is important to be able to predict the need for certain types of workers ahead of an actual crisis. The most pressing shortage among the healthcare industry's professional occupations is for nurses. There has been a 30-year decline in interest in nursing as a profession.[23] In addition to the adverse working conditions, the nursing shortage has been attributed to the poor state of physician–nurse relationships, demeaning media stereotypes, and hospitals' cost-cutting strategies.[24] Physicians often do not appreciate the fact that, although they may have more knowledge of disease processes, nurses have more in-depth nursing knowledge and a "local" understanding of how each patient is coping with the treatments he or she is receiving. Television shows and movies often portray physicians positively, as authority figures and as spokespersons. Few nurses are portrayed in the same way. Hospital cost-cutting tactics, such as the introduction of hospital reengineering and the development of clinical pathways intended to re-duce headcounts and substitute less skilled personnel wherever possible, have also contributed to the ongoing nursing shortage.

Because of this declining interest and lack of new nursing recruits, the nursing profession is one of the top 20 occupations that will be affected by the baby boomers' retirement.[23] The aging of the baby boomers will also in-crease the need for nurses, especially in long-term care settings.[1] The Bureau of Labor Statistics reports that employment of registered nurses is expected to grow faster than the average for all occupations through 2012.[1] Besides problems related to the low growth rate for the nursing workforce, health-care organizations have struggled to retain nurses. Job satisfaction among nurses is low. Nurses are frustrated with having little control over different aspects of their jobs.[23] Additionally, nursing wages have not kept pace with inflation, and the primary way for nurses to increase their salaries is to gain more education and leave the field to take on administrative jobs.[23] Suggestions for both recruitment into the nursing profession and improved retention include enhanced career ladders, better wages, flexible hours, and the provision of child care.[23] The real key, however, may lie in a better physician–nursing relationship and management recognition of nurses' pri-mary (rather than subsidiary) role in healthcare delivery.

Determining the future need for professionals has been made even more difficult by the tremendous specialization that has taken place among professional occupations, which is most obvious in the growing abundance of allied health professionals.[1] Allied health professions have begun to license their scopes of practice, requiring expanded time in pre-professional curricula, and exert tighter control over the accreditation processes for training programs.[1] This increased specialization, in combi-nation with the adoption of new technology (which may have been made possible by the increased specialization), have made the allied health pro-fessions the fastest-growing occupational group in the United States, with a 144% growth rate from 1970 to 1990.[1] In response to this intense spe-cialization and the costs that it brings, the healthcare system has made an effort to train multiskilled healthcare providers.

One driver of the growth in the allied health professions is the trend for clinical work to move to the least costly practitioner. This shift has resulted in increased employment of nonphysician clinicians. In the past decade, the number of patients seeing a nonphysician provider has increased; however, this trend seems to reflect more patients seeing both a nonphysician and a physician.[25] The use of nonphysician clinicians was supposed to address a shortage of physicians for underserved populations. In reality, this does not appear to be the case, as those patients who are more likely to see nonphysician clinicians tend to be white, be wealthy, and have insurance.[25]

Assessing physician shortage or surplus, achieving an appropriate mix of primary care and non–primary care physicians, a maldistribution of physicians between urban and rural areas, and a lack of minority physicians are critical health manpower issues that medicine has struggled with for the past 25 years.[26]

Physician Shortage/Surplus

In 1980, the Graduate Medical Education National Advisory Committee (GMENAC) concluded that the United States had a current surplus of physicians.[26] This surplus was expected to become even greater with the beginning of managed care and its emphasis on primary care providers and gate-keeping. In 2000, there were 780,000 physicians in the United States, about 140,000 more than the GMENAC had predicted.[26] However, even with the overabundance, a physician surplus does not seem to exist; indeed, there are indications that a shortage may exist.[6] The shortage is especially pronounced for those uninsured, publicly insured (particularly Medicaid), and under-insured. Unfortunately, just training more physicians is unlikely to resolve this shortage.

The initial concern regarding a shortage of physicians in the 1980s was accompanied by worries about the ratio of primary care physicians to specialists due to the expected impact of managed care. This concern led to numerous federal and state policies designed to encourage doctors to choose primary care and resulted in an increase of primary care physicians, although the ratio never stabilized at the proposed 50/50 split.[26] The United States still lags behind other industrialized countries when it comes to having a balanced primary and specialist care physician workforce, despite growing evidence linking primary care to better population health and specialist focus to adverse health outcomes.[27–35]

Provider Maldistribution

For the past 70 years, the ratio of physicians in rural areas versus urban locations has steadily declined.[36] This trend has been attributed to the social and cultural isolation of practicing in a rural location, the greater availability of hospitals and technology in urban areas, and physicians' desire to enjoy urban affluence.[36] In rural communities of about 10,000 people, there is a physician-to-person ratio of 6/100,000. In urban areas, this ratio is 300/100,000.[37] Physicians who were raised in a rural area or who received training from a medical school with a mission to train rural physicians are more likely to practice in rural areas.[37] This awareness has led to a call for medical schools to recruit more rural medical students and include rotations in rural areas.[37] Additionally, osteopathic physicians are more likely to practice in rural locations.[37] In another effort to encourage rural physicians, the National Health Service Corps offers loan repayment for medical graduates who practice in underserved areas, called health professional shortage areas (HPSAs). Some HPSAs are also located in urban areas.

Provider Diversity

In 1999, African Americans and Hispanic Americans each accounted for approximately 12% of the population in the United States; however, they made up only 2.6% and 3.5%, respectively, of the physician workforce. Native Americans are even more disproportionately represented; they account for 0.7% of the population but only 0.1% of all physicians.[38] Diversity in the physician workforce is important because it improves cultural competency. Cultural competency is the ability to understand how cultural and ethnic backgrounds affect the reasons patients come in for care, their perceptions and views about disease and treatment, and their interactions with the medical care setting. Another important reason for increasing the number of minorities in the physician workforce is that African American, Hispanic American, and Native American physicians are more likely to treat large numbers of minorities.[38] Given that the majority of the United States' designated HPSAs have large minority populations, it is reasonable to assume that an increase in the number of minority physicians would decrease the shortage of physicians in critical areas.

Emphasis on Efficiency

In the midst of the increased demand, staff shortages, and supply distribution issues, there has been an increasing demand for the healthcare system to become more efficient and productive. The impetus to achieve greater efficiency is driven by the desire to reduce the costs of health care. "A technically efficient healthcare system would only deliver care that improves health status and in a way that minimizes the use of society's resources."[39] In our market-based system, providers, insurance companies (including the government), and even patients all have an incentive to reduce costs.

Use of Electronic Medical Records

One trend related to efficiency is the greater reliance of electronic medical records (EMRs). EMRs are supposed to reduce paperwork, eliminate lost or misfiled medical records, ensure accuracy, and reduce medical errors.[40] The use of EMRs, however, has created concerns about the privacy of health information. To ensure that privacy is protected in this information era, Congress enacted the Health Insurance Portability and Accountability Act of 1996. Besides computerized medical records, technology has sought to improve efficiency and quality by installing error-prevention capabilities in pharmacies and using clinical reminder systems.

Medical Errors

The quality of our healthcare system has been put into doubt by medical errors that harm millions of Americans each year. Although some errors are due to incompetence of individual providers, the vast majority of errors are attributable to system deficiencies. In the drive for efficiency, systems still need to include checks to catch human errors. Maintaining quality care has become increasingly difficult as knowledge and technology have expanded, requiring the provider to know and do more. The Institute of Medicine, in its report, *Crossing the Quality Chasm: A New Healthcare System for the 21st Century,* has suggested six aims for improvement: safety, effectiveness, patient-centeredness, timeliness, efficiency, and equitable provision of care.[19] The human resources manager must address these tasks.

THE LEGAL ENVIRONMENT

To understand the legal and regulatory environment facing healthcare sector human resources, it is necessary to be aware of the laws and regulations that apply to the various human resources functions.

Federal Equal Employment Opportunity Laws

Title VII of the Civil Rights Act of 1964 prohibits employment discrimination based on race, color, religion, sex, or national origin. The Civil

Rights Act of 1991 amended Title VII to allow for recovery of compensatory and punitive damages for violations of Title VII and the Americans with Disabilities Act.

The Americans with Disabilities Act of 1990 requires employers of more than 15 employees to provide individuals with disabilities an equal opportunity for employment-related benefits. This act prevents discrimination in recruitment, selection, compensation, promotion, and social activity. It also mandates that employers make accommodations for physical and mental disabilities unless it results in undue financial and administrative hardships.

The Equal Pay Act of 1963 prohibits sex-based wage discrimination for male and female employees of the same company performing similar functions.

The Age Discrimination in Employment Act of 1967 prohibits employment discrimination against potential or current employees over the age of 40. It especially protects workers from being fired or forced to retire simply due to their age.

General Employment Laws

The Fair Labor Standards Act of 1938 established minimum-wage, overtime pay, record-keeping, and child labor standards. This act applies to both full- and part-time workers in both the private and public sectors. It sets the minimum wage at $5.15 per hour for nonexempt employees and mandates payment of 1.5 times an employee's regular salary for time worked over 40 hours.

The Social Security Act of 1935 provided the mechanism for a social insurance program funded through a dedicated payroll tax. After workers retire, they are eligible for a monthly payment that depends on their cumulative earnings record. The act also provides for continued payment for surviving spouses and/or children of deceased workers and a graduated payment due to loss of earnings due to disability. In 2005, the tax was 6.2% of the first $90,000, paid by the employee, and a matching contribution paid by the employer.

The National Labor Relations Act of 1935 protects the right of employees to organize and bargain collectively with their employer. The act prohibits discrimination in hiring, compensation, or promotion based on membership in a union and establishes rules of conduct for both the employer and the union. In health care, these requirements include a mandatory advance notice of strike or picketing to ensure that the healthcare organization has time to organize for continued patient care.

Benefits

The Employment Retirement Income Security Act (ERISA) of 1974 sets minimum standards of protection for pension and health plans voluntarily established by private industry. ERISA requires employers to provide comprehensive information about the plans, gives responsibilities to those who manage the plans, and allows employees to submit grievances and sue based on a breach of those responsibilities.

The Consolidated Omnibus Budget Reconciliation Act (COBRA) of 1986 gives employees and their health dependents the right to continue their health benefits for a limited amount of time. Qualified individuals may be required to pay up to 102% of the cost of benefits. Voluntary or involuntary loss of a job, transition between jobs, reduction in hours worked, death, and divorce qualify as events that would allow for the continuation of health benefits.

The Family and Medical Leave Act of 1993 requires employers to grant up to a total of 12 weeks of unpaid leave during any 12-month period. The following reasons qualify an employee for leave: birth and care of a newborn child, placement of a son or daughter for adoption or foster care, care for an immediate family member with a serious health condition, or medical leave when the employee is unable to work due to a serious health condition.

Safety

The Occupational Safety and Health Act of 1970 requires employers to provide a place of employment that is free from hazards that are known to cause death or serious harm, such as exposure to toxic chemicals, excessive noise levels, mechanical dangers, heat or cold stress, and unsanitary conditions. The act also mandates that the Secretary of Labor establish and regularly review work safety standards.

Worker's compensation laws provide compensation to employees who are injured, disabled, or killed while performing a job. Some of these laws also provide for reimbursement for medical care following a work-related injury or disability and eliminate the liability of co-workers. Worker's compensation laws are the domain of state governments and therefore vary between states.

Health-Related Regulations

The Health Insurance Portability and Accountability Act (HIPAA) of 1996 protects coverage for members of group health plans. It prevents discrimination against employees based on health status and allows for the purchase of individual insurance after COBRA benefits have been exhausted. The act also required medical records to be computerized by October 2003 to better ensure the privacy of patients' health information.

MAJOR HUMAN RESOURCE'S ISSUES IN THE HEALTHCARE SETTING

The preceding sections dealt with human resources and legal issues facing the healthcare sector globally. This section highlights human resources challenges for specific healthcare settings, which will be discussed in-depth in later chapters of this book.

The Public Sector (Chapter 4)

The public sector (including federal, state, and local levels) has traditionally played a subsidiary role to the private sector in healthcare delivery. This position has caused the federal and state governments' involvement to consist of "stop-gap" programs that are not rationally developed. Because these programs are implemented as add-ons to private sector programs, there is a lack of coordination, both between the private sector and the government and among the government programs themselves, which occasionally results in the duplication of certain services and in attention to most other needed services. This lack of coordination is partly caused by the turnover in key staff with each change of the presidential administration. In addition, these programs are susceptible to funding cuts in times of economic downturns, as public health is generally considered a low-priority area.

The Public Health Sector (Chapter 5)

Public health departments at the state and local levels are responsible for a multitude of diverse issues. While certain public health problems require constant attention, others are deemed important due to a sudden outbreak or for a political reason. The federal government, through both regulation and funding, sets many of the state and local public health departments' priorities. State and local public health departments are also considered low priority and often find their funding cut. As a consequence, state and local public health workers are poorly paid, which makes recruitment and retention difficult. This issue will emerge as an even greater problem in the next few years, when the majority of the public health workforce will reach retirement age.

Integrated Delivery Systems (Chapter 6)

For integrated delivery systems (IDS) to be effective, strategic planning is paramount. If IDS hopes to be financially viable and improve the coordination of patient care, the various aspects of the healthcare system must work together efficiently. This working relationship is determined by the level of functional, clinical, and physician integration and the presence of an integrated information system. Achieving such a level of integration will be costly and difficult to obtain. In addition, maintaining a cost-cutting focus while ensuring effective staffing and a supportive organizational structure can be difficult.

Managed Care Organizations (Chapter 7)

Managed care providers assume financial responsibility for their patients' care and, therefore, have an incentive to provide quality care at the lowest cost possible. However, there has been a backlash against heavily regulated care models. In response, managed care organizations (MCOs) are reworking their structures to support patient decision making about cost. This revised role might include copayments and premium shifts or the use of preferred provider organizations (PPOs) rather than health maintenance organizations (HMOs). In another effort to reduce costs, MCOs also try to use the lowest-cost provider to deliver services, such as non-clinician providers. Many MCOs are also using nurses in nontraditional roles to design wellness and disease management programs in an attempt to reduce the costs of treating chronic diseases.

Hospitals (Chapter 8)

Hospitals have long been the cornerstone of the healthcare industry. The majority of healthcare expenses are incurred in hospitals, and the majority of healthcare workers work in hospitals. Simply because of the sheer number of staff required in these facilities, professional staffing shortages—especially nursing shortages—are a major issue facing hospitals. Nurses often leave the hospital to work in less stressful environments that allow them to have more professional autonomy, such as outpatient clinics. Hospitals are also concerned about the transfer of many types of procedures and care to these outpatient settings, and many are partnering with outpatient clinics in an effort to increase their revenues.

Long-Term Care Facilities (Chapter 9)

An aging population will require greater assistance for individuals as they lose some of their functional capacity. In the past, this care was provided primarily by nursing home services that would house, feed, and deliver nursing care to their clients. Recently, because of the high cost of care, limited insurance coverage, and perceived quality-of-care issues, many new types of long-term care have emerged. These new delivery arrangements include adult day care, home health care, assisted living services, and hospice services. Nursing homes must compete with these new providers for clients. However, these new providers have also encountered financial pressures, as Medicare has capped the number of visits and reimbursement levels.

Community Health Centers (Chapter 10)

Community health centers are safety-net providers offering primary care to vulnerable populations, such as uninsured or underinsured individuals, racial and ethnic minorities, and low-income patients. These health centers face unprecedented challenges as public funding sources dry up while the demand for care from a growing indigent population increases. In addition, recruiting and retaining healthcare providers to work in underserved areas is a constant battle. To continue serving vulnerable populations, health centers must work to identify new funding sources, continuously improve the quality of health care, deliver health care in a cost-effective manner, and ensure that their compensation packages for providers are competitive.

Physician Practices (Chapter 11)

A physician practice is a group of three or more physicians who share operating expenses and income. This type of collaboration is seen as a necessity, given that reimbursement rates have been on the decline and malpractice insurance costs are rising, which has decreased physicians' income. Additionally, the cost of operating a physician's office is increasing due to the trend for more complicated procedures to be performed in outpatient settings; such procedures involve more staff and require more expensive equipment. Pooling of resources and sharing of these overhead costs are, therefore, major benefits of a physician practice arrangement.

Public Health Clinics (Chapter 12)

Public health clinics are operated by local public health departments or municipality governments and are the only health agencies to heavily emphasize prevention of disease and disability. Recently, these facilities have begun to offer bioterrorism-related programs in response to pressure from local government officials. It is also the responsibility of public health clinics to provide emergency screening or care in the event of an emergency. However, public health clinics are also finding that they are serving more of a transitional role in care due to expansions in Medicaid and the State Children's Health Insurance Program. Unfortunately, because of state and local budget constraints, many of the facilities have stopped offering primary clinical services. These local clinics are attempting to partner with a variety of other organizations to help provide care.

THE FUTURE OF HEALTHCARE DELIVERY

Human resources management is an important component of healthcare delivery. In large and small healthcare organizations alike, human resources personnel are being asked to coordinate or participate in strategic planning exercises to address and anticipate problems with the delivery of healthcare. More and more, the importance of human capital is being recognized as essential for the success and stability of healthcare organizations.

Human resources management is needed to prepare for the anticipated demands of the baby boomer generation. The aging of this cohort will most likely place an increased burden on the healthcare system, with an increased number of chronic diseases being thrown into the case mix. To successfully treat these patients, especially those with more than one chronic condition, healthcare providers must stay current on evidence-based guidelines, and healthcare organizations must have systems in place to ensure that these evidence-based guidelines are implemented for each patient. Human resources management will also need to promote healthcare settings that encourage self-management skills for patients. This might involve increasing the number of nonphysician clinicians. Nonphysician clinicians' time is less costly, and their focus tends to be more on patient education. Additionally, the patient (especially the older patient) will view this extra time and "caring touch" positively.

Another important issue human resources must address is the increasing dissatisfaction of healthcare providers. Healthcare organizations need to become more politically active in addressing the issue of malpractice insurance for physicians. Besides encouraging governmental regulation, healthcare organizations could offer to pay part or all of practicing physicians' malpractice insurance. These organizations also need to find ways to encourage both the recruitment and the retention of nurses. A nursing shortage currently exists because of discontent with wages, which makes it difficult to recruit new nurses, and because of difficulty in holding on to nurses, who are often frustrated with the lack of career advancement opportunities and the job's long hours. Increasing pay for nurses, instituting career ladders, creating a more collaborative environment between physicians and nurses, and offering flexible schedules are all ways human resources managers in healthcare settings could try to improve nurse recruitment and retention.

Rural and urban area healthcare organizations face recruitment and retention problems for both nurses and physicians. To persuade physicians to practice in these areas, healthcare organizations need to encourage medical schools to recruit from rural and urban areas. This trend would improve the physician supply in these areas, as physicians born or raised in rural or urban areas are more likely to practice in these settings. It would also improve the diversity of the physician workforce, as recruiting in urban areas would primarily recruit African American and Hispanic American medical students.

The healthcare system must address all of these problems within an increasingly strict regulatory and legal environment. It is paramount that human resources management be involved in any change to ensure that the change satisfies the legal and regulatory boundaries. There is much opportunity for change in the healthcare system, but such change will require the appropriate vision and the right human capital.

REFERENCES

1. U.S. Department of Labor. Bureau of Labor Statistics. 2005. Available at: www.bls.gov. Accessed July 20, 2005.

2. Pew Health Professions Commission. Critical Challenges: Revitalizing the Health Professions for the Twenty-First Century. 1995. Available at: www.futurehealth.ucsf.edu/compubs.html. Accessed July 30, 2005.
3. Sultz HA, Young KM. *Health Care USA: Understanding Its Organization and Delivery.* Sudbury, MA: Jones and Bartlett; 2004.
4. Evans M. Healthcare inflation plateaus. *Modern Healthcare.* 2005; 26:8–9.
5. Pauly MV. Should we be worried about high real medical spending growth in the United States? *Health Affairs.* 2003; 3:15–27.
6. Cooper RA. Weighting the evidence for expanding physician supply. *Annals of Internal Medicine.* 2004; 141:705–714.
7. Garber AM, Sox HC. The U.S. physician workforce: serious questions raised, answers needed. *Annals of Internal Medicine.* 2004; 141:732–734.
8. Dohm A. Gauging the labor force effects of retiring baby-boomers. *Monthly Labor Review.* 2000; 123:17–25.
9. Stanfield PS. *Introduction to the Health Professions.* Boston: Jones and Bartlett; 1995.
10. American Osteopathic Association. 2005. Available at: www.osteopathic.org. Accessed August 15, 2005.
11. American Dental Association. 2005. Available at: www.ada.org. Accessed August 15, 2005.
12. Knapp KK, Quist RM, Walton SM, Miller LM. Update on the pharmacist shortage: national and state data through 2003. *American Journal of Health-System Pharmacy.* 2005; 62:492–499.
13. Hooker RS, Berlin LE. Trends in the supply of physician assistants and nurse practitioners in the United States. *Health Affairs.* 2002; 5:174–181.
14. Fitzgerald MA, Jones E, Lazar B, McHugh M, Wang C. The midlevel provider: colleague or competitor. *Patient Care.* 2005; 29:20–37.
15. Cooper RA, Laud P, Dietrich CL. Current and future projected workforce of nonphysician clinicians. *Journal of the American Medical Association.* 1998; 25:140–154.
16. Anderson GF, Shea DG, Hussey PS, Keyhani S, Zephyrin L. Doughnut holes and price controls. *Health Affairs.* 2004; W4:396–404.
17. Foyce GF, Keeler EB, Shang B, Goldman DP. The lifetime burden of chronic disease among the elderly. *Health Affairs.* 2005; W5:18–29.
18. Wagner EH, Austin BT, Davis C, Hindmarsh M, Schafear J, Bonomi A. Improving chronic illness care: translating evidence into action. *Health Affairs.* 2000; 20:64–78.
19. Institute of Medicine. *Crossing the Quality Chasm.* 2001. Available at: www.iom.edu. Accessed October 10, 2005.
20. U.S. Census Bureau. Health Insurance Data. 2004. Available at: www.census.gov. Accessed October 6, 2005.
21. Mendelson DN, Abramson, RG, Rubin RJ. State involvement in medical technology assessment. *Health Affairs.* 1995; 14:83–98.
22. Mello MM, Studdert DM, DesRoches CM, Peugh J, Zapert K, Brennan TA, Sage WM. Caring for patients in a malpractice crisis: physician satisfaction and quality of care. *Health Affairs.* 2004; 23:42–53.

23. Sochalski J. Nursing shortage redux: turning the corner on an enduring problem. *Health Affairs.* 2002; 21:157–164.
24. Gordon S. *Nursing Against the Odds: How Health Care Cost Cutting, Media Stereotypes, and Medical Hubris Undermine Nurses and Patient Care.* Ithaca, NY: Cornell University Press; 2005.
25. Druss BG, Marcus SC, Olfson M, Tanielian MA, Pincus HA. Trends in care by nonphysician clinicians. *New England Journal of Medicine.* 2003; 348:130–137.
26. Salsber ES, Forte GJ. Trends in the physician workforce, 1980–2000. *Health Affairs.* 2002; 21:165–173.
27. Shi L. Primary care, specialty care, and life chances. *International Journal of Health Services.* 1994; 24:431–458.
28. Shi L. Balancing primary versus specialty care. *Journal of the Royal Society of Medicine.* 1995; 88:428–432.
29. Shi L, Starfield B, Kennedy B, Kawachi I. Income inequality, primary care, and health indicators. *Journal of Family Practice.* 1999; 48:275–284.
30. Shi L, Starfield B. Primary care, income inequality, and self-rated health in the United States: a mixed-level analysis. *International Journal of Health Services.* 2000; 30:541–555.
31. Shi L, Starfield B. The effect of primary care physician supply and income inequality on mortality among blacks and whites in U.S. metropolitan areas. *American Journal of Public Health.* 2001; 91:1246–1250.
32. Shi L, Macinko J, Starfield B, Wulu J, Regan J, Politzer R. The relationship between primary care, income inequality, and mortality in U.S. states, 1980–1995. *Journal of the American Board of Family Practice.* 2003; 16:412–422.
33. Shi L, Macinko J, Starfield B, Xu J, Politzer R. Primary care, income inequality, and stroke mortality in the United States: a longitudinal analysis, 1985–1995. *Stroke.* 2003; 34:1958–1964.
34. Shi L, Macinko J, Starfield B, Xu J, Regan J, Politzer R, Wulu J. Primary care, infant mortality, and low birth weight in the states of the USA. *Journal of Epidemiology and Community Health.* 2004; 58:374–380.
35. Shi L, Macinko J, Starfield B, Politzer R, Wulu J, Xu J. Primary care, social inequalities, and all-cause, heart disease, and cancer mortality in U.S. counties, 1990. *American Journal of Public Health.* 2005; 95:674–680.
36. Colwill JM, Coltice JM. The future supply of family physicians: implications for rural America. *Health Affairs.* 2003; 22:190–198.
37. American Academy of Family Physicians. Rural Practice, Keeping Physicians in. 2002. Available at: www.aafp.org/x16635.xml. Accessed October 7, 2005.
38. Cohen JJ, Gabriel BA, Terrell C. The case for diversity in the health care workforce. *Health Affairs.* 2002; 21:90–102.
39. Nichols LM, Ginsburg PB, Berenson RA, Christianson J, Hurley RE. Are market forces strong enough to deliver efficient health care systems? Confidence is waning. *Health Affairs.* 2004; 23:8–21.
40. Himmelstein DU, Woolhandler S. Hope and hype: predicting the impact of electronic medical records. *Health Affairs.* 2005; 24:1121–1123.

CHAPTER 2

The Practice of Human Resources Management in the 21st-Century Healthcare Organization

Steven D. Berkshire

While the opening chapter has provided an overview of human resources in the healthcare sector, this chapter concentrates on some current issues affecting the practice of human resources management, discusses the challenge of finding and retaining competent people, and points to where human resources go from here.

CURRENT ISSUES

People are at the heart of any healthcare organization, whether that organization is a major research teaching hospital, a primary healthcare clinic in the inner city, the county public health office, or a health maintenance organization. All too often, administrators, third-party payers, government, and even boards of directors see only the patients and technology. In reality, as all healthcare professionals know, it is the people behind the technology, treatment protocols, services, and activities of the organization who ensure quality care. How healthcare organizations manage and invest in their human capital truly impacts the quality of care and services provided.

The way in which healthcare organizations structure and manage human resources is probably more important as we enter the 21st century than it has ever been. The world of the 21st century affects the management of human resources as much as it does the practice of medicine or the provision of public health services to the citizens of a community. How managers respond to employment issues, compensation planning, performance management, and employee relationship issues is affected by changes in the economic and social environments that healthcare organizations find themselves in. Obviously, third-party reimbursements come to mind as a major contributor to managing people—how many people, of what skill level and profession, are needed to cost-effectively deliver care and services without adversely affecting quality. Medicare and Medicaid reimbursement and quality standards have much to say about the numbers of professionals needed and the skill levels at which they must perform. Consumer demands on healthcare facilities and organizations often dictate response times and services that must be provided to stay competitive. Political leaders at the local, state, and national levels influence policy that impacts staffing levels, both in healthcare facilities and public health agencies. The balance between staying within approved budgetary boundaries and maintaining adequate staffing to ensure quality lies at the heart of many disagreements between management and clinicians. In addition, the competition for scarce skills and abilities within the pool of available professionals remains a troublesome issue for healthcare executives.

Third-party reimbursement practices are increasingly affecting the way healthcare providers staff hospitals, long-term care facilities, clinics, and public health agencies. Most expenses in healthcare organizations are related to people, as health care is a people-intensive industry. If an organization's competitors can provide a particular service at a lower cost, the quickest way to look for savings is to scrutinize the type, quality, and efficiency of the people providing care. In the late 1980s and the 1990s, for example, healthcare facilities looked for ways to reduce their dependence on people, especially higher-cost professionals such as registered nurses. Several projects examined ways to "right-size" hospitals, and long-term care facilities considered how to use nursing assistants more. The late 1990s brought a negative reaction to these moves, prompting healthcare executives to reverse these efforts to find lower-cost people to provide care. Both physician groups and other professional organizations recognized the need for higher levels of professionals and technicians to provide services and care. Accrediting bodies, such as the Joint Commission on Accreditation of Healthcare Organizations (JCAHO), published specific standards and criteria related to the expertise and skill levels of people involved in providing care and treatments.

Today, the emphasis is on working more productively and efficiently, rather than on substituting one level of caregiver for another. Managed care organizations (MCOs), health maintenance organizations (HMOs), and third-party payers are creating new models for tracking nursing hours per patient visit, supply costs, technology expenses, and the types and amounts of services clinicians use in their practice. Organizational leaders must respond to all of these pressures, making the human resources manager a major player in allowing healthcare organizations to operate successfully in the community.

Besides seeking to improve the efficiency of people, healthcare managers are trying to improve efficiency in delivery structure. One development in health care that illustrates this trend is the creation of integrated healthcare systems. While some physicians and others have begun or renewed the effort to form "niche" provider organizations, integrated systems have been a more popular model used to bring efficiencies into the system. They combine lateral and vertical integration of services, including how those services are delivered and by whom.

Demands on government in the early years of the 21st century to fund anti-terrorism projects and programs and to support a rapidly changing economy are putting pressure on both the U.S. Congress and state legislatures to find ways to reduce expenditures in domestic programs and not increase taxes. Medicare and Medicaid will again be in line for either reductions in their growth rates or actual reductions in funding. In 2004 and 2005, many state governments looked to their Medicaid programs as places to reduce state expenditures. As governmental programs cut expenditures and healthcare organizations are forced to look for additional savings, people become an attractive target. The "war on terrorism" in the early 2000s and the national deficit are likely to have long-term impacts on federal and state funding of welfare and healthcare programs, for example. "Pay for performance" and other models for reimbursing or paying for healthcare services are already being examined for their ability to ensure provision of high-quality care, but in more efficient ways. As in employee compensation programs that pay for individual or group performance, payers—including the government—are considering whether healthcare providers can be reimbursed based on quality and cost performance. The better one exceeds an expectation for care based on quality outcomes while simultaneously controlling expenses, the higher the payment rate. This higher payment comes from a pool of dollars generated by savings to third-party payers and government. The adoption of such systems will necessitate better management of both human capital and technology.

Managing human capital is also important, as there are currently shortages in many healthcare professions, including nurses, physical therapists, occupational therapists, and technologists. The nursing shortage is expected to last until at least 2010, if not beyond. Demographic statistics suggest that there are probably a sufficient number of licensed nurses to meet most of the need, but many of these nurses are finding employment outside the healthcare system because of professional equity issues or simply because they are "burned out" and are seeking more fulfilling careers elsewhere. Nursing schools are having trouble finding enough students to meet both current and future needs. Professional nurses have also become more specialized in the past few decades, adding to the demand and shortage. In the past, most registered nurses (RNs) graduated from diploma programs after two or three years; few had college degrees. In the 21st century, the required entrance card in many locations is a bachelor's degree. The skills and knowledge required by a professional nurse today are vastly more complex than they were 50 years ago. As these technical and quality demands increase, so do the requirements for nursing experience and background. Besides needing a bachelor's degree, many RNs are seeking advanced training and education and becoming nurse specialists in obstetrics, oncology, emergency care, cardiac care, psychiatric care, and many other fields. Because of the distribution of medical professionals, RNs have also gone on to become nurse practitioners, with the ability in some locations to practice independently. Indeed, several institutional settings use the services of these professionals instead of employing physicians for routine care. The changing environment for nurses and the greater demand for their skills simply makes the shortage more intense.

For at least a decade, if not longer, there has been a movement away from generalization in health care to specialization, whether in medicine, nursing, therapy modalities, or institutions. In part, this trend reflects the expansion of technology, which requires ever more specialized skills from technologists and professionals. Once upon a time, a radiological technologist could operate multiple machines; now, however, MRI technicians, PET technicians, and nuclear medicine technicians are required. Laboratory technicians have also become more specialized. To be a physical therapist in the 21st century, one must have a doctoral degree in physical therapy. Recently, pharmacy schools have decided to turn the traditional five-year bachelor's or master's degree program into a new doctor of pharmacy degree program. The list goes on in mental health and counseling professions, and even in administration. Where once only physicians specialized, now almost everyone in health care needs to have advanced training.

This specialization can be profitable, offering the ability to increase market share while controlling costs. Some areas of the United States have seen the expansion of "boutique" providers, facilities that specialize in one or two organ systems or surgical practices. These providers serve a segment of the population that previously was admitted to general hospitals. While the more traditional hospitals and clinics continue to have needs for workers in these areas, the new facilities have increased the competition for those professionals.

Along with specialization, increased governmental and accreditation body oversight, advanced technology, and better techniques for treating people, the healthcare industry must cope with increased liability for almost everything healthcare providers do. Liability concerns are also driving the agenda to find and retain qualified and effective people. Having just anyone fill a position is no longer a real option; healthcare organizations need to find that "right" person with the unique combination of professional skills and education, as well as a commitment to quality care and customer service. "Bedside manner" does count, whether in a hospital, a nursing home, a clinic, or a community health clinic run by the county health department.

To keep pace with the changes in professional qualifications and skills, changes in technology, and changes in expectations from the public, the field of human resources management is changing rapidly. Human resources is now at the executive table in most organizations, joining as a partner in strategic planning and management of the organization.

Back in the 20th century, human resources professionals were content with managing personnel policies, developing benefit programs, making sure the hiring process worked, and providing employee development programs. While the functional aspects of human resources management remain in place, these professionals are being asked to step up and become change managers, organizational development consultants, compliance managers and advisors to other executives and first-line supervisors, researchers, and quality assurance experts. Between the 1970s and 1990s, employers saw an ever-increasing number of legislative and regulatory actions that affected the way organizations relate to their employees. The courts have taken a bigger role in defining what Congress meant in passing laws affecting civil rights, disabilities, age, gender, and other issues. Also, in the early years of the 21st century, questions about corporate ethics and values have taken center stage, placing more emphasis on what human resources executives must monitor and control in the organization.

The chief human resources officer is now as vital to the executive management team as the chief executive, chief financial officer, chief nursing officer, and chief medical officer. Human resources professionals are expected to have advanced education and certification in their areas of expertise, whether as Senior Professionals in Human Resources (SPHR), Certified Compensation Professionals (CCP), or members of other specialties. Many are members of the American College of Healthcare Executives (ACHE), Medical Group Management Association (MGMA), and other professional groups. Understanding the healthcare environment, including reimbursement, accreditation, clinical programs, legal issues, and patient care, is just as important as understanding compensation and benefits programs, employment law, union relations, employee relations, training and career development, recruitment and hiring, and health and safety programs.

THE CHALLENGE OF FINDING AND RETAINING COMPETENT PEOPLE

Shortages of competent healthcare professionals—primarily nurses—ranked third among issues confronting hospital executives, according to a 2004 report published by the American College of Healthcare Executives.[1] In the same report, 87% of the participants in the survey said that finding nurses continued to be the number one recruiting issue (Table 2-1). Twenty-nine percent of the respondents also identified complying with staffing ratios as a problem.[1] Technical fields appear also to pose a hiring problem for hospital executives, especially in the area of imaging technicians and pharmacists.

The Bureau of Labor Statistics reports that by 2012 there will be a growth of more than 623,000 new positions for registered nurses from

Table 2-1 Personnel Shortages, 2004

Registered nurses	
Imaging technicians	66%
Pharmacists	54%
Physicians—surgical specialists	44%
Therapists	41%
Lab technicians	39%
Physicians—medical specialists	31%
Nurse anesthetists	30%
Complying with staffing ratio requirements	29%
Licensed practical nurses	29%
Worker dissatisfaction	24%
Entry-level support staff	22%
Physicians—generalists	21%
Succession planning for boards, managers, clinical leaders	16%

Source: American College of Healthcare Executives. Top Issues Confronting Hospitals. http://www.ache.org/pubs/research/ceoissues.cfm.

2002, as well as 343,000 new positions for nursing aides, orderlies, and attendants, mostly in long-term care settings.[2] The same report notes that the fastest-growing occupations include medical assistants, physician assistants, social and human service aides, home health aides, health information professionals, physical therapy assistants, and occupational therapy aides.[2] According to the Bureau of Labor Statistics, 20% of all employment in 2002 was in education and health services.[2]

Between January 2004 and January 2005, there was an increase of 15.1% in employment in the healthcare sector of the U.S. economy, with a slight decrease only in employment in nursing and residential facilities (Table 2-2).[3]

The data from the Bureau of Labor Statistics suggest that health care continues to be "the place" to look for employment. At the same time, shortages continue to plague the industry, making the recruiting job much more competitive, especially for highly competent people. Between 1986 and 2006, the Bureau of Labor Statistics expects jobs in the health assessment and treating occupations, as well as the health technician and technologist occupations, to grow by 44%. The Bureau states that this growth is twice the growth in all occupations.[4]

Table 2-2 Seasonally Adjusted Employment in Health Care (100,000s)

	Jan. 2004	Sept. 2004	Oct. 2004	Nov. 2004	Dec. 2004	Jan. 2005	Change from Dec. 2004 to Jan. 2005 (%)
Total healthcare[1]	11,931.7	12,106.0	12,135.3	12,153.6	12,174.1	12,189.2	15.1
Ambulatory health services[2]	4,867.1	4,975.0	4,996.9	5,006.7	5,023.8	5,035.0	11.2
Physician offices	2,027.8	2,064.5	2,074.2	2,077.7	2,084.4	2,084.7	0.3
Outpatient care center	437.6	448.7	449.5	449.8	450.1	451.7	1.6
Home healthcare	755.0	779.5	782.7	789.2	793.5	797.4	3.9
Hospitals	4,267.9	4,306.0	4,311.2	4,319.7	4,323.1	4,327.6	4.6
Nursing and residential[3]	2,796.7	2,825.0	2,827.2	2,877.2	2,827.2	2,826.6	−0.6
Nursing care facility	1,572.5	1,576.6	1,576.8	1,576.4	1,575.5	1,572.8	−2.7

1. Total healthcare includes social assistance.
2. Includes physician offices, outpatient centers, and home health.
3. Includes nursing care facilities.
Source: Bureau of Labor Statistics News. Employment Situation Jan. 2005. USDL05-178. http://www.bls.gov/news.release/pdf/empsit.pdf.

The contingent workforce, while not just a healthcare issue, is a significant worry for healthcare executives. Hospitals and long-term care facilities have always used temporary nurses, "floaters," fly-in nurses, and others. Managing such contracts is a major issue for human resources and nursing managers. Agencies representing such professionals are typically required to ensure that individuals meet professional standards, are licensed, and are competent; however, each facility must assure itself that its contingent workforce meets those standards to avoid potential medical liability and to avoid violating federal and state laws. Each facility must also negotiate a contract with these workers, attempting to get the best deal possible. In addition, many healthcare facilities are outsourcing various functions, including housekeeping, maintenance, food service, therapy services, payroll, and benefits management. Human resources managers are often called upon to manage or monitor such agreements. Federal tax laws, worker compensation, Fair Labor Standards Act (FLSA) regulations, and other laws and regulations must be monitored whenever an employer uses contingent workers.

Performance management—always a challenge to supervisors—becomes even more important when quality and safety are vital to patient care and community health. Human resources professionals must ensure that the appropriate models are used and that the criteria can be validated. Such activity starts with the task of determining the essential functions of the jobs performed. Beyond that, performance management often has tort liability implications. Healthcare providers are at risk if the wrong person is performing a treatment, procedure, intervention, test, or service. Accrediting bodies as well as the government require that facilities ensure that healthcare professionals are competent to perform the duties assigned. Early identification of problems and deficits is essential for risk control. And when deficits in any of these areas are identified, training, development, and behavior modification must be provided. Human resources plays a significant role in identifying training needs; indeed, while the actual training may be provided by a clinical area, the tasks remain a human resources function.

COMPENSATION AND BENEFITS ISSUES

Compensation affects the ability of healthcare organizations—including public health clinics and agencies, hospitals, and nursing homes—

to recruit and retain qualified professionals and workers. It was not that long ago (the 1970s) that healthcare workers were paid at or near the minimum wage, the assumptions being that such jobs served the public good and that people working in these fields did so as a vocation, much like religious orders. The introduction of Medicare and broader financing from third parties meant that more dollars became available for these positions. There were also increased expectations regarding the qualifications, education, and training that nurses, technicians, and other healthcare workers should have. Wages and salaries have increased significantly since the 1970s; there is, however, an ongoing debate about whether the compensation paid to healthcare workers and professionals has reached the appropriate level yet, considering the American public's expectations regarding these individuals' skills and expertise. Unions use compensation as one vehicle for gaining support among employees. And competition for people puts pressure on managers and boards to consider raising both the pay scale and the benefits offered. Many hospitals still offer "signing bonuses" and incentives to get people with specific skills to come to the institution.

Besides dealing with the pressure on wage and benefit levels, human resources professionals are looking at which methods and models are best for compensating employees. Should performance-based systems be introduced to encourage more productive and efficient work? Many healthcare organizations use competency-based hiring and selection models that then translate into compensation levels. Should all nursing personnel be paid the same, or should there be recognition for educational attainment, specialty credentials, and other factors? If the latter, how do we go about determining and assessing those factors?

Human resources is primarily accountable in the organization for researching and developing the compensation philosophy and policy for the organization. While the chief executive and the board make the final decision, human resources personnel must understand the organizational goals and the environment, and then translate that understanding into a philosophy regarding how to compensate the employees of the organization fairly. It is not sufficient just to know that the competition is paying $40,000 for a starting nurse with a bachelor's degree and three years of experience; human resources must also know what that means to its own organization, based on the services, market placement, types of skills needed, and whether the organization wants to be the market leader. Benefits are much the same: Why is the organization offering them, and which mix is best to attract the "right" person with the "right" skills and knowledge? Retention of needed people is also a significant aspect of the compensation policy. Are there some positions where significant turnover is acceptable because the skills can easily be found in the community? Are there other skills that are difficult to find, so that it is vital to retain people who have those skills? Obviously, money is only one factor in creating a working environment that attracts people who want to stay. A true compensation philosophy integrates all of these factors.

LEGISLATIVE AND REGULATORY ENVIRONMENTS

In the early years of the 20th century, most organizations probably had a personnel clerk who handled paperwork, ensured that payroll was completed, and perhaps did recruiting. Often, labor disputes were handled by the courts if the employer and the employee could not negotiate an agreement. Then came the 1920s and 1930s and the passage of several labor-relations laws, including the National Labor Relations Act (NLRA), the Fair Labor Standards Act (FSLA), and the Social Security Act. For most healthcare human resources professionals, FLSA plays a significant role, because it regulates overtime pay for nonexempt workers, hours worked, child labor, and other pay-related activities. Only in 2004 did the federal government finally modify the 70-year-old rules. Should a healthcare facility classify nurses as professional employees who are exempt from the overtime limits? If the facility does, what happens when people need to be sent home because the patient load on a particular day declines? Until the late 1970s, nursing salaries did not need to meet the minimum wage standard set for other industries; now nursing salaries in many cases are competitive with other jobs in the community. What happens when an adolescent treatment center sends staff on wilderness adventures? Is the staff on duty 24 hours a day while out on the trip, hence meeting the overtime rules, or can the center reasonably state that the staff is not required to be on the job 24 hours a day?

Another major healthcare-related law, the Health Insurance Portability and Accountability Act (HIPAA), was passed in 1996. Healthcare human resources professionals have a special relationship with HIPAA because it affects not only the portability of health insurance from one employer to another, but also the privacy of health information. Healthcare professionals and workers have access to reams of personal information about patients and clients. There is an obligation to protect that information. How often can an outsider sit in the hospital cafeteria and listen as professionals talk about "old Mrs. Jones" and her ailments? That may be a violation of patient health information privacy. Then there is always the possibility that Sam, down in housekeeping, may end up as a patient. How does the hospital protect his privacy?

The Employee Retirement and Income Security Act (ERISA) has changed the way human resources looks at the organization's retirement plans. The widespread adoption of 401(k) plans and 405 plans has changed retirement from a defined-benefit to a defined-contribution plan, making employees responsible for investing their retirement dollars, rather than the employer. Is there some ethical or moral obligation on the part of the healthcare organization to assist employees in making wise decisions?

The healthcare organization, while providing care to the community, also must provide health coverage for its own employees. If the organization is part of a system, should it self-insure; act as a health maintenance organization for its employees, requiring them to seek all services through the HMO; or purchase a third-party contract?

As mentioned in Chapter 1, COBRA has brought changes such that employers must now meet certain deadlines in notifying terminated employees that they have the right to continue their health insurance or a divorced spouse that he or she may have some rights to continued coverage. As part of a healthcare organization, human resources personnel advise recently unemployed patients that they should continue their coverage under COBRA, but as an employer do we really want that potential risk in our own insurance plan?

Unionization

Once upon a time, nurses, house staff, maintenance workers, housekeepers, and office staff were not interested in forming unions in "their" work environment. Since the late 1970s, however, unions have become a reality that human resources must face when negotiating with workers. In the early 1970s, the nurses' union in Seattle effectively closed down all hospitals in that region because all of the hospitals belonged to one bargaining unit. The idea behind this structure was to prevent the leap-frogging of wages and benefits. Unfortunately—or fortunately, depending on one's perspective—the nurses' union used that cooperative to win significant concessions. The infamous Local 1199 was quite effective at intimidating hospital managers until the mid-1990s. The threat of a nursing strike alarms not only management, but also physicians and the community. The media often give favorable exposure to the union, putting pressure on management to settle in favor of the nurses, or the housekeepers, or whomever. Human resources professionals need to be ready to handle such situations and are under pressure to develop effective employee relations programs so that unionization is not an issue or, if there is already a union, so that the organization maintains good relationships with union leaders. Human resources must ensure that the employer does not cross the line in what it can or cannot say, nor allow management to commit an unfair labor practice.

At the AFL-CIO convention in the summer of 2005, a dramatic change took place. Three major unions left the umbrella of the larger organization to go it alone. During the last quarter of the 20th century, the AFL-CIO relied heavily on its political influence in Washington, D.C., to support laws giving employees more rights and benefits. Union leaders believe that this strategy is what caused the dramatic decline in union membership in the latter part of the century. Could the latest move be the beginning of a renewed effort to increase union membership among employees? Or could it mean the demise of unions as management have come to know them over the years? We won't know the final answer for several years. In the meantime, this trend likely means increased efforts to win professionals over to union membership with promises of job security and stable pay and benefits. United Airlines' "dumping" of its pension obligations and threats from other major employers to do the same will likely fuel the fire.

Human resources managers and professionals need to understand the causes and reasons professionals in the health field might want to join a union as well as ways to counter such unionization efforts. There are always some managers who are happy to have a union, because it defines the working relationship in a formal contract: Everyone knows where they stand and how to behave. Others believe that it is important for management and employees to work collaboratively to effect change and quality in the organization. Union contracts can limit and restrict the ability of the organization to change and meet new challenges. Some unions and management work well together; Southwest Airlines is one such example. For the most part, however, having a union means that there is a third party between management and workers. Human resources is normally charged with the responsibility for developing programs that encourage good employee relationships. This includes working with managers to ensure that they treat the people working with and for them with respect and understanding. In today's work environment (and health care is certainly in the forefront of this movement), empowerment and collaboration in the work environment are vital. It is important to quality care and efficient operation that physicians, nurses, and others on the "team" work effectively together and that all opinions and recommendations be given equitable weight when making decisions. Certainly, pay and benefits are important in building relationships, but research study after research study suggests that working conditions are far more important considerations—"how am I treated."

Assuming the organization is unionized (and it makes no difference whether the union is a public union representing public health agency employees or the nurses' union at a hospital), human resources needs to be effective in guiding relationships and understanding what can and cannot be done when making work assignments, handling grievances, and changing working conditions. In a changing environment, especially one affected by government and third-party reimbursement, having excellent union relationships will go far in ensuring that the organization can change when it needs to. Recent research into management–employee relationships in health care suggests that, for the organization or agency to operate effectively, empowerment, the ability for both parties to gain from the relationship, and two-way communication are vital.[5, 6]

Title VII and Other "Rights"

In 1867, Congress passed the first civil rights legislation and amended the U.S. Constitution. However, not much attention was paid to ensuring individual civil rights until President Lyndon Johnson's Great Society of the 1960s. Title VII of the Civil Rights Act came into force in 1965, and later amendments further defined the rights of women and minorities. Title VII affects healthcare organizations providing services to patients and clients and is meant to ensure that all people receive equal care and services within their ability to pay. For human resources professionals, Title VII defines how people are treated in the workplace. It affects employee testing and placement, recruitment and hiring practices, promotion and assignments—whether genders are being treated equally in the workplace, when the organization can or cannot require Mary Sue to retire, and whether that 60-year-old lab technician was illegally denied a promotion because a 35-year-old got the promotion instead. Sexual harassment is a continuing issue that human resources professionals must deal with in the workplace. Today the quid pro quo violation, where a supervisor demanded sexual favors in return for better assignments or promotions, has largely given way to the concept of a hostile workplace, making prevention and human resources intervention more difficult.

Gender discrimination is always a reality that must be confronted in the workplace, and, with health care being primarily a female industry, it is even more important to be aware of such discrimination's implications. Healthcare organizations need to seek out and promote qualified women candidates for administrative positions rather than simply assuming the only executive position is the chief nursing officer. Not only has there been a glass ceiling for women in health care, but the same ceiling has affected the mobility of minorities as well. Organizations such as the American College of Healthcare Executives (ACHE) and others have appointed commissions to increase awareness and opportunities for minority candidates. Human resources personnel must take a leadership role in developing and implementing affirmative action policies that will seek out, recruit, and hire qualified women and minorities for higher-level positions. This often requires human resources departments to work with educational institutions to develop and implement programs that will prepare people for positions in the field.

Harassment is another problem in the workplace. Indeed, it ranks among the top reasons for lawsuits brought against employers. Healthcare organizations present a unique challenge, because not all harassment occurs between supervisors and subordinates. Physicians may be guilty of harassing nurses, therapists, or technicians. Vendors may be a problem; employers are also liable for the actions of these "nonemployees." It is vital that healthcare organizations have effective sexual harassment policies and procedures that employees, medical staffs, and vendors are aware of, and that these rules be enforced. Just like the annual fire safety training and infection control training, harassment policies need to be communicated often.

The Americans with Disabilities Act (ADA) presents unique challenges in healthcare organizations. Determining essential job functions for various positions within the organization is vital in treating people with disabilities fairly when recruiting and selecting people for jobs within the sector. Just because a person is in a wheelchair or has a significant health problem, such as HIV, does not mean that person cannot successfully meet patient care needs.

In 2004, the Equal Employment Opportunity Commission (EEOC) reported that 79,432 charges were filed against employers for possible violations of Title VII and other employment discrimination statutes.[7] While there has been a slight decrease in these lawsuits since 2002, they remain a significant issue for employers. Of these charges, 35% were related to race complaints, 30.5% to sexual harassment, 22.5% to age discrimination, and 19% to ADA complaints.[7] Settlements of EEOC complaints in 2004 amounted to $251.7 million.[8] These numbers have stayed fairly constant over the years, demonstrating that human resources has a long way to go in educating management and supervisors about the consequences of violating civil rights and anti-discrimination statutes.

According to reports from the EEOC in 2002 (the latest data available), 52% of the U.S. workforce was male; 37% were white males, and 33% were white females.[9] The same report shows that, of professional employees (including many of the healthcare professions), 39% are white males and 41% are white females.[9] The report shows disproportionately fewer blacks and Hispanics in professional occupations, while the percentage of Asia/Pacific Islanders in professional occupations is about double their participation rate.[9] Based on these numbers, it appears human resources professionals have much to do to bring equity to the job market.

Immigration presents another challenge to healthcare organizations. Obviously, healthcare organizations must request documentation that immigrants are in the United States legally. As more immigrants fill housekeeping, food service, and maintenance positions, however, HR must be even more diligent in ensuring that Title VII rules are upheld while ensuring compliance with the Immigration Reform and Control Act.

Compliance Functions

The Sarbanes-Oxley Act, the False Claims Act, medical fraud and abuse laws, and other compliance rules and regulations do not necessarily affect human resources directly. Nevertheless, human resources professionals must be aware of these statutes and regulations. Sarbanes-Oxley came about after the 2001–2002 accounting and financial scandals. The False

Claims Act places special emphasis on filing accurate claims for services. Human resources must take an active role in setting an example of honesty and fair dealing in performing its own work and in leading organizational change. Training programs that emphasize compliance, like harassment training and infection control, must be scheduled periodically so that people know what is expected. Beyond compliance is a preference for basic ethical behavior that human resources can help instill in the organization.

The aftermath of September 2001 brought passage of the Patriot Act, which affects travel, immigration, national internal security, and emergency response to local and national disasters and events. How this particular piece of legislation will eventually play out in health care is still being determined, but it is known that healthcare organizations—especially public health and hospitals—are central in any response plan. In the past, these entities worked closely with local and state emergency response agencies. Now the U.S. Department of Homeland Security is taking the lead in both funding and planning responses. Human resources professionals play a role in doing background checks on employees, planning staffing to meet specific needs, recruiting, and ensuring compliance with the law.

Safety

Although most hospitals employ a separate risk manager and safety officer, human resources is integral in any planning and implementation of workplace safety programs. Workplace violence is a significant concern not just in relation to the Patriot Act, but to prevent violence from other sources. Gang violence that spills over into emergency rooms, demonstrators outside on the street, domestic violence that follows employees to work, and the disgruntled employee who comes back that afternoon to do harm—all of these situations, and more, must be planned for and evaluated.

State and county public health agencies have a new and vital role in the prevention or remediation of terrorist activities within the United States. Bioterrorism is a threat, and the most likely candidates for dealing with such a threat are public health professionals. This recognition changes the focus from immunization programs, water purity, sanitation, well-baby clinics, disease prevention, HIV prevention, and other programs to ways to prevent harm from attacks on the public health. Public health agencies are responsible for working with law enforcement and security agencies to protect those water systems and determine what can be done if they are attacked. Human resources professionals must not only consider the professional skills of workers in traditional fields of public health, but also ensure that professionals are available who can counter any bioterrorist attack, whether it is poison in the water system, gas in the subway system, contaminants let loose in the airways, dirty diseases that might infect the population, or the after-effects of a bomb. Disaster training and preparedness have taken on a new priority in the 21st century. Public health may be shifting from primary care and disease prevention to a population model focused on prevention of a whole new set of concerns. The skills and credentials that are now required and the way public health agencies find these professionals pose new problems for the human resources professional who is charged with locating and recruiting such individuals.

WHERE DOES HUMAN RESOURCES GO FROM HERE?

Rondeau and Wagar suggest that human resources management practices play a significant role in patient care quality and operational effectiveness: The more progressive the human resources practices, the more likely the healthcare institution is to have better patient care quality, higher patient satisfaction, better employee morale, higher physician satisfaction, improved operating efficiencies, and more organizational flexibility.[10] Oakland and Oakland also found that investing in employees makes a difference in world-class organizations.[11] Treating people with respect and having good human resources management practices fit nicely into what managers have learned from leadership and management research since World War II and what is increasingly being talked about in recent research on servant leadership, transformative leadership, and spiritual leadership. Human resources professionals can be at the leading edge in healthcare organizations in bringing good management practices to bear on human resources programs.

   These professionals obviously need to be proficient and competent in the many functional areas of human resources practice; otherwise, the organization will not meet both employee and management expectations for an efficient and effective healthcare organization. However, the human resources professional cannot stop at just being an expert in human resources law and programs. He or she must also step up and be a leader in the modern healthcare organization, bringing together knowledge and skill in human resources management practices, as well as knowledge and ability in organizational change, financial management, strategic planning, and leadership.

REFERENCES

1. American College of Healthcare Executives. Top Issues Confronting Hospitals. Available at: http://www.ache.org/pubs/research/ccoissues.cfin.
2. Bureau of Labor Statistics, U.S. Department of Labor. *Occupational Quarterly.* Winter 2003–2004.
3. Bureau of Labor Statistics, U.S. Department of Labor. News BLS: Employment Situation, January 2005. Available at: http://www.bls.gove/news.release/pdf/empsit.pdf. Accessed February 4, 2005.
4. Bureau of Labor Statistics, U.S. Department of Labor. *Occupational Outlook Quarterly.* 1999; 43:1. Available at: http://www.bls.gov/opub/oog/ooghome.htm.
5. Boselie P, Paauwe J, Richardson R. Human resource management, institutionalization and organizational performance: a comparison of hospitals, hotels and local government. *International Journal of Human Resource Management.* 2003; 14:1407–1429.
6. Bartram T, Cregan C. Consultative employment relations in human resource management environments with union presence. *Journal of Industrial Relations.* 2003; 45:539–545.
7. U.S. Equal Employment Opportunity Commission. Charge Statistics: FY1992 through FY2004. Available at: http://www.eeoc.gov/stats/charges.html.
8. U.S. Equal Employment Opportunity Commission. All Statutes: FY1992 through FY2004. Available at: http://www.eeoc.gov/stats/all.html.
9. U.S. Equal Employment Opportunity Commission. Occupational Employment in Private Industry by Race/Ethnic Group/Sex, and Industry, United States, 2002. Available at: http://www.eeoc.gov/stats/jobpat/2002/us.html.
10. Rondeau KV, Wagar TH. Reducing the hospital workforce: what is the role of human resource management practices. *Hospital Topics.* 2002; 80:12–18.
11. Oakland S, Oakland JS. Current people management activities in world-class organizations. *Total Quality Management.* 2001; 12:773–788.

CHAPTER 3

Essential Components of Human Resources Practices and Management

Mark Burns

- Jamail Washington, Director of Nursing for a medium-sized clinic in St. Louis, is pondering what to do about Nurse Vinez Robinson. Nurse Robinson, an older white woman, is becoming increasingly hostile in her relationships with other employees, particularly minorities.
- Spenser Martin, CEO of a small hospital in rural Georgia, is still recovering from his shock that a union organizer has been conducting secret meetings with lower-level employees of the Building and Grounds and Dietary Services Departments. "I never would have thought we'd be dealing with a labor union here," he thinks to himself, weighing his options.
- Anne Minzenty, Assistant Administrator of a large long-term care facility in Omaha, is considering whether to recommend that her organization start an in-house day care center. Some members of her staff are pushing for one, but she wonders whether such a service would pay off in the long run.

All three of these busy healthcare administrators face problems involving aspects of human resources administration. Healthcare organizations are fundamentally people-centered organizations, and successful actions in this area are a vital component of their everyday organizational life.

In terms of their mission, healthcare institutions have their roots in the ancient traditions of philanthropy and kindness to strangers. Moreover, these labor-intensive enterprises revolve around the intimacy of the patient–caregiver relationship, with services being delivered by a higher portion of women than in many other industries, and in many cases serving a substantial number of low-income and/or minority group patients.[1, 2] Given the people-centered nature of the healthcare field, it is not surprising that excellence in human resources practices correlates closely with general organizational excellence among healthcare organizations.[3]

This chapter reviews the organizational elements of human resources activities and discusses the vital functions that human resources staff can perform in the healthcare organization.

ORGANIZATIONAL ELEMENTS OF HUMAN RESOURCES IN HEALTHCARE ORGANIZATIONS

Healthcare organizations have some unique properties due to their substantive functions, mostly stemming from their high percentage of professional staff (i.e., physicians, nurses, allied health workers). The high educational level and greater autonomy of these staff call for organizational structures and supervision strategies that are substantially more challenging for administrators than those of most organizations.

Despite their substantive differences, healthcare organizations also share certain characteristics that are generally found in all organizations. For example, they have leaders who must work to motivate their employees. Intentionally or unintentionally, they develop their own unique organizational culture. They must communicate with their employees and process information flowing from inside and outside the organization. And they function in an environment for which they may or may not be well designed, an environment typified by increasing diversity.

Leadership

"If you're spending all your time in your office, then you're looking for problems in the wrong place!"

—*Hospital administrator*

Traditionally, the healthcare administrator was portrayed as a bold individual who was almost single-handedly carrying the organization toward success. Terms such as "power broker" were applied to these assertive, forceful individuals.[4] This concept fitted well with the idea that healthcare institutions had an intimate relationship, both moral and financial, with their local community. It also fitted well with a less complicated healthcare system, in which it was thought feasible for a single individual to be cognizant of the entire sweep of the total activities of even a large hospital.[5]

In the modern, highly complex healthcare organization, such roles are no longer widely applicable. In recent years, the healthcare system has become more fragmented, more regulated, more technologically complex. Even small local clinics find themselves dealing with reimbursement sources whose headquarters may be in a far state, or with radiological consultants based in another country. In this complicated, ever-changing system, the administrator has of necessity become more of a "team leader" or "facilitator." This person is capable of balancing many complex interests and points of view—those of medical staff, nurses, other administrators, clients, the community at large—and leading not so much through force of personality as through reconciling these diverse interests while weaving from them an inspiring, progressive vision of the future.[6]

Such a team leader, whether the CEO or the director of the human resources department, must be proactive in his or her orientation, seeking to anticipate crises in the organization and preempt them before they can occur, or at least in their earlier stages. This quality also means that the team leader must remain constantly alert for new information sources, such as Internet-based professional journals or even Web "blogs." He or she must be ready to seek out leads on new innovations and new opportunities to learn and facilitate learning in the organization.[7]

Motivation

A key factor in mobilizing the human resources of the healthcare organization is motivation. Employees first of all need to have their material needs met—such as basic salary, minimal benefits, and reasonably comfortable working conditions. Once these fundamental needs are met, however, they seek to satisfy higher, more abstract needs—such as group fellowship, peer recognition, and status.[8]

To the extent that organizational leaders can persuade employees that they can meet their needs by fulfilling the needs of the organization, a more effective organization results.[9] Setting a vision for the healthcare organization can be a critical need, but so can such simple day-to-day tasks as an administrator making himself or herself highly available to employees and practicing daily rounds, popularly called "management by walking around."[10] In some cases, such less tangible motivators may actually be more effective methods for motivating employees than financial incentives.[11]

Organizational Culture

"My staff is practically like family to me."
—*Clinic administrator*

Fundamental to both leadership and motivation is the nurturing of an appropriate organizational culture.[12] Organizational culture can be defined as the loose collection of social artifacts within organizations. Although it is mostly an informal phenomenon, it has been shown to affect such areas as commitment to the organization and job satisfaction.[13] It is also an important component of the development of strategic human resources management (SHRM), as discussed later in this chapter.

An organization's culture manifests itself in numerous ways, both obvious and subtle. Healthcare organizations, for example, rely heavily on technical language, acronyms, badges, and technologies that may be difficult for the average person to comprehend. Culturally, such specialized language not only serves as a unifying tool within a particular professional group (e.g., neurosurgeons), but also can actually influence the attitudes and behaviors of the group using it.[14]

The variety and complexities of such languages present a daunting barrier to the average patient or family member. Some large healthcare organizations inadvertently add to these barriers by installing less than optimal signage, leaving bewildered visitors to lament, "I can't find *anything* in this place!"

From the viewpoint of the human resources administrator, specialized languages can present both a communicative obstacle and a social barrier. Suppose for example, in an employee grievance situation, the employee retorts, "You wouldn't understand; you're not a nurse!" Making an appropriate response may require either a substantial knowledge of the language of nursing on the part of the administrator reviewing the grievance or the involvement of a "translator" in the form of another nurse.

There are less tangible manifestations of organizational culture as well. Office décor and artwork can send subtle signals, ranging from warm to officious. Even informal organizational stories told over coffee breaks and around the water cooler can be powerful signals of the morale of the organization, furnishing a positive or negative indication of the larger organizational culture.[15]

The extent to which organizational culture can be molded by leadership has been the subject of much debate. Because culture's roots go deep in the human psyche, it cannot be changed quickly. At the same time, it is not completely static. Sometimes dramatic action (or *dramaturgy*) by an administrator can influence organizational culture.[16] For example, a new hospital CEO who replaces a more aloof predecessor may promote the perception of cultural change by announcing an "open door" policy, dropping in to chat with staff working the "graveyard shift," redecorating/rearranging his or her office in a more informal décor, or instituting more frequent opportunities for informal social interaction among managers and employees.

Communication and Information Processing

"I love my Blackberry. The whole management team at our medical center has them now."
— *Administrator of an outpatient surgicenter*

Healthcare organizations are linked together through webs of communication, both formal and informal, written and verbal, printed and electronic. Communication goes both up and down the administrative hierarchy, out from the center, and in from the periphery. Although it is easy to visualize communication in the "top-down" mode, with orders flowing down an organizational hierarchy, of equal or greater importance is communication flowing up from the lower levels of the organization ("bottom-up" mode), conveying vital information to its higher levels. The pace of communications in modern health care is becoming faster and faster, thanks to e-mail, instant messaging, and Internet-linked cellphones.

With this constant tidal wave of information, the problems of communication distortion become increasingly more serious. In fact, an unfortunate downside of speedier electronic communications is that it becomes much easier to send out rumors, personal notes, games, even "bootleg software"—all of which clogs up the organization's overall communications system. It also becomes easier to send hasty communications without thinking them through for such matters as tone and confidentiality. A hasty message dashed off without careful thought can lead to anything from hurt feelings to an employee grievance, or even to a lawsuit or violation of federal regulations.

In an effort to restore some clarity and order in their internal communications systems, healthcare organizations have adopted such strategies as banning instant messaging and restricting Internet access. They have also sought to conserve valuable bandwidth by limiting the transmission of large graphics and audio files unrelated to the mission of the organization. Modern healthcare organizations must also take care that electronic communications involving patient information adhere to the extensive privacy and confidentiality standards set forth in the 1996 Health Insurance Portability Act (HIPAA). HIPAA covers such areas as restricting access to patient records, both paper and electronic, standards for document retention, and compliance administration.[17] Smaller healthcare organizations may find these requirements especially challenging.[18]

Environmental Influences

"You don't dare come on like gangbusters. The moment you pick up the Good Book and hit it a few times, you are in trouble."
                                                                    —*Healthcare planner*

Organizations dwell in a sea of other organizations, and healthcare organizations are no exception. Even nonprofit healthcare organizations have competitors, in the form of both similar organizations and not-so-similar organizations seeking to make inroads on their markets. A nursing home, for example, may compete not only with other nursing homes but also with assisted living facilities and even hospitals seeking to acquire a skilled nursing facility (SNF) offering a full range of medical care, nursing care, or rehabilitation services.[19] The question of whether healthcare organizations face an environment that is more significantly uncertain than the environment faced by other organizations is open to interpretation. Some authors consider the healthcare environment to be almost chaotic in nature—so dynamic, in fact, that making predictions about it is highly unlikely.[20, 21] Others would contend that healthcare environments are no more chaotic and unpredictable than those in which other complex organizations operate. Nevertheless, no one denies that the healthcare environment is challenging and difficult.[22] Assessing and monitoring this complicated environment becomes an important adjunct to developing appropriate organizational strategies, including strategic use of human resources.

In this kind of highly competitive atmosphere, it becomes extremely important for individual organizations to seek allies and reduce at least the most negative effects of competition. One strategy for doing so involves forging a *domain consensus,* a broad agreement with other neighboring organizations as to what the core organization is trying to accomplish and the values it upholds. Reaching such an agreement about its sphere of operations may bring an organization useful allies that can provide needed expertise, resources, or power.[23] Like seeking change in organizational culture, fashioning a domain consensus is best undertaken by constant low-level, informal efforts rather than by fiat.[24] Moves toward creating greater transparency in healthcare organization operations may also contribute positively to this effort.[25]

In facing the concerns of their environment, healthcare organizations must also cope with pressures from government regulatory sources and legal decisions. As will be detailed later in this chapter, an increasing number of such organizations are hiring a corporate compliance officer for assistance with this important area.

Design

Design issues were one of the first subjects discussed by writers on organizations, beginning with Max Weber's classic efforts to outline which design makes for the most effective bureaucracy.[26] Successful design is a direct response to the demands placed on the organization, both internal and external. For example, better RN staffing patterns can have a direct impact on improving quality of care in the nursing home setting.[27]

Healthcare organizations must maintain an appropriate chain of command, whose scope depends in part on the size of the organization. In structuring that chain of command, the span of control must also be considered: How many units should report to a supervisory administrator or supervising group? Some modern organizations, especially small ones, have a rather flat chain of command, with large spans of control; traditional bureaucracies tend more toward the opposite extreme.[28]

Issues of delineating line and staff also arise. Who does the actual substantive work of the organization, directly interacting with clients? Who works with services central to the organization, such as budgeting, information technology, and human resources? Whose duties mix both aspects?

Finally, just as some modern big businesses "outsource" jobs abroad to cut costs, many healthcare organizations have undertaken their own "outsourcing" through contracting. Increasingly, services such as security, laundry, and even management are being performed by outside organizations having a contractual relationship with the core organization.[29] Such relationships further complicate the task of human resources departments.

Human Resources and Diversity Issues

"Addressing diversity really isn't all that complicated. Basically it's just treating everyone decently."

—*Equal Opportunity officer*

Healthcare organizations and their human resources managers must deal with an American society that is increasingly rich in religious, ethnic, generational, and social differences. Furthermore, as new groups move into the American mainstream, it is becoming apparent that even those groups are somewhat fractured by their own complicated divisions. For instance, the term "Hispanic" is now being rejected by some of the very people it was once thought to characterize, whereas others in that group find this term entirely appropriate.[30]

Pressures on healthcare organizations to be more cognizant of diversity matters are increasing concomitantly. Although cultural competence has been identified as a key component of achieving better quality of care, unfortunately healthcare managers are not always sensitive to its importance.[31] Achieving such competence involves developing an individual's sensitivity to factors such as the culture, history, and behavior of a particular population.[32]

Government, although rejecting the idea of outright "quotas" in most cases as an unfair imposition on the rights of individuals, maintains efforts to provide open access to all.[33, 34] Increasingly, however, prodiversity efforts are stemming from basic marketing concerns: If your market is one-third Haitian Americans, it makes good business sense to make some effort to reach that market, preferably in French! From an organizational standpoint, having a multiethnic staff is just one more way for an organization to increase its chances of survival by making responses to its environment as varied as the challenges of the environment itself.[35]

HUMAN RESOURCES FUNCTIONS

On a day-to-day basis, all healthcare organizations must perform several basic functions in their human resources activities. First, ideally these activities should be aligned with the larger strategy of the healthcare organization. Furthermore, the organization must recruit new members as it expands, or simply to counteract attrition due to retirement, transfer, or firing. The organization also must have a legal, contractual relationship with its employees. Its employees must receive initial orientation in their duties with the organization, to be augmented with further training and education as their job responsibilities change and evolve. Because the healthcare organization does not want to squander the investment it has made in its employees, a retention program is of vital importance. Finally, employee performance must be evaluated from time to time to ensure the employee has the best "fit" with the organization, and this evaluation should be reflected in the employee's compensation.

In carrying out human resources functions, healthcare organizations must be cognizant of appropriate legal, regulatory, and compliance issues. Relevant state, federal, and local laws must be taken into account.

In addition to their direct functions, human resources activities can supplement the organization's other operations. Knowledge of the human resources situation is important to such aspects as planning for change in the organization. Continuous improvement efforts also rely on the human resources component.

STRATEGIC HUMAN RESOURCES MANAGEMENT

Ideally, the human resources mission of the healthcare organization should be aligned with its broader, strategic aims in a process known as *strategic human resources management*.[36] Tompkins notes that SHRM is

> a continuous process of determining mission-related objectives and aligning personnel policies and practices with those objectives. The personnel department plays a strategic role to the extent that its policies and practices support accomplishment of the organization's objectives.[36] (p. 1)

Under this concept, human resources administration becomes an important part of the healthcare organization's business plan, and the human resources department analyzes the organization's human resources in terms of their fit to that plan. At the same time, this unit directs attention to those aspects of the organization's culture and environment that may be crucial to the success of the business plan.[37]

The most common variant of thinking about SHRM draws analogies between the organization and the world of biology, stressing that the "successful" organization (or organism) must rise above the mere need to survive to also grow and prosper. This contention resembles that discussed earlier in regard to diversity issues. Specifically, healthcare organizations should seek to promote two types of congruity or "good fit":

- Congruity among the various human resources components of the organization, so that they support each other
- Congruity between human resources actions and the other components of the organization's strategic plan[38]

As a practical matter, then, SHRM mandates that human resources programs in healthcare organizations look at broader concerns than the mechanics of the traditional functions covered in the following sections. In addition to issues related to culture and environment, these concerns would include keeping the organization abreast of technological change, assessing the appropriateness of its organizational structure, and scrutinizing its managerial philosophy.[37] Employee empowerment may be a vital component of this process.[39]

RECRUITMENT AND SELECTION

All healthcare organizations eventually need new employees. Finding them begins with human resources planning. Administrators must ask what the current personnel needs of each unit in the organization are, what growth is planned, and which vacancies have occurred or may be likely to occur, whether through attrition, removal, or retirement. New positions must be carefully designed to avoid poor "fit" between potential employees and the needs of the employing organization.[40] Ideally, such design will be based on a careful job analysis of the actual tasks of a given position, which can then be used to appropriately screen applicants for relevant knowledge, skills, and abilities.[41]

Next to be considered is what forms of advertising for the position are appropriate. These venues may include in-house newsletters and bulletin boards, plus the organization's intranet—its internal, private version of the Internet—if it has one. If not, in-house e-mail may be used. To reach potential applicants outside the organization, it may be necessary to place advertisements in print media, the Internet, and relevant professional publications. It is also important to consider publication outlets of relevance to potential minority applicants—for example, advertisements in smaller African American–oriented newspapers, which may publish only once a week.[1]

Eventually, applicants will begin contacting the organization. It is important that the staff with whom the applicant will make first contact be properly trained to receive inquiries courteously and knowledgably. For example, if a particular degree is mandatory for the position, applicants may be notified by the staff at the initial point of contact, saving valuable time in the screening process.

The next step is to have potential applicants fill out an application form. This document may be used as a further screening device. In fact, some organizations include simple discussion essays on their forms to further facilitate screening.

Next, the candidate participates in an interview. In the interview, one or more staff members discuss the potential job with the applicant, ask questions, record the applicant's responses, and make judgments about the applicant's suitability for the position. Depending on the nature of the position, the interview may be structured or unstructured. Generally, the higher the position, the less structured the interview.

For medium- to high-level positions, an increasing number of health-care organizations have begun to administer personality testing in an effort to determine whether an applicant "fits" the organizational culture of the facility. This practice has stirred up considerable controversy. Although properly administered personality testing may possibly save users from losses of as much as $1 million annually from hiring inept or ill-suited employees, even proponents of such testing concede that many firms conducting these tests fall short in such areas as poor test construction and weak validation. A more focused variant that is growing in popularity is "situational" testing, in which an applicant is asked his or her reactions or proposals for a specific hypothetical case related to the functioning of the position.[42]

Toward the end of the hiring process, the human resources department attempts to verify the references of the applicant. Thanks to the increasingly litigious tendencies occurring in the United States, this process may not be as enlightening as was once the case. Many organizations now seek to protect themselves from lawsuits by stating only, "Yes, Mr. Allen worked here from 1998 to 2001," and decline further comment. However, such terse remarks at least verify the reality of "Mr. Allen's" employment, a nontrivial consideration given that some career advice books recommend that applicants dissemble if necessary to cover up negative aspects of their backgrounds.[43] One alternative to traditional efforts at reference checking may be to outsource the process to a commercial agency.[44]

Assuming the reference checks uncover no problems, final aspects of the recruitment process usually include a required physical examination and drug screening. The applicant then becomes a new employee.

CONTRACT/AGREEMENT

With hiring concluded, the employee and the organization enter into a binding legal relationship, an employment contract. But what is the nature of this relationship?

Generally, contracts specify such matters as term of service and salary, and set basic responsibilities for the employee and the hiring organization. Disciplinary or grievance procedures usually stem from clauses in the written contract. In many healthcare organizations, the contract provides for a probationary period, after which the employee cannot be dismissed without going through a more elaborate review procedure. Typically, employment contracts also include outlines of grievance procedures in the event of disagreement between employee and organization; these grievance procedures describe which mechanisms have been established to allow an offended employee to formally protest or appeal his or her treatment by the healthcare organization.

Labor issues may be another factor governing the contract between the employee and the healthcare organization. If a union is present in the facility, it will have established some sort of legal relationship with the organization that must be acknowledged in the contract. For instance, if a *closed shop* is in effect, potential employees must join the union to be hired. If a less restrictive *union shop* is in place, the employee has a set number of days to join the union. In certain states having right-to-work laws, where both closed and union shops are illegal, there may still be an *agency shop* in which the employee does not have to join the union but must pay certain professional dues to it. Finally, if there is an *open shop,* the employee does not have a compulsory relationship with the union and joins it only if he or she wishes to do so.

As the employee enters into a new legal relationship with the organization, a key doctrine of the law should be kept in mind. *Respondeat superior* states that the organization is legally responsible for the actions of its employees. An employee's incompetence can directly result not only in frustration for his or her supervisors, but also in potential harm to clients, who increasingly show little hesitancy in filing lawsuits for redress.[45]

Sometimes, the employee's failure to adhere to the terms of the contract may lead to disciplinary action. This usually starts at the informal level, with encouragement from a supervisor to do better and correct a pattern of inappropriate behavior. More formal action may involve verbal corrections recorded in an employee's file, written corrections likewise recorded, or even suspension or removal. In each of these instances, maximum effort must be made to observe due process and fully respect employee rights, both as a matter of ethical behavior and as a way to avoid claims of wrongful termination.[46]

Similarly, the organization should develop a mechanism for processing employee grievances. Not only should an employee have the right to complain to a supervisor but, if the supervisor is the source of the problem perceived by the employee, an alternative channel should be available for lodging complaints. For example, a female employee who is seeking to charge her supervisor with sexual harassment should not find that her first level of complaint is expected to be to that same supervisor!

Of course, the ideal way for a healthcare organization to deal with conflict is to avoid it if possible, or at least to minimize its deleterious efforts. One method of addressing this matter in advance is through appropriate attention to developing a constructive organizational culture. Hader, for example, urges that "We must infuse into our healthcare culture zero tolerance for actions that threaten, intimidate, or harass."[47] Furthermore, staff should be encouraged in the development of appropriate and positive types of communication to minimize interpersonal conflict.[47]

TRAINING AND EDUCATION

Education of employees begins with their basic orientation in the organization after being hired and ideally should continue throughout their tenure in the healthcare organization. A "learning" organization cannot be structured without constantly "learning" employees. Moreover, medical professionals must participate in a set number of *continuing education units (CEUs)* each year to maintain their licensure. Such units must be approved by relevant state or national boards of the particular profession. Their goal is to ensure that physicians, nurses, and other healthcare providers maintain appropriate and current levels of professional competence.[48]

Even for staff who are not medical professionals, ongoing updating of their skills is important. New types of equipment, new administrative techniques, and new computer programs all present a challenge to supervisors who want to help their staffs stay current and to stay current themselves.

Three basic types of employee education exist: passive, active, and experiential. In *passive education* (the most basic form), the "student" simply sits quietly receiving the information. Lectures are the classic illustration of this type, if not necessarily the most enjoyable; manuals are another traditional form of passive education. More sophisticated techniques include demonstrations, video tapes, and "self-taught" course materials. In addition, some large healthcare organizations are putting training materials on their intranets, which may include sophisticated graphics and even video.[49]

Active education techniques feature students interacting with one another in the learning process. Simulations and games are one example, as are group discussions. Other possibilities are case studies and the many options offered by organization development techniques.[50]

Somewhere in between the activity levels of these two alternatives are *experiential education* methods, which involve learning through the work process. Basic on-the-job training of a new employee is the most common example. Another is rotation, in which an employee is temporarily placed in a different job setting so that he or she can acquire new knowledge and techniques used by that unit.

RETENTION

In an effort to retain employees within the organization and deal with problems that may interfere with their effectiveness, many healthcare organizations have instituted employee assistance programs (EAPs). Such programs may advise employees about better personal health habits, family relationships, career counseling, substance abuse problems, and financial difficulties.[51]

One reality of employee relations in the modern world is the need for a drug testing policy, which must be made clearly known to all employees. In fact, institutions receiving federal funds are required to do so by the Drug-Free Act of 1988. A variety of approaches to such policies are possible:

- *Pre-employment testing* before the employee joins the organization
- *Random testing* conducted periodically on a cross section of employees
- *Reasonable suspicion testing* when an employee exhibits specified unusual behavior
- *Post-accident testing* after any accident with a vehicle during working hours
- *Blanket testing* involving the (expensive) testing of all employees within the organization

Human resources departments must carefully weigh the virtues of the many drug tests available, which differ in sensitivity and expense. Simple urinalyses, for example, will detect only recent drug use. Hair tests, by contrast, can detect drug use dating much further back, even exposure to drugs from secondhand smoke.

PERFORMANCE EVALUATION

Healthcare organizations periodically evaluate their employees on some regular basis. At the most informal level, just a comment from a supervisor may be both evaluative and motivational (*"Great* job on the Benning report, Keisha!"). More formal evaluations should be held on at least an annual basis.

Such evaluations fall into two categories: structured and unstructured. A *structured evaluation* entails use of the same evaluation form for all employees, with a simple check-off or numerical rating in a series of categories (e.g., attitude toward the job, promptness in completing projects). *Unstructured evaluations,* which rely more on a general line of questioning and support more latitude for variation by the interviewer, tend to be used for higher-level employees. Even in those areas, however, more structure is starting to appear, due to legal considerations.

Typically, at the end of the process, the employee is asked to sign a form indicating that he or she has undergone the evaluation, whether agreeing with its observations or not. Usually a space is provided for comments by the employee, who may choose to register agreement or dissent.

Some evaluations include a section for the supervisor to specify areas in which the employee should seek improvement before the next evaluation.

Both supervisor and employee can find value in the evaluation experience. From the supervisor's perspective, this process offers a chance to review the employee's work during the period, offer corrective suggestions if needed, and, where required, build a case for disciplinary action if negative behaviors continue. From the employee's point of view, the experience provides a chance to review his or her work from a broader perspective than day-to-day activities and to better understand the supervisor's concerns. Used properly, evaluation can be a positive experience for both parties.[52]

COMPENSATION

Compensation in 21st-century America can involve a variety of forms, of which salary is only one. Other possible types of compensation include the following:

- Health insurance
- Retirement plans
- Day care
- Coverage for professional conferences
- Use of company facilities, such as discounted memberships in on-site health clubs
- Special "Employee of the Week" parking

Regardless of which form it takes, an organization's compensation program should be structured around two basic forms of equity. *Internal equity* means that two employees who perform the same job for an organization at the same rate of skill must receive similar compensation. *External equity* means that an employee who performs a particular job should receive compensation similar to an equivalent employee who works in a similar job elsewhere in the local area or region, depending on the market served by the organization.

Compensation matters fall under the purview of the Fair Labor Standards Act (FLSA), which regulates such matters as the minimum age of employees and overtime. Furthermore, the Wage and Hour Division of the U.S. Department of Labor can review wages and salaries of employees.

Careful administration of an employee benefits program can be one of the most challenging tasks for a human resources department. With rising medical and retirement costs, such benefits are increasingly seen as a major issue in employee compensation, and developing more efficient means to process and monitor them is a vital concern of human resources administrators in health care.[53] Among mechanisms that may be of use to these administrators in monitoring and controlling benefits are setting quality performance standards for benefits providers and offering employees a wide choice of options within specific plans.[54]

LEGAL/REGULATORY ISSUES AND COMPLIANCE

Numerous federal, state, and even local regulations and laws govern human resources administration in healthcare organizations. Among the chief federal roles are establishing regulations and laws in the areas of equal opportunity, safety, and labor relations.

A major factor in concerns about equal opportunity is the 1964 Title VII of the Civil Rights Act, which prohibits discrimination based on such criteria as ethnic identity, gender, and religion. Subsequent amendments to the act have extended it to cover a broad range of organizations, including healthcare organizations. In addition, the 1967 Age Discrimination in Employment Act prohibits unequal treatment based on age. Another major anti-discrimination act, the 1990 Americans with Disabilities Act, seeks to ensure fair treatment of the disabled, including alcoholics, people with emotional illnesses, the learning disabled, and those with attention-deficit disorder. One area not yet covered by federal anti-discrimination law is discrimination based on sexual preference, which currently is addressed only in some state and local ordinances.

Safety in working conditions of employees is the major concern of the 1970 Occupational Safety and Health Act. Under that law, the *Occupational Safety Administration (OSHA)* of the U.S. Department of Labor specifies standards for such areas as bio-safety and physical plant operations. OSHA has the power of inspections to enforce its standards. Because many healthcare organizations use radioactive substances in diagnosis, treatment, or both, those aspects fall under the purview of the Nuclear Regulatory Commission (NRC) under the 1954 Atomic Energy Act.

The keystone of federal labor law is the 1935 National Labor Relations Act (NLRA), also called the Wagner Act, which provided employees with basic rights of organizing for collective bargaining. The earliest version of the law put proprietary healthcare organizations under its jurisdiction but excluded public institutions. The status of private, nonprofit healthcare organizations was left to the courts for interpretation.

In 1959, a Republican-dominated Congress amended the NLRA through the Taft-Hartley Act in an attempt to plug what were perceived as loopholes too favorable to labor. Among other provisions, it specifically exempted nonprofit healthcare institutions from the NLRA. Section 14B of Taft-Hartley allowed states to pass "right-to-work" laws prohibiting any bargaining agreements that forced employees to join unions.

In 1967, a Congress more favorably inclined toward the labor side of the labor–management equation formally brought nonprofit healthcare organizations under the NLRA by passing Public Law 93-370. However, P.L. 93-370 did exempt smaller institutions (e.g., "mom and pop" nursing homes) from its provisions.

To ensure adherence to federal regulations, and in response to relevant court cases, proactive healthcare organizations are increasingly moving to establish *corporate compliance programs,* which aim to prevent and detect criminal violations of federal law.[55] Most hospitals, for example, either have such plans in place or are moving to establish them.[56] Such programs are headed by a *corporate compliance officer* who has direct access to the CEO of the organization but is removed from the organization's direct chain of command to facilitate employee confidence in reporting violations.[57]

THE ROLE OF HUMAN RESOURCES ADMINISTRATION IN SUPPORTING FUNCTIONS

Human resources administration plays a key role in supporting most major planning activities of a healthcare organization. Physical resources, programs, and human resources all must be coordinated to allow the organization to grow and flourish.

In organizational change efforts, the human resources department can facilitate the testing, implementation, and continuation of programs for organization development. Given the lengthy time period needed for such programs to take hold (as even organization development experts stress), on-site human resources personnel can continue to shepherd progress in the organization development initiative long after outside consultants have left the scene.[50]

The human resources staff can play a valuable role in continuous process improvement, helping to guide work groups and "brainstorming" teams. Also, quality assessment is at least partially the assessment of employees and their interactions, and human resources staff can be of help in this area as well. Inventorying the nature of the organizational culture may even give indications of crucial cultural barriers that can hinder the implementation of initiatives in total quality management or continuous quality improvement.[58]

Finally, because a healthcare organization's most valuable component is its people, the human resources staff can help with the continuing identification and nourishment of employee potential. The lower-level clerical assistant of today, properly identified and encouraged, may be the department head—or even CEO—of tomorrow.

CONCLUSION

Healthcare organizations share a variety of basic organizational characteristics with many other types of organizations. Their human resources components also perform basic functions, which, though similar at the most general level, have to be implemented in a great variety of specific organizations. The chapters that follow will examine how these functions are carried out in particular types of healthcare organizations.

REFERENCES

1. Dreachslin JL. *Diversity Leadership.* Chicago: Health Administration Press; 1996.
2. Williams DR, Rucker TD. Understanding and addressing racial disparities in healthcare. *Healthcare Finance Review* 2000; 21:75.
3. Zairi M. Managing human resources in healthcare: learning from world class practices—part I. *Health Manpower Management.* 1998; 24:48–58.
4. Johnson RL. The power broker—prototype of the hospital chief executive. *Health Care Management Review.* 1978; 3:67–73.
5. McGibony JR. *Principles of Hospital Administration.* 2nd ed. New York: G. P. Putnam's Sons; 1969.
6. Axelsson L, Kullén-Engström A, Edgren L. Management vs. symbolic leadership and hospitals in transition—a Swedish example. *Journal of Nursing Management.* 2000; 8:167–173.

7. Robinson DF, Savage GT, Campbell KS. Organizational learning, diffusion of innovation, and international collaboration in telemedicine. *Health Care Management Review.* 2003; 28:68–78.

8. Maslow AH. A theory of human motivation. *Psychological Review* 1947;50: 370–396.

9. Barnard C. *The Functions of the Executive.* Cambridge, MA: Harvard University Press; 1938.

10. Peters TJ, Waterman RH, Jr. *In Search of Excellence.* New York: Harper and Row; 1982.

11. Franco LM, Bennett S, Kanfer R, Stubblebine P. Determinants and consequences of health worker motivation in hospitals in Jordan and Georgia. *Social Science & Medicine.* 2004; 58:343–356.

12. Collins J. *Good to Great: Why Some Companies Make the Leap . . . and Others Don't.* New York: Harper Business; 2001.

13. Nystrom PC. Organizational cultures, strategies, and commitments in healthcare organizations. *Health Care Management Review.* 1993; 18:43–49.

14. Ott JS. *The Organizational Culture Perspective.* Chicago: Dorsey Press; 1989.

15. Mitrof I, Kilman R. On organization stories: an approach to the design and analysis of organizations through myths and stories. In: Kilman RH, Pondy LR, Slevin DP, eds. *The Management of Organization Design: Strategies and Implementation.* New York: North-Holland; 1976:189–207.

16. Thompson V. *Modern Organization.* Tuscaloosa, AL: University of Alabama Press; 1977.

17. Roach WH, Jr. Access to protected health information: a HIPAA primer. *Topics in Health Information Management.* 2002; 22:17–34.

18. Proctor PE, Davis N, Rosenblum B. Rightsizing HIPAA security compliance for smaller organizations. *Journal of Healthcare Information Management.* 2003; 17:34–40.

19. Longtermcareeducation.com. F150 Definition SNF, NF, resident rights overview §483.5; 483.10. Accessed July 10, 2005.

20. Richardson M, Schneller ES. Out of the box: health management education in the 21st century. *Journal of Health Administration Education.* 1998; 16:87–97.

21. Stefl ME. Editorial. *Frontiers of Healthcare Management.* 1999; 16:1–2.

22. Begun JW, Kaissi AA. Uncertainty in healthcare environments: myth or reality? *Health Care Management Review.* 2004; 29:31–39.

23. Hudson B. Joint commissioning across the primary healthcare–social care boundary: can it work? *Health and Social Care in the Community.* 1999;7: 358–367.

24. Burns M. Domain consensus in Alabama health systems agencies: an empirical assessment. *Administration and Society.* 1982; 14:319–342.

25. Grayson M. The open organization: an interview with the AHA chair-elect Richard Umbdenstock. *Hospitals & Health Networks.* 2004; 78:36–44.

26. Weber M. *From Max Weber.* New York: Oxford University Press; 1946.

27. Weech-Maldonado R, Meret-Hanke L, Mor V. Nursing staffing patterns and quality of care in nursing homes. *Health Care Management Review.* 2004;29: 107–116.
28. Mintzberg H. *The Structuring of Organizations.* Englewood Cliffs, NJ: Prentice Hall; 1979.
29. Hoppszallern S. Contract management survey 2002. *Hospitals & Health Networks.* 2002; 76:51.
30. Falcón A, Aguirre-Molina M, Molina CW. Latino health policy: beyond demographic determinism. In: Aguirre-Molina M, Molina CW, Zambrana RE, eds. *Health Issues in the Latino Community.* San Francisco: Jossey-Bass; 2001:3–22.
31. Aries N. Managing diversity: the differing perceptions of managers, line workers, and patients. *Health Care Management Review.* 2004; 29:172–180.
32. Resnicow K, Braithwaite RL. Cultural sensitivity in public health. In: Braithwaite RL, Taylor SE, eds. *Health Issues in the Black Community.* 2nd ed. San Francisco: Jossey-Bass; 2001:516–542.
33. Legal Q and A. *Hispanic Times Magazine.* 2000; 22:44–47.
34. Fried BJ. The legal environment. In: Fried BJ, Johnson JA, eds. *Human Resources in Healthcare.* Washington, DC: AUPHA Press/Health Administration Press; 2001:59–85.
35. von Bertalanffy L. *General Systems Theory: Foundations, Development, Applications.* New York: Braziller; 1968.
36. Tompkins J. Strategic human resources management in government: unresolved issues. *Public Personnel Management.* 2002; 31:1–10.
37. Tokesky GC, Kornides JF. Strategic HR management is vital. *Personnel Journal.* 1994; 73:115–118.
38. Niehaus R. Strategic HRM. *Human Resource Planning.* 1995; 18:53–60.
39. McWilliam CL, Coleman S, Melito C, et al. Building empowering partnerships for interprofessional care. *Journal of Interprofessional Care.* 2003; 17:363–377.
40. Adams A, Bomkamp R, Lopis R. Plan to recruit the right director of managed care. *Healthcare Financial Management.* 1995; 49:72–73.
41. Fottler MD. Job analysis and job design. In: Fried BJ, Johnson JA, eds. *Human Resources in Healthcare.* Washington, DC: AUPHA Press/Health Administration Press; 2001:87–115.
42. Emmett A. Snake oil or science? That's the raging debate on personality testing. *Workforce Management.* 2004; 83:90–92.
43. Molloy JT. *Live for Success.* New York: William Morrow; 1981.
44. McInerney T. Approaching physician recruitment systematically. *Healthcare Financial Management.* 1998; 52:83–84.
45. *Black's Law Dictionary.* 8th ed. St. Paul, MN: West; 2004.
46. Lind EA, Greenberg J, Scott KS, Welchans TD. The winding road from employee to complainant: situational and psychological determinants of wrongful-termination claims. *Administrative Science Quarterly.* 2000; 45:557–590.
47. Hader R. Collaboration paves the way for better care. *Nursing Management.* 2005; 36:4.

48. Harrison RV. The uncertain future of continuing medical education: commercialism and shifts in funding. *Journal of Continuing Education in the Health Professions.* 2003; 23:198–209.

49. Austin CF, Boxerman SB. *Information Systems for Healthcare Management.* Ann Arbor, MI: AUPHA Press/Health Administration Press; 2002.

50. Bennis WG. *Organization Development.* Reading, MA: Addison-Wesley; 1969.

51. Gerstein L, Bayer G. Employee assistance programs: a systematic investigation of their use. *Journal of Counseling and Development.* 1988; 66:294–297.

52. McGraw S. Do's and don'ts to motivate your staff. *Review of Opthalmology.* 2002; 9:26–27.

53. Moynihan JJ, Kibat G. EDI for human resources saves money and time. *Healthcare Financial Management.* 1994; 48:72–76.

54. Titlow K, Emanuel E. Employer decisions and the seeds of backlash. *Journal of Health Politics, Policy and Law.* 1999; 25:941–948.

55. Nolan W. Corporate compliance/corporate culture. *Behavioral Health Management.* 1998;18.

56. McAvoy SG, Schillaci A, Jr. Compliance crunch. *Trustee.* 1998; 51:12–16.

57. Willging PR. Corporate compliance isn't just "more government." *Nursing Homes Long Term Care Management.* 2004; 53:18–21.

58. Huq Z, Martin TN. Workforce cultural factors in TQM/CQI implementation in hospitals. *Health Care Management Review.* 2000; 25:80–93.

CHAPTER 4

Human Resources Practice in the Public Sector

Harold R. Griffin

VIGNETTE

Dana Griffin, a Marine Corps veteran and accomplished human resources practitioner with more than 10 years of experience, has recently accepted a position as Director of Human Resources for a local Veterans Affairs Medical Center (VAMC). Prior to accepting this position, Griffin's experience was limited to private sector health service organizations. Most recently, she was Director of Human Resources at Valley General, a 425-bed acute care facility with nearly 2,400 employees.

The VAMC is an acute care facility that operates 500 licensed beds in a large metropolitan area. Currently, it has more than 2,900 employees who serve the healthcare needs of 150,000 to 175,000 patients per year. The American Federation of Government Employees is the local union and is the exclusive representative of all employees, with the exception of management and a few other key positions that are excluded from the collective bargaining agreement. The relationship between the union and management can be characterized as "adversarial" at times, which has led to mutual feelings of distrust and apathy. Although the VAMC has been moderately successful in stabilizing the labor force in certain departments, such as Social Work, Nuclear Medicine, Engineering, and Laboratory Services, the turnover in other departments, such as Nursing, Pharmacy, and Physical Therapy, has consistently exceeded industry averages.

Strict governmental rules and regulations apply with regard to the hiring, disciplining, and retaining of employees. These rules and regulations are intended to ensure consistency and equity in the management of personnel, but they can also present a unique challenge to the recruitment and retention of new talent. This chapter provides insight into and approaches for successfully navigating these and other frequently encountered challenges facing healthcare human resources departments that operate in the public sector.

INTRODUCTION

During the 1990s, the U.S. economy underwent significant changes that required organizations to improve their performance and customer service, empower employees to get results, and reduce costs. These changes challenged human resources management (HRM) practitioners in both the private and public sectors to help organizations—both large for-profit companies with declining profit margins and federal and state agencies funded by shrinking tax revenues—to address these issues successfully. In the public sector, human resources managers work to serve not shareholders or owners, but rather the people as a whole. They also seek to further the interests of the community, whether that community is as small as a city or as large as the nation.

Downsizing, new approaches to human resources (HR) development and labor–management partnerships, and redirection of the HRM function have also affected public sector HRM in recent years. Downsizing occurred 25 to 30 years after a period of growth in the federal government and resulted in a reduction of 351,000 positions between 1993 and 1998.[1] Such reductions were accomplished by targeting highly paid employees and supervisors and offering buyouts that appealed mainly to employees who were eligible to retire.

While downsizing achieved the primary goal of reducing the federal payroll, it produced some unanticipated negative results as well. Organizations discovered that downsizing actually increased costs for training, overtime, contingent workers, and salaries. Furthermore, it engendered long-term morale problems for the remaining employees that resulted in a loss of organizational intellectual capacity and skill imbalances.[2]

Increasingly, successful managers were required to understand their HRM responsibilities (hiring, firing, developing, and evaluating employees) and to take on more of these duties as part of their jobs. HRM professionals' responsibilities shifted to advising and supporting managers and helping them provide a work environment where employees were treated with respect and dignity—functions that have been traditionally associated with the private sector.[3] This trend led to an increased focus in the public sector on developing and using HRM tools and techniques to implement real changes in HRM.

This chapter focuses on HRM in the public sector, examining how it functions relative to the areas of recruiting and retention, compensation and benefits, performance management, training and education, and collective bargaining. Where appropriate, applications are made to public health and health care in general. Strategic HRM and current HRM challenges are also discussed.

OVERVIEW OF THE SETTING

Public sector HRM is concerned with giving the people who make up the public sector workforce the tools, practices, strategies, and leadership needed to carry out the policies of government effectively and efficiently.[4] This section discusses the qualifications of public sector HR administrators and the unique challenges that they face in their public sector work.

QUALIFICATIONS OF HUMAN RESOURCES ADMINISTRATORS

HR administrators perform a number of functions, depending on their level, as determined by the employee population in the department, agency, or bureau in which they are employed.[5] At the managerial level, the HR administrator may be responsible for the following tasks:

- Administering the entire personnel program, excluding collective bargaining and labor relations, in the central office of a department, bureau, or commission that has decentralized operations, or in a department of administrative services in the HR division

- Planning and directing the activities of one or more statewide HR programs or operating units or sections
- Supervising the activities of HR analysts and/or managers at lower levels[5]

HR administrators must be knowledgeable about business and human resources and public administration; civil service laws, rules, and policies; procedures and provisions of collective bargaining contracts; supervisory principles and techniques; speech and effective communication techniques; public relations; and budgeting. In addition, they must have good computer skills.[6] They must be able to define problems, collect data, establish facts, and draw valid conclusions; write complex reports and position papers; counsel others on sensitive and controversial matters; and establish a friendly atmosphere as a supervisor. Among the educational and experience requirements are a minimum of a bachelor's degree in business, human resources, or public administration; several years' experience in business, human resources, or public administration; and supervisory principles and procedures.[7]

Issues in HRM Administration

During the 1990s, when the public sector experienced significant downsizing, some agencies that reduced or eliminated their HRM functions relied on employees in other specialties to perform HR work as collateral duties. These employees often did not receive sufficient training to enable them to perform this work accurately and efficiently. Also, many transaction-based activities, which are generally administrative and routine in nature, began to be automated and moved to a shared-delivery system. At the same time, as HRM staffs were being reduced, they were being asked to perform such higher-level responsibilities as managing change, leading strategic planning, and resolving conflicts.[3]

Federal agencies' ability to respond to the downsizing challenge was severely limited by both perceived and actual barriers that existed in the HRM system. Managers considered the systems to be too complex and inflexible, and accountability for performing major HRM functions such as hiring, handling issues related to classification and pay, supervising performance management, nurturing human resources development, and enforcing discipline was unclear.[3]

By the end of the 1990s, however, organizations began recognizing that people were the key component needed to achieve strategic goals and objectives and that HRM had to be redefined in terms of results. In pragmatic terms, this understanding meant that managers were free to adjust work and people to meet agency goals and objectives in a cost-effective manner; create and maintain a quality, diverse workforce; lead and train employees and develop their talents; foster a quality work environment that let employees manage work and personal responsibilities; and promote cooperative relationships with employees and unions.[8]

To achieve these goals, a report by the National Performance Review (NPR), created by President Bill Clinton in 1993, proposed comprehensive civil service reform legislation and HRM reform.[9] The NPR, now known as the National Partnership for Reinventing Government, was an intervention led by a task force of approximately 250 career civil servants and a few consultants, a few state and local government employees, and leaders in organizational change from business and government. Their aim was to create a federal government that "works better, costs less, and gets results Americans care about."[10] (p. 1) This effort, guided by Vice President Al Gore, saved taxpayers $136 billion, reducing the per capita cost of government spending for the first time since the Eisenhower administration, downsizing the federal workforce by 17%, and prompting the passage of 90 laws intended to streamline government.[10]

These changes had limits, however. Created more for legions of clerks rather than for the more sophisticated workforce of the 21st century, the hierarchy of employees in the federal government is based on a system of occupational pay levels, or "grades." Federal civil service workers begin their employment at an entry grade level and initiate a climb up a "career ladder." Each rung represents a serial promotion. Some of these promotions are noncompetitive and are awarded at regular intervals as long as the employee's job performance meets expectations.

The NPR recommended that the Office of Personnel Management (OPM) take steps to "dramatically simplify the current classification system and give agencies greater flexibility in how they classify and pay employees" so that agencies could more effectively recruit and retain quality staff.[9] (p. 59) It was recommended that the OPM propose legislation to "remove all grade-level classification criteria from the law"[11] (p. 25) and to adopt the broad-band approach to classification.[12]

Despite these and other efforts, civil service reform legislation has not been passed. Nevertheless, many federal agencies have taken vigorous action to reform and reinvent HRM within the structure of the current system by using existing flexibilities or solutions to a greater extent and by removing unnecessary barriers created by the agencies themselves. For example, the classification system has been identified as a major barrier to structuring work responsibilities to accomplish agency objectives. An interim broad-band model was proposed as one solution for overcoming this barrier.[13] In addition, the OPM has taken several steps to reform federal HRM systems, such as decentralizing and deregulating performance management. Some agencies have also delegated the authority for classifying positions to managers.

Revamping HR practices to improve government operations at the state and local levels is now under way as well. More than 11 million people are currently employed by local governments throughout the United States, an increase of more than 20% in the past 10 years.[14] According to Hays, the continued delegation of federal power to the state and local levels will mean continuing growth of the state and local sectors.[15] The literature reveals not only a concern with the administrative aspects of HRM at the state and local levels, but also with the "people" aspects, such as job satisfaction and creating a climate based on principles of merit, fairness, and openness.

HRM researchers and practitioners have devoted much study to the reasons people give for why they are satisfied or unsatisfied in their jobs.[16] Practical reasons for understanding and explaining job satisfaction—such as increasing productivity and organizational commitment, lowering absenteeism and turnover, and, in the long run, increasing organizational effectiveness—have been at the heart of these investigations of job satisfaction. More humanitarian reasons—for example, the principle that employees deserve to be treated with respect and to work in an environment that maximizes their psychological and physical well-being—have also been part of the focus on job satisfaction.[17] Research has shown that satisfied workers tend to go "above and beyond the call of duty,"[17] whereas dissatisfied workers tend to show counterproductive behaviors, including withdrawal, burnout, and workplace aggression.[18]

Some studies have begun to emerge that focus specifically on job satisfaction of government employees at the federal, state, and local levels. At the federal level, the Partnership for Public Service and American University's School of Public Affairs' Institute for the Study of Public Policy has published *Best Places to Work in the Federal Government 2005*.[19] Findings are based on a government-wide survey of almost 150,000 federal employees working at 250 agencies. Performed by the OPM, the survey found that the Office of Management and Budget, the National Science Foundation, and the Nuclear Regulatory Commission were the top-rated agencies, with all registering scores of 75% or higher in employee satisfaction.[19] Conversely, sounding an alarm just a few years ago about dwindling interest among graduates of public policy and public administration schools in working for government was Paul Light,[20] who reported that the percentage of new graduates seeking employment in the federal government fell between the early 1970s and 1993 from 21% to 15%. In a survey of 1,000 graduates, researchers found that only 65% of those working in government were "very satisfied" with their work, falling behind the 66% working in the private sector and the 75% working for nonprofit agencies who said they were "very satisfied."[20]

Despite the fact that in *The Best Places to Work in the Federal Government 2005,* the private sector scores in employee engagement and employee satisfaction overall remained higher than overall scores in the federal government, the difference between them shrank between 2003 and 2005: 3% of federal agencies had a higher overall score than private companies in 2003, but 20% beat the private sector score in 2005.[19] Longitudinal studies, including the biennial reports in the *Best Places* series, may with time identify whether this upturn in satisfaction indicates a meaningful trend.

One of the more recent studies of local government is Ellickson and Logsdon's[21] investigation of job satisfaction, which found that job satisfaction of municipal government employees is significantly influenced by perceptions of employee satisfaction with promotional opportunities, pay, and fringe benefits, with promotional opportunities being a major consideration.

Selden, Ingraham, and Jacobson[22] identified emerging trends and innovations in state personnel systems using data collected from a national survey conducted by the Government Performance Project. These researchers compared states in the areas of personnel authority, workforce planning, selection, classification, and performance management. Results showed that many states are modernizing their HR practices by delegating authority for personnel functions to agencies and managers, shifting their HR missions to being more proactive and collaborative with agencies, and adopting performance management systems that integrate organizational and individual goals. Proactive and collaborative HR operations seek a viable connection between employees' skill sets and the agency's organizational mission; they also recognize that such a connection promotes employee engagement and discourages job shifting, which is expensive for the employer.

Wisconsin has been a leader in acknowledging that government HR systems and processes must become more responsive, flexible, and efficient. The Wisconsin Department of Employment Relations has modernized state civil service laws, delegated decision making to operating agencies, developed creative ways to assess job applicants, made greater use of technology, expanded recruiting activities and affirmative action efforts, created more flexibility in compensation, and developed partnerships with public employee labor unions. These reforms have resulted in faster hiring, well-qualified job candidates, a more diverse workforce, and better ways to reward and retain talent.[23]

RECRUITMENT AND SELECTION

Both private and public sector organizations compete to employ the same people. Indeed, their ability to function depends on having enough people who possess the needed skills and knowledge.[4] In the public sector and particularly in public health, there has been a long-held assumption that health professionals are motivated by intrinsic rather than extrinsic factors, which has influenced both recruitment and retention policies.[4] The World Health Organization, however, notes that other factors motivate public sector health workers, including flexible working schedules, a safe work environment, and continuing education and career development opportunities; also, like all workers, public health workers are motivated by equitable and timely pay.[24]

In the public sector, the flow of high-quality new hires has decreased dramatically while the average age of workers has risen. Today many managers are attempting to rebuild a pipeline of entry-level employees in the most competitive labor market of the last 40 years.[1]

Current federal hiring methods have not kept pace with the private sector. While federal departments and agencies have the authority to conduct their own recruiting and examining for most positions, and although central registries and standard application forms have been abolished, agencies must still use the same rules and regulations as before. Therefore, hiring at the federal level remains a slow and tedious process.

RETENTION

According to Soni,[25] the current rigid command and control system—in which a manager has power over all equipment, personnel, procedures, and communications necessary for the planning, coordinating, and executing of a strategic tactical operation—restricts managers and workers to such an extent that individuals are not encouraged to work or act creatively. Advances in technology require a new kind of public sector employee: the knowledgeable worker with an entrepreneurial spirit.

The State of Texas has experienced the same recruitment and retention issues that exist at the federal level. Demographic trends and the demand for higher skills present major workforce challenges for Texas. For example, it was estimated that turnover would cost the state $345 million in 2004. At that time, almost half of all state employees had fewer than five years of experience with their current agencies. Another segment of the workforce was rapidly reaching retirement age, which was expected to result in the loss of state and institutional knowledge.[26] These career civil servants had entered state employment in the 1970s, committed their careers to their agencies, and were nearing retirement in 2004. Frequent job shifting by workers who entered the ranks of state employment—as well as federal employment—late in the 20th century meant that the government workforce might be broad but not deep and that the sweep of retirements scheduled as baby boomers leave employment (32% are expected to be eligible between 2001 and 2005) could result in what has been termed "an erosion of institutional memory."[27] (pp. ix, 6)

COMPENSATION

The federal compensation system was established at the end of the 1940s, when more than 70% of federal white-collar jobs consisted of clerical work.[28] Today, government work is highly skilled and specialized "knowledge work." Yet despite the obvious technological advances, pay and job evaluation systems that were designed for file clerks in the 1940s are still in use.

As noted earlier, the federal system is based on a hierarchy of occupational pay levels, or "grades." At entrance into the federal civil service, workers are assigned a grade according to their occupation, and throughout their career they move up in grade at promotions. If they meet performance standards, they receive promotions at regular intervals, but not usually more than once annually. Sometimes, however, two-grade increases are awarded. Pay is tied to grade, and each occupation's grade has its own pay level and its own steps within the grade.[29]

Physicians or lawyers, for example, might be hired at grade 11 or 12, and might be paid somewhat higher pay—entering at a step higher than step 1—if it was difficult to attract applicants.[30] Those who have master's degrees might be hired at grade 9, and those with bachelor's degrees are likely to be hired as professionals at grade 5, 6, or 7. Grade 4 is for those who have technical training or experience and skills as technicians. If a beginner has a high school diploma or some training, he or she might begin employment at grade 2 or 3. Grade 1 is reserved for beginners without a high school diploma and without experience (e.g., clerks).

After federal workers who are not supervisors reach the highest rung on their career ladder, they can still obtain pay increases (step increases) for performance that meets the standards of their agency or for outstanding performance.[30] Promotions, however, are typically competitive, based on merit, and depend on vacancies occurring.

Supervisors and managers are eligible for promotions, bonuses, and longevity increases. At the very top of these leadership positions is the Senior Executive Service (SES), an elite corps of leaders who are at a higher level than most other civil servants but below those who are nominated by the Executive Branch and approved by the Senate. Few civil servants are classified as SES workers. These positions elicit considerable competition, and pay increases are more likely to be based on performance than are pay increases for lower-level positions.

Applicants for this elite group are expected to demonstrate their competencies in five areas: (1) leading change, (2) leading people, (3) producing results, (4) demonstrating business acumen, and (5) building coalitions and communications.[31] Degrees earned or experience is not enough. An SES employee in health care or a related field might be a Veterans Affairs medical center controller, the chief of a center for medical biotechnology, or the director of an office of biohazardous materials management.

To remain competitive, employees are expected to expand and upgrade their skills by participating in continuing education programs. Acquiring new knowledge and skills can mean career advancement, increased responsibility, and rising pay. While universities and the annual meetings of professional associations have long offered such education, online education programs, including some sponsored by traditional providers, have become a substantial industry, representing a $7 billion market nationally and a $25 billion market globally.[32]

The persistent gap between the pay systems of the public and private sectors has led to calls for a more flexible compensation and benefits system—one that better supports the strategic management of human capital and allows government agencies to tailor their pay practices to recruit, manage, and retain the talent needed to accomplish their objectives. A more responsive compensation system would be characterized by performance- and results-driven reviews and would recognize competitive employment sectors with increases in base and ceiling pay as well as benefit offerings that match those in the specific market. In the current federal white-collar pay system, pay increases are not tied to performance; thus, performance is a secondary consideration when setting compensation rates.[28]

Another aspect of the federal compensation system that makes it increasingly irrelevant in the modern world is its emphasis on internal equity at the expense of external equity and individual equity.[28] The system does not permit federal agencies to allow nonclassification factors—for example, the importance of the work to the employing agency, salaries paid by competing employers, and turnover rates—to influence base pay.[28]

Merit system principles, such as equity, procedural justice, and openness, which were the foundation of the modern idea of a civil service,[5] remain important today. Agencies that have already moved outside the mainstream pay and job evaluation systems continue to use these principles effectively. The federal government as a whole can likewise be guided by merit system principles as it considers modernizing its compensation systems.[28]

Some have argued that performance of government employees, particularly in light of the terrorist attacks on the United States on September 11, 2001, is critically important.[1, 25, 33] In the narrowest terms, government operations that prevent terrorist attacks before they happen, governmental interagency teams that detect and dismantle arms systems that could deliver weapons to terrorists, and other federal initiatives that work to keep Americans and American interests safe have been accorded a more prestigious status, and so have the federal employees that make them successful.

In practical terms, the U.S. Department of Health and Human Services obtained permission from the OPM to hire health workers immediately as needed in the event of such public health crises as a terrorist attack or an infectious disease outbreak.[34] In a modernized organization, the government would require a results-oriented compensation system in which performance truly made a difference. Daley[33] asserts that if the federal government is to recruit, manage, and retain the human capital needed to accomplish and sustain this transformation, its white-collar pay system would need to (1) incorporate the principle of providing equal pay for work of equal value, (2) give agencies the authority and resources to offer competitive salary levels, (3) recognize individual and organizational competencies and results, and (4) link employee efforts and pay to accomplishment of objectives.

BENEFITS

In addition to initiatives undertaken to reduce the number of workers through downsizing, reorganizations, mergers and consolidations, elimination of middle management, forced early retirements, and outsourcing, there have been widespread initiatives to decrease benefits. Benefits in the public sector, like those in the private sector, have also been affected.[7, 35] Two decades ago, federal government jobs were considered better than average when compared to those of the typical American worker. Not only were salaries generally higher and health benefits better, but there was excellent job security and an outstanding retirement system, the Civil Service Retirement System (CSRS).[35]

In the mid-1980s, the CSRS was replaced with the Federal Employees Retirement System (FERS), which pays less in defined benefits at retirement. Further, the Civil Service Reform Act (CSRA), combined with recent changes in federal personnel regulations and practices, has taken away the job security federal workers once enjoyed. Enacted in 1978 and prompted in part by the Watergate scandal, the CSRA was the most dramatic civil service legislation in almost 100 years. Under CSRA, the Civil Service Commission was abolished, and its functions were assumed by the OPM, the Merit System Protection Board, and the Federal Labor Relations Authority, created to monitor labor–management relations. Subsequently, the environment in the public sector workplace has become more like that of a private sector firm. As in private sector organizations, these changes have largely hurt the average and lower-level federal employees, but not high-level executives, political appointees, or elected officials.[7]

The reductions in the number and level of benefits of public sector workers have contributed to the growing schism between the rich and the poor and the gap between the pay of workers and of top management. Job security has also decreased, as layoffs and firings can now occur at management's discretion. This trend was reflected in increases in anxiety about job insecurity among government employees, including white-collar employees, in the 1990s.[36] Health insurance takes an increasingly larger bite out of workers' pay, and a growing number of Americans cannot afford it.[5]

A recent survey conducted by the International Public Management Association for Human Resources, which encompassed responses from 324 public sector employers, found that over the most recent three-year period, double-digit increases in health insurance costs occurred.[37, 38] Almost 90% of the public entities reported making changes to the health benefits plan; one of the most common changes implemented was shifting a greater share of the cost of health benefits to the employees. Of the respondents, 99% offered health insurance to full-time employees, 67% provided health insurance to part-time employees, and 92% offered dental insurance. Costs to the public sector employer of providing health insurance ranged from greater than 40% of annual base payroll (12% of respondents) to 31–40% (32%), 21–30% (38%), and 20% or less (18%).

A trend that has gained momentum in both the private and public sectors is outsourcing of benefits. Outsourcing benefits functions can offer many advantages for public sector employees, such as improved communications, faster feedback, and rapid problem solving. These elements can also help boost employee morale and raise service levels.

The federal government's HR agency, the Office of Personnel Management, has reportedly been evaluating the outsourcing of some HR functions, according to a Conference Board report, *HR Outsourcing in Government Organizations,* published in 2004.[39] The Conference Board, a nonprofit global organization working in the public interest, conducts research and sponsors conferences to support business and to help it serve society. Federal government options include both classic outsourcing organizations and lift-and-shift operations that take an agency's existing HR personnel, technology, and processes and move them off site and into the vendor's environment. The complexity of some HR functions makes them particularly appropriate choices for outsourcing. Other processes besides benefits suggested as potential HR targets for outsourcing include call centers, Web sites, and staffing and recruitment.

A review by the U.S. General Accounting Office (GAO) of such outsourcing by eight federal agencies found that drug and alcohol testing, employee assistance programs, and health screening and wellness programs have been outsourced by some federal agencies. Other, more complex activities outsourced were strategic human capital management and workforce planning, organizational assessments, and benchmarking.[40] In addition to private outside companies, other government agencies that provide reimbursable services were selected for outsourcing initiatives. Benefits included freeing up agency staff to pursue strategic planning and introducing staff to new areas of expertise. Conclusions, or lessons learned, from using the alternative service delivery (ASD) options included the following:

- The importance of grasping the complexity of the activity before attempting to outsource it
- Setting measurable objectives as outcome measures
- Engaging in a meaningful relationship with the ASD vendor that helps both parties through any contractual or performance problems

An outcome of the GAO review was the establishment of communication between the council of chief human capital officers with the OPM, so that information about ASD could be shared, cost efficiencies achieved through ASD could be maintained or expanded, and accountability issues could be addressed.

A local government entity, the Detroit Public Schools (DPS), offers an illustration of the advantages of outsourcing. This school system was plagued with a decaying infrastructure, dwindling enrollments, and a $70 million deficit. After several failed attempts at educational reform, officials recognized that educational reform and fiscal reform needed to go hand-in-hand if they were to succeed in improving the school system. The first step was to overhaul DPS's benefits program. In addition to struggling with the program's complexity of databases, staff, and variability in benefits, employees routinely were bounced back and forth between the benefits office and insurance carriers, each of which promised—but did not always deliver—answers to the employees' questions. The unsurprising result: employee frustration and an erosion of trust.

Stephen Hill, the executive director for risk management for DPS, demonstrated that outsourcing would offset existing expenses to the tune of $3.5 million to $5 million by eliminating the exorbitant late fees and administrative costs; eventually, it would enable DPS to negotiate competitive plan rates. Hill was authorized to sign a five-year, $12.5 million vendor contract.[41]

While the unions were at first apprehensive about outsourcing (mainly because of DPS's past history of poor handling of employee claims and problems), job losses were not a concern because the DPS benefits department was understaffed. When union leaders understood the new system and, in particular, the new benefits employees would receive, they switched their position to support outsourcing.

DPS realized three major advantages of outsourcing the benefits program: cost savings, better union–management relationships, and better customer (employee) service. DPS has saved $1 million each year in carrier overpayments, eliminated late frees, reduced its annual health insurance costs by 4%, and negotiated premium increases that are 7% below the average (13% versus 20%). Union–management relations have improved because the new system has restored DPS's credibility and given DPS greater bargaining power in labor negotiations. By improving customer (employee) service, DPS has significantly reduced the number of benefits-related grievance calls unions would normally receive.[41]

Benefits are becoming more important for state employees and are accounting for an increasing proportion of the total compensation package. Kearney's[42] study attempted to identify factors that account for variations across the states in individual and family health insurance contributions, pension benefits, paid leave, child and elder care, and average salary. According to Kearney, the level of union representation was the most consistent and important determinant of compensation. Cost of living was also predictive of some compensation factors.

Roberts[43] surveyed 118 New Jersey local governments on their employee benefits practices. The survey results indicated that these governments are competitive with the private sector in terms of traditional benefits (health, pensions, dental coverage, and so on). However, local governments lag behind the private sector in the deployment of key family-friendly benefits, such as child care, elder care, flexi-place, flextime, and job sharing.

PERFORMANCE MANAGEMENT

In today's world, the public sector clearly needs a results-oriented, performance-based compensation system. The success of a performance-oriented compensation system, however, depends on the quality of the underlying performance management system.[44] A major and ongoing challenge in performance management is establishing and communicating credible and reliable measures of performance, whether at the organizational, work unit, or individual level.

A number of experts[9, 33, 44–46] agree that the standards for and quality of federal agency performance management and measurement are inconsistent. The OPM believes it may be time to establish a government-wide framework for making pay distinctions based on performance.[28] According to Daley,[33] the government needs to send a message to its employees: "Performance matters." However, unless this message is supported by a compensation system that bases pay increases on performance according to rigorous and realistic standards, it will likely be viewed as hollow rhetoric.

In the private sector, pay is linked to performance as a matter of principle.[11, 47] In the public sector, linking pay to performance will focus agency and employee attention on performance management, which could create a strong (and much-needed) incentive for agencies to improve how they measure and manage performance.[33]

In the area of differentiating levels of performance, which is already done in private sector organizations, the federal government needs considerable reform. Many agencies have applied "outstanding" ratings to so many members of their workforce that the term has been rendered meaningless;[44] other agencies have inflated performance ratings altogether.[12] Performance rated as better than fully successful starts as low as the 20th percentile in many agencies.[12] The ingrained policies of general increases, within-grade increases, and career ladder promotions also contribute to the ineffectiveness of the current public sector system.[46]

Little research has been conducted to answer the basic question of how effective performance appraisals are in public sector organizations. Longenecker and Nykodym's[48] research examined which specific functions were performed by the formal appraisal process in a public sector organization, whether managers and subordinates differed in their perceptions of appraisal effectiveness, and how the formal appraisal process might be improved. Their survey was administered to 357 members of the professional staff of a large multipurpose public sector service organization located in the Midwest. This organization had a professionally developed appraisal system, provided rater training, and required managers to conduct annual reviews of subordinates who reported directly to them.

The results of the study revealed that both managers and their subordinates believed that the appraisal process encourages employees' input about their jobs, informs employees of where they stand, helps clarify employees' performance and objectives, and facilitates the discussion of employees' development. By contrast, the appraisal process was perceived as being less than effective by both parties as a vehicle for improving employee motivation/performance and linking merit pay to the employee performance.

These findings are particularly noteworthy, because two of the most frequently cited justifications for doing performance appraisals are merit pay administration and improvements in employee motivation and performance. In each scenario, the appraisal system received disastrous ratings, especially from the subordinates' perspective. Managers believed the appraisal process was reasonably effective in both areas, while subordinates viewed the process as ineffective. Given the importance of manager–subordinate working relationships and effective manager–subordinate communications, the findings suggest that managers might not be aware that the appraisal process is not meeting the needs of their subordinates.

By its very nature, the appraisal process forces the manager to communicate with the subordinate, but the converse is not necessarily true. The advantages of the appraisal process as a tool to improve manager–subordinate relationships and communications are thus called into question by the very individuals whom the process is supposed to benefit.

In state and local governments, the use of performance measures is being driven by increased citizen demands for government accountability, greater interest on the part of local legislators in performance-related information to assist in program evaluation and resource allocation decisions, and the efforts of various organizations and professional associations to make governments more results-oriented.[49] A progressive pressure system used in Dallas County, Texas, which makes performance measurement and comparison with targets a daily instrument of shared management, shows how these concerns can be addressed satisfactorily.[50]

Dallas County began regular quarterly performance reporting in the early 1990s. By 1998, every county department was trained in outcome measurement and was required to submit outcome measures as a part of the budget process. These measures and targets have been reported quarterly since their development.

Nonthreatening, nonpunitive, progressive pressure is applied to managers to focus their operations on outcomes. Dallas County has developed a pattern of sending six to ten letters each quarter to department heads whose measures fail to meet their targets. Approximately twice that many nonperforming programs or programs with goals unrelated to the departments' outcome measures are assigned to "watch list" status. Thus far, there has been complete positive compliance with the requests for additional information. As a result, programs whose merit has come into question are discussed informally at least once during the year at a performance forum.[50]

Ammons[51] examined how various municipalities define duties and corresponding performance outcomes of city clerks, whose responsibilities vary from community to community. The following examples illustrate the measures used, along with performance benchmarks:

- Providing advance materials for upcoming meetings (e.g., delivering agenda packets at least four days prior to the meeting, as the city of Sunnyvale, California, does. The same task is to be performed 15 working days beforehand in Overland Parks, Kansas).
- Promptly indexing council documents and actions (e.g., within five working days, as is done in Anaheim, California).
- Promptly processing official documents (e.g., execute/publish/file 90% of official documents within 10 days of adoption/receipt/authorization, as the local government does in Oak Ridge, Tennessee).
- Promptly retrieving records and information (e.g., 80% within 24 hours, as is done in Peoria, Arizona).

Within a domain such as health, city officers might set a benchmark to meet or exceed the national rate for childhood vaccinations in their own community.

TRAINING AND EDUCATION

Federal government educational requirements are similar to private sector educational requirements for most major occupational classes. As might be expected, four-year college degrees are required for most professional occupations. These positions are considered grade 5 or 7, and in 2003 paid between about $23,400 and $37,700.[52] Within the federal government, managers are usually drawn from the professional occupations. The grades below them include office and administrative support workers, whose work typically requires only a high school diploma. The grades above them include personnel whose work may require additional training—physicians, lawyers, and scientists with doctoral degrees. For any of these jobs, relevant work experience is an asset. For jobs that do not require even a two-year college degree, for example, most departments and agencies would choose workers with vocational training or previous experience over those without.[29]

Training requirements vary between agencies and departments, but most offer opportunities for employees to acquire or improve their job skills so as to qualify for a new position or advance in an existing one. Schooling outside the agency may be made more accessible by tuition assistance or reimbursement. Executive or management training, as in the private sector, may be offered within the walls of employment or supported in business schools at nearby university campuses. Seminars and workshops are available to workers as well.[5]

UNIONIZATION

Nearly 17% of all union members in the United States are public sector employees. More than 6% of all union members work in the federal government, and more than 10% have jobs in state and local governments.[53] Approximately 37% of all government workers belong to unions.[1] Of this number, about 60% are federal employees, and 43% are state and local government employees.[1] U.S. federal, state, and local governments must deal with many different unions, as well as numerous individual bargaining units.

At the federal level, the largest union is the American Federation of Government Employees (AFGE), which represents about 600,000 federal employees.[54] The National Treasury Employees' Union, founded in 1938, has about 150,000 members in 30 government agencies.[55] The largest independent union for nonpostal government workers, it organizes workers from the Department of Health and Human Services, a government agency that encompasses the Public Health Service, the National Institutes of Health, and the Centers for Disease Control and Prevention.

The oldest union representing federal government employees is the National Federation of Federal Employees, which was founded in 1917.[56]

Although public sector employee organization efforts date back to the early 19th century, a major landmark occurred with the passage of the Lloyd-LaFollette Act in 1912, which first allowed federal government employees to organize. Even with this and other new rights to organize and collectively bargain on issues such as salaries, hours, and working conditions, governments on all levels have continued to resist the rights of their employees to use the ultimate weapon at their disposal: the right to strike.[1]

In 1935, the National Labor Relations Act (NLRA) was passed by Congress, based on its power to regulate interstate commerce and to govern the employer–employee bargaining and union relationship on a national level. When the NLRA was being drafted and debated in the 1930s, a central question was whether compulsory unionism should apply to government employees. The growing pool of government employees drew the attention of union organizers, but they faced great opposition for a number of reasons.

First, opponents of mandatory collective bargaining for government employees argued that compulsory union membership would threaten public safety. For example, they argued that forcing military leaders to bargain collectively with armed forces personnel unions would pose a serious threat to the effectiveness of the national defense. Second, critics argued that there is a major difference between government and the private economy in the areas of competition and consumer choice. For example, private sector businesses that negotiate union contracts with extravagant wages and inefficient work rules would soon be forced to drive up their prices and sacrifice customer service to meet the demands of their labor agreement. Recognizing these and other potential problems with public sector compulsory unionism, Congress exempted government employees from mandatory collective bargaining until 1978, when federal legislation mandated collective bargaining for many federal employees.[57]

The NLRA was amended by the Labor Management Relations (Taft-Hartley) Act in 1947, which in part defined six unfair labor practices, and by the Labor Management Reporting and Disclosure (Landrum-Griffin) Act in 1959, which protected the rights of members of employees' unions from unfair practices by unions. The employees and agencies in the federal public sector are currently subject to the Federal Service Labor-

Management Relations Act (FSLMRA), which is administered by the Federal Labor Relations Authority.[58]

While there is general acknowledgment that unions have proved useful in addressing many of the salary and working conditions issues of previous eras, some believe that today unions are an obstacle to reform in the public sector.[35, 59, 60] For example, technology has made many former rote, tedious jobs obsolete. Budgeting and personnel administration activities in the public sector need more thoughtful, flexible workers who both use the new technologies and create continuously improving public services. Traditional boundaries between production and management are breaking down, despite the unions' traditional us-versus-them position toward management.[25]

In the public sector, HR strategy needs to consider the range of different constituent perspectives and focus on both national and lower organizational tiers. This complexity precludes autonomous management actions in many instances. If these characteristics of public sector HRM are ignored, unrealistic HR strategies may be formulated that are destined to fail.[8]

CONCLUSION

This chapter discussed HRM in the public sector, including how it functions relative to the areas of recruiting and retention, compensation and benefits, performance management, training and education, and collective bargaining. Strategic HRM moves away from the traditional focus on management–trade union relations, workforce control, and organizational policies and toward a view of the people in the organization as important assets, or human capital. Public sector human resources administrators face many challenges in today's rapidly changing environment. Some of the more significant challenges relate to recruiting qualified individuals into public sector employment, finding meaningful career paths for these individuals, and accepting the necessity and challenge of culture change.

In the federal government, hiring remains a slow and tedious process as compared with hiring in the private sector, even in a competitive labor market. The number of high-quality new hires has decreased, while the average age of federal workers has risen. Furthermore, rapid technological change has required hiring of workers with corresponding skills, but federal agencies are unable to make compelling offers to attract appropriately skilled employees.[44] Even with a reduced federal workforce, more than 100,000 hires will be required annually just to make up for attrition. More than 20,000 of those hires will be for technical and administrative professional positions where competition is most intense. Because years of downsizing have resulted in more internal selection and less selection from employees from outside federal agencies, human resources administrators will have to refresh their recruiting skills and develop creative approaches to attracting and retaining talent.[4]

Efforts to reform the current outdated and inflexible position classification system must be made, not only to eliminate artificial and inefficient hierarchical organizational structures, but also to ensure that talented individuals remain in federal service. These challenges must be dealt with in other public sector areas as well. Most cities and counties use a single classification system for all employees, although many (like the federal government) use different classification plans for different kinds of employees, such as clerks, trades people, professionals, and executives. The smaller the jurisdiction, the more likely it supports multiple classification systems.[57] Position classification systems work very well for a hierarchical command-and-control environment. Advances in technology, however, require that workers be cross-trained and allowed to move across rigid positive classification systems.[1]

Labor market conditions have also had implications for succession planning. While many public agencies have reexamined their approach to recruiting, retaining, and managing workers, there has been a strong lack of focus on succession planning. Currently, overall turnover rates are relatively low—around 6%; in the future, however, the aging workforce and skills imbalance will result in a retirement surge and fewer available younger workers. At the same time, the nature of the employment relationship in public service is changing. Contrary to the traditional notion that a career in public service is a career for life, a growing number of employees no longer want to spend their entire work life with the same employer or occupation.[61]

Public sector agencies can pursue many strategies for change without altering existing law or government-wide policy; however, true change involves a fundamental shift in attitudes, culture, and values regarding the civil service system and employment in the public sector. Such a shift will require agreement among the stakeholders on the fundamental context and content of the changes, champions to provide the leadership, and a coalition of the key players to make it happen.[4]

In today's workplace, paternalistic cultures are being replaced by cultures that foster greater equality and adult relationships.[4] These changes will require employees to take more responsibility for their own competence, performance, and development.[44] Meanwhile, executives and managers at all levels must take responsibility for providing challenging work opportunities and creating a culture that fosters learning, teamwork, and accountability for results. Significant civil service reform should begin with an articulation of values reflecting these culture changes. Current merit system principles can provide guidelines; they should be retained to the extent that they support the overarching values.[3, 13]

REFERENCES

1. Hays SW, Kearney RC (eds.). *Public Personnel Administration.* 4th ed. Upper Saddle River, NJ: Prentice Hall; 2003.
2. National Academy of Public Administration (NAPA). *Downsizing the Federal Workforce: Effects and Alternatives.* Washington, DC: 1997.
3. National Academy of Public Administration (NAPA). *Human Resource Management Responsibilities of Line Managers.* Washington, DC: 1997.
4. Berman EM, Bowman J, West J. *Human Resource Management in Public Service: Paradoxes, Processes, and Problems.* Thousand Oaks, CA: Sage; 2000.
5. Shafritz JM, Rosenbloom DH, Riccucci NM, Naff KC, Hyde AC. *Personnel Management in Government.* 5th ed. New York: Marcel Dekker; 2001.
6. Elliott RH, Tevavichulada S. Computer literacy and human resource management: a public/private sector comparison. *Public Personnel Management.* 1999; 28:259–264.
7. Pynes JE. *Human Resources Management for Public and Nonprofit Organizations.* San Francisco: Jossey-Bass; 1997.
8. Nigro LG, Nigro FA. *The New Public Personnel Administration.* Ithaca, IL: FE Peacock Publishers; 2000.
9. National Performance Review (NPR). 1993 Report: From Red Tape to Results. Creating a Government That Works Better and Costs Less. 1993. Available at: http://govinfo.library.unt.edu/npr/library/nprrpt/annrpt/redtpe93/2342.html. Accessed October 31, 2004.
10. National Partnership for Reinventing Government. FAQs: National Partnership for Reinventing Government. 2000. Available at: http://govinfo.library.unt.edu/npr/library/papers/bkgrd/q-n-a.html. Accessed October 17, 2005.
11. National Academy of Public Administration (NAPA). *Modernizing Federal Classification: An Opportunity for Excellence.* Washington, DC: 1991.
12. National Academy of Public Administration (NAPA). *Federal Classification: Operational Broad-banding Systems Alternatives.* Washington, DC: 1995.

13. National Academy of Public Administration (NAPA). *Innovations and Flexibilities: Overcoming HR System Barriers.* Washington, DC: 1997.
14. U.S. Census Bureau. *Statistical Abstract of the United States.* Washington, DC: U.S. Census Bureau; 2003.
15. Hays SW. Trends and best practices in state and local human resource management: lessons to be learned? *Review of Public Personnel Administration.* 2004; 24:256–270.
16. DeCenzo DA, Robbins SP. *Human Resource Management.* 6th ed. New York: Wiley; 1999.
17. Dessler G. *Human Resource Management.* 9th ed. Upper Saddle River, NJ: Prentice Hall; 2003.
18. Spector, P. *Job Satisfaction: Application, Assessment, Causes and Consequences.* Thousand Oaks, CA: Sage; 1997.
19. *The Best Places to Work in the Federal Government 2005.* Washington, DC: Partnership for Public Service and the Institute for the Study of Public Policy Implementation, School of Public Affairs, American University; 2005. Available at: http://www.bestplacestowork.org. Accessed October 18, 2005.
20. Light P. *The New Public Service.* Washington, DC: Brookings Institute; 1999.
21. Ellickson MC, Logsdon K. Determinants of job satisfaction of municipal government employees. *State and Local Government Review.* 2001; 33:173–184.
22. Selden SC, Ingraham PW, Jacobson W. Human resource practices in state government: findings from a national survey. *Public Administration Review.* 2001; 61:598–605.
23. Lavigna RJ. *Best Practices in Public-Sector Human Resources: Wisconsin State Government.* New York: Wiley; 2002.
24. Buchan J, Adams O. Health sector reform and human resources: lessons from the United Kingdom. *Health Policy and Planning.* 2000; 15:319–325.
25. Soni V. From crisis to opportunity: human resource challenges for the public sector in the twenty-first century. *Review of Policy Research.* 2004; 21:157–163.
26. Texas State Auditor's Office. A Summary of the State of Texas Workforce for Fiscal Year 2004. 2004. Available at: http://www.sao.state.tx.us/Reports/report.cfm/report/05-704. Accessed December 30, 2004.
27. U.S. Merit Systems Protection Board. *The Federal Workforce for the 21st Century: Results of the Merit Principles Survey 2000.* Washington, DC: U.S. Merit Systems Protection Board; 2003.
28. U.S. Office of Personnel Management (OPM). *A Fresh Start for Federal Pay: The Case for Modernization.* Washington, DC: U.S. Office of Personnel Management; 2002.
29. McKinney A. *Real Ksas—Knowledge, Skills, and Abilities—for Government Jobs: Improve Your Chances of Gaining Federal Employment by Preparing Top-notch Ksas.* West Fayetteville, NC: Prep Publishing; 2003.
30. Trautman KK. *Federal Resume Guidebook: Write a Winning Federal Resume to Get In, Get Promoted, and Survive in a Government Job.* Indianapolis, IN: JIST Works; 2004.

31. U.S. Office of Personnel Management (OPM). *Guide to Senior Executive Service Qualifications.* Washington, DC: U.S. Office of Personnel Management; 1998.

32. Bleak J. Insulated or integrated: for-profit distance education in the non-profit university. *Online Journal of Distance Learning Administration.* 2004; 5. Available at: http://www.westga.edu/~distance/ojdla/summer52/bleak52.html. Accessed November 1, 2005.

33. Daley DM. *Performance Appraisal in the Public Sector.* New York: Greenwood Press; 2002.

34. Sontag E. Testimony on Federal Hiring Reform before the Subcommittee on Oversight of Government Management, the Federal Workforce and the District of Columbia Committee on Governmental Affairs, U.S. Senate, 2004. Available at: http://www.hhs.gov/asl/testify/t040720.html. Accessed October 7, 2005.

35. Ban C, Riccucci NM. *Public Personnel Management: Current Concerns, Future Challenges.* 3rd ed. New York: Longman; 2001.

36. Aaronson D, Sullivan DG. The decline of job security in the 1990s: displacement, anxiety, and their effect on wage growth. *Economic Perspectives.* 1998; 22:17–43.

37. Thigpen J, Phillips JD. *Trends in Public Sector Human Resources.* Alexandria, VA: International Public Management Association for Human Resources; 2005.

38. International Public Management Association for Human Resources. 2005 IPMA-HR Benchmarking Committee Report: Healthcare Benefits Cost Management. 2005. Available at: http://www.ipma-hr.org/index.cfm?navid=128. Accessed November 1, 2005.

39. National, state governments join companies in outsourcing HR and other functions. *PA Times* (September 2004):7. [The *PA Times* is published by the American Society for Public Administration.]

40. U.S. General Accounting Office (GAO). *Human Capital: Selected Agencies' Use of Alternative Service Delivery Options for Human Capital Activities.* Washington, DC: U.S. General Accounting Office; 2004.

41. Koch J, Dell D, Johnson LK. *HR Outsourcing in Government Organizations.* New York: Conference Board; 2003.

42. Kearney RC. The determinants of state employee compensation. *Review of Public Personnel Administration.* 2003; 23:305–322.

43. Roberts GE. New Jersey local government benefits practices survey. *Review of Public Personnel Administration.* 2001; 21:284–307.

44. Daley DM. *Strategic Human Resource Management: People and Performance Management in the Public Sector.* Upper Saddle River, NJ: Prentice Hall; 2001.

45. Atkinson A, McCrindell JQ. Strategic performance measurement in government. *CMA—the Management Accounting Magazine.* 1997; 71:20–31.

46. U.S. General Accounting Office (GAO). *Federal Personnel Management: Views on Selected NPR Human Resource Recommendations.* GAO\GGD-95-221BR. Washington, DC: U.S. General Accounting Office; 1996.

47. *Private Sector Compensation Practices.* Booz Allen and Hamilton Report to the U.S. Office of Personnel Management. Washington, DC: 2000.

48. Longenecker CO, Nykodym N. Public sector performance appraisal effectiveness: a case study. *Public Personnel Management.* 1996; 25:151–163.
49. Condrey SE (ed.). *Handbook of Human Resources Management in Government.* 2nd ed. San Francisco: Jossey-Bass; 2004.
50. Scheps PB. Linking performance measures to resource allocation. *Government Finance Review.* 2000; 11–15.
51. Ammons DN. *Municipal Benchmarks: Assessing Local Performance and Establishing Community Standards.* Thousand Oaks, CA: Sage; 1997.
52. U.S. Department of Labor. Career Guide to Industries, 2004–05: Federal Government, Excluding the Postal Service. 2004. Available at: http://www.bls.gov/oco/cg/cgs041.htm. Accessed October 19, 2005.
53. Spengler AW. *Collective Bargaining and Increased Competition for Resources in Local Government.* New York: Quorum; 1999.
54. American Federation of Government Employees (AFGE). *The American Federation of Government Employees, AFL-CIO.* Washington, DC: AFGE; 2005. Available at: http://www.afge.org. Accessed October 19, 2005.
55. National Treasury Employees Union (NTEU). Washington, DC: NTEU; (no date). Available at: http://www.nteu.org. Accessed October 19, 2005.
56. National Federation of Federal Employees (NFFE). *NFFE-IAM: Pride—Unity—Strength.* Washington, DC: NFFE; 2005. Available at: http//www.nffe.org. Accessed October 19, 2005.
57. Henry N. *Public Administration and Public Affairs.* 6th ed. Englewood Cliffs, NJ: Prentice Hall; 1995.
58. Carrell M, Heavrin C. *Labor Relations and Collective Bargaining.* Upper Saddle River, NJ: Prentice Hall; 2001.
59. Buell J. The future of unions. *Humanist.* 1997; 57:41–42.
60. Candaele K, Drier P. Labor's growing pains. *Commonweal.* 1996; 123:9–10.
61. Wilkerson B. *Public Sector Succession Planning.* Denver, CO: WisdomNet; 2002.

CHAPTER 5

General Principles of Human Resources Management in Public Health Settings

Lloyd Greene

VIGNETTE

Robert Lewis sat back at his desk in the Human Resources (HR) Department of the Maryland State Department of Health and Mental Hygiene, pondering the past few years. National events such as the terrorist attacks of September 11, 2001, and anthrax scares had created a growing awareness of and need for public health services. This trend had amplified the importance of his job, especially with the current and projected labor shortages; complex regulatory, jurisdictional, and legal requirements; and movement toward generic core competencies for public health workers. There were certainly more challenges ahead, especially in the diverse and unique work environment of state public health—challenges he had better get back to work on.

INTRODUCTION

Public health settings lend themselves to rich and complex applications of human resources strategies, skills, and practices. Often, 24-hour-a-day, 7-day-a-week demands on highly specialized, professionally diverse teams functioning in a truly "open system" environment, typically in multiple geographic locations, require consistent and thoughtful attention to human resources issues. Added to this work environment are the special values, such as altruism, concern for social justice, and caring for the underserved, that many public health professionals bring to and find in their daily work life.[1]

Effective HR management (HRM) should help create an environment that provides equity, encourages productivity, organizes people to achieve goals and desired results, and meets individual needs for achievement, recognition, and growth. Best practice HRM is able to accomplish these goals. While very little literature is devoted to this subject, and professional organizations such as the American Hospital Association and the American Society for Healthcare Human Resources Administration have largely focused on HRM in more generic healthcare settings, this chapter examines those issues and practices associated with HRM in public health organizations. It covers the scope and work environment of public health settings and the functions essential to an HRM role in public health settings. The fully developed HR function typically includes policies, procedures, and programs for recruitment and employment, benefits, compensation, employee relations, training, employee safety, and strategic leadership. These functions are highlighted in each section of this chapter. The goal is to illuminate those issues and practices that are germane to public health organizations and their stakeholders. Given the importance of creating interdependence between these functions, some overlap between sections is inevitable. The chapter also describes generic issues and practices as well as examples of specific applications in public health environments.

To be of the greatest value, HR functions need to be aligned with and connected as directly as possible to the business and strategic objectives of an organization, department, or unit. To paraphrase David Ulrich, human resources needs to be connected to the real work of an organization.[2] Furthermore, the major HR functions should be integrated with and supportive of one another. In this sense, HR can take an important leadership role in helping organizations achieve success.

OVERVIEW OF THE SETTING

Roles

According to the first enumeration of the public health workforce in more than 20 years, 448,254 professionals work in this field at the federal, state, or local level.[3] Approximately 75% are employed as nurses or in allied health roles.[4] Some of the roles performed by these professionals are nurse, medical assistant, nursing aide, social worker, physician, respiratory therapist, home health aide, pharmacist, and physical therapist.[5] In addition, nonmedical roles include administrative support personnel, technicians such as software and hardware experts, managers and administrators, inspectors, and epidemiologists. While approximately 67,500 of these workers are employed at the federal level, chiefly by the Department of Health and Human Services, the majority are employed by state or local governments.[6]

The Work Environment and Public Health Programs

Communicable diseases, bioterrorism preparedness, immunizations, septic systems and wells, and restaurant inspections are just a few of the issues with which public health professionals deal.[7] A review of the Austin/ Travis County (Texas) Health and Human Services Department identified public health services as including Environmental and Consumer Health, Communicable Disease Unit, Emergency Medical Services, Healthy Neighborhood Unit, Health Promotion and Disease Prevention Unit, Public Health Emergency Preparedness and Response, and Community Health Centers.[8] Examples of specific work sites for nurses and allied health professionals include community clinics, mobile outreach units such as vans, schools, and wherever emergency response is needed. Tasks that these professionals often perform include health assessments, treatment, education, diagnosis, triage, referral, follow-up visits with patients, pharmaceutical and nutritional counseling, and patient transport. This work environment and programmatic diversity provide many excellent opportunities for HRM to creatively and progressively perform its role in support of organizational goals and outcomes.

Trends in Public Health Human Resources Management

Human resources management in healthcare settings such as hospitals and, more recently, public health settings has been slowly evolving from a traditional, isolated personnel department to a more proactive HR function that is linked as directly as possible to an organization's operational and strategic needs.[9] A high-level view identifies public health challenges as including labor shortages, the growth of managed care, an enhanced role for prevention, the growing number of uninsured persons, shifting public expectations, and restructuring at all levels.[10]

More detailed information about the labor shortage will be covered in the "Recruitment and Selection" section of this chapter. As an overview, however, it is noteworthy that the overall labor force in public health has been shrinking over the last 30 years even though the U.S. population has been growing. The number generally reported as the size of the public health labor force for decades was 500,000 but, as noted earlier in this chapter, is now 448,254. With population growth, this dwindling of the workforce has resulted in a significantly changed ratio of public health workers per individual, up from 457:1 to 635:1.[11] This trend has critical implications for the nation's health and the public health system's capacity to respond to crises such as the attacks on the World Trade Centers and Pentagon and the later anthrax threats. Clearly, it heightens the need for thoughtful, strategic HR actions and plans.

Growth of managed care seems to be a way of life in any healthcare setting. Increases in healthcare costs, charges, insurance premiums, and individual out-of-pocket expenses have forced more employers, individuals, and governments into some kind of contractual relationship with providers, including public health medical facilities. These arrangements typically result in reduced revenue for healthcare providers in relation to charges. For example, Medicare and Medicaid continue to reduce their reimbursement amounts. Combined with rapidly increasing costs of providers driven by a steady rise in the cost of labor, the escalating cost of pharmaceuticals, rapidly developing diagnostic and therapeutic technology, increased demand for services, and reduced or minimally increased budgets for public health, it is not difficult to see that creative and insightful management of human capital is essential in these settings.

As employers eliminate or significantly increase the cost of health insurance for their employees, and as public assistance programs are eliminated or drastically reduced, the number of uninsured persons in the United States continues to rise. While most uninsured seek care at a crisis level through emergency departments, often the burden of providing that care falls to public health facilities, which further increases their financial pressures.

As a result of terrorist threats including public infrastructure sabotage, bioterrorism, and violence, the U.S. public now expects greater response capability, surveillance, planning, and coordination from all levels of public health. In summary, all of these trends have important implications for thoughtful, consultative, and strategic HRM.

What would a more proactive and organizationally aligned HR role look like in this environment, and how would this vision differ from the more traditional personnel office approach? The HR role traditionally included record keeping and technical attention to policies, benefits, and compensation administration; tended to be reactive and unaligned with organizational objectives or strategies; and tended to function in a closed system model. That is, "personnel" did not need to respond to—nor were they significantly affected by—external forces. The needs of public health organizations, as outlined earlier in this section, would most likely be reacted to, not planned for, and almost certainly not managed by HR professionals partnering with senior leaders. Partly because of external trends and challenges, and partly because the evolution of the HR profession has created a role that fully partners with stakeholders including leaders and employees, the approach to HRM has begun to change. The role has evolved toward a strategic business partner in both a programmatic and a consultative sense.[2]

Predictions about future directions for HR roles indicate a change from less programmatic to more consultative application of HR principles. This shift will be driven, in part, by reengineering of the HR role to reduce costs and focus on customer needs. Past criticisms of "personnel offices" focused on their staff's excessive concern with strict compliance with rules and procedures rather than results.[12] More recent shifts in the terminology—if not the emphasis—of the HRM function include the "human capital" approach. Human capital is defined as the know-how, skills, and capabilities of individuals in an organization; it is seen as the most important resource, particularly for knowledge-based organizations.[13]

These trends have been the basis for three models of HRM reform in public health organizations: customer service, organization development and consulting, and strategic HRM.[14] In brief, the customer service model exhorts HR departments to do what they do better and faster, recognizing that the manager is the key customer. The organization development and consulting model suggests that HR professionals facilitate resolution of large-scale organization problems and serve as internal consultants on human resources and a wide range of organizational problems and issues. This approach is often coupled with the HR department giving up some traditional HR functions—for example, benefits administration. In the strategic HRM role, HR professionals help create and support an organization's mission, vision, and strategic stance through HR alignment, planning, and actions. Each of these roles requires a differentiated set of competencies, such as managing for customer service, reengineering, process consultation, and creating a shared vision. It is probably most useful for HR professionals to think of these models as polarities rather than as absolute choices. Each can be useful and appropriate, given organizational culture and needs.

Managing polarities requires "both/and" (not "either/or") thinking.[15] This is particularly true of public health settings, which are characterized by significant diversity in operating unit services, missions, goals, job classifications, and HR needs in general. Getting clarity about the HR needs of an operating unit is a basis for determining which model(s) may be appropriate at any given time. For example, given the previously described trends facing public health, HR professionals could use the consultant model to help organizations think about restructuring; assist managers in responding to the shift in public expectations through patient relations and cultural sensitivity training design and delivery; use the strategic model to help address the labor shortage challenge; and use the customer service model to help reduce costs, increase flexibility, and improve response time to organizational problems.

The next part of this chapter deals with the basic HR functions. It defines their meaning, describes their legal basis where applicable, and discusses practical issues related to application in public health settings.

RECRUITMENT AND SELECTION

The recruitment function is intended to expedite attracting well-qualified applicants to organizations. It must do so within an increasingly complex legal and regulatory environment that starts with defining and understanding the employer–employee relationship.

Regulatory and Legal Issues in Employment

The legal basis for most employer–employee relationships is known as "employment at will." This concept defines the relationship between employee and employer to exist "at the pleasure" of either. Fundamentally, this can be described as a noncontractual relationship, either implicitly or explicitly. However, in terminating the employment relationship, most organizations have adopted methods that allow for grievance hearings and progressive discipline for involuntary terminations. In public health settings, this approach is typically amplified because of statutory requirements.

For example, public sector employers, unlike their private sector counterparts, deal with constraints imposed by constitutional guarantees, including greater rights of due process and free speech, as well as privacy protections incorporated into the U.S. Constitution and corresponding to more expansive rights provided under state and local constitutions or statutes.[16] Both the U.S. Constitution and state constitutions protect citizens from "government action." Specifically the Fourth Amendment to the U.S. Constitution protects against "unreasonable searches and seizures" by the government or under government authority, and the Fifth Amendment protects against self-incrimination (which deals with crimes—and all criminal law is based on the government's power to enact criminal statutes). In short, the U.S. Constitution and most state constitutions are designed to protect citizens from the government (the founding fathers did not want a strong government in this sense). The exception is the concept of privacy, which is not really spelled out in the U.S. Constitution (but is in some state constitutions). Where the courts have deemed that citizens have a right to privacy under the constitution (U.S. or state), this ruling applies across the board, although the U.S. Supreme Court has held that employees have a lesser expectation of privacy in the workplace than at home or even in their cars. In short, public employers need to be cognizant of these distinctions and generally be aware of the enhanced protections due to their employees.

Human resources managers in public health settings need to pay particular attention to these rights and are advised to seek legal council in establishing their HR policies. Likewise, HR managers in public health deal with a statutory framework that differs in key respects from the framework facing private employers.[16] Thus managers and supervisors in the former settings find themselves dealing with rules and regulations that are unique to local labor contracts and/or employment practices for all public entities in their jurisdiction, not just the public health providers. This multiplicity of legal, jurisdictional, and contractual relationships greatly complicates the relationship between employees and employers. It is advisable to create, wherever possible, a single basis for the employment relationship. The "Employee Relations" section of this chapter will expand on this point and give some operational examples of this complexity.

Design and Implementation of Recruitment Processes

It is incumbent on HR departments to provide leadership in the design and implementation of recruitment processes. In public health environments, this often must be done with civil service laws relating to hiring in mind. These laws often detail the manner in which individuals are hired, procedures for making promotion decisions, evaluation processes, and disciplinary/termination procedures. Many of these requirements vary substantially from state to state and sometimes even by locality within those jurisdictions.[16] This multiplicity of rules again adds to the complexity of HRM in public settings, but should not prevent HR professionals from adopting "state of the art" procedures. For example, one public health clinic is considering the use of computer software to screen job applicants as a way of expediting the employment process, improving quality, and reducing costs.[17]

Recruitment processes typically start with a needs analysis coupled with a position-control, budget-driven system. They then move to various levels of approval before HR people become involved. Position control should link human resources and finance in the recruiting process. A position-control system prevents attempts to fill positions for which no budget dollars are available and therefore stops the recruiting process at its inception. For example, if a manager wanted to fill a vacant position, he or she would send a requisition (often via an automated system) to the HR department. However, if the manager's personnel budget has been cut, the position has been eliminated, or, for some other reason, no funding is available to support hiring a new employee, the position-control system would be aware of this fact and would prevent the requisition from going forward.

Ideally, line managers should have the greatest involvement in the hiring process, and HR professionals should help with coordination, policy oversight, strategic leadership, and monitoring effectiveness and efficiency. Having metrics that assess the quality of hires, the cost of the hiring process, and the time it takes to fill a position is an example of a value-added role that human resources can take in the recruitment process. Anticipating and addressing a labor shortage, establishing employment policies, and educating staff about legal issues in the employ-ment process are other examples of HR roles in recruitment.

Recruitment Challenges and Opportunities in Public Health Settings

Like organizations in most contemporary healthcare settings, public health organizations are challenged to fill many clinical positions. Nurses, imaging professionals, lab technicians, respiratory therapists, emergency medicine technicians, medical assistants, medical social workers, and physicians are examples of these sorts of caregivers. These professions are plagued by a current and chronic labor shortage. For example, recent pre-dictions indicate a shortage of 400,000 registered nurses by 2010.[18] While this number includes nurses who work in all major practice settings, including public health, it indicates the difficult recruiting chal-lenge for healthcare providers. In fact, 30 out of 37 reporting states indi-cated that nursing is the occupational class most affected by the workforce shortage; nursing shortages are twice the shortages noted in the next lead-ing class, epidemiologists.[19] In addition, states report labor shortages for laboratory workers, environmental health specialists, public health man-agers, and microbiologists.

In addition to these current shortages, the Bureau of Labor Statistics, as indicated in Table 5-1, predicts that the greatest growth in healthcare em-ployment by 2010 will include medical assistants (50% increase), physi-cian assistants (50% increase), respiratory therapists (33.3% increase), physicians and surgeons (22.2% increase), and registered nurses (15% in-crease).[20] This trend will clearly amplify an already existing problem!

Coupled with this demand for new staff is the increasing national va-cancy rate for RNs (11%), and other healthcare professions, such as phar-macists (21%) and imaging technicians (18%).[21] Another significant variable affecting this labor challenge is the average age of public health workers. According to the Association of State and Territorial Health Officials (ASTHO), the average age of state public health workers is 46.6 years, while the average age of the U.S. workforce is 40 years.[19] Because the largest portion of the U.S. working population is starting to move into retirement age, this trend toward an aging workforce creates new challenges for filling vacant positions in public health.

Unless significant changes are made in our ability to educate clinical professionals or healthcare delivery is restructured in significant ways, the

Table 5-1 Employment of Selected Hospital Occupations, 2000–2010

Occupation	Projected Percent Change, 2000–2010
Total (includes public and private and all occupations)	9.8
Registered nurses	15.1
Nursing aides	11.1
Physicians and surgeons	22.2
Medical assistants	50.0
Respiratory therapists	33.3
Home health aides	33.3
Surgical technologists	16.9
Cardiovascular technicians	32.0
Respiratory therapy technicians	33.3
Physical therapists	15.9
Public health social workers	22.2
Computer support specialists	66.7
Health information specialists	22.2
Physician assistants	50.0
Social and human service assistants	33.3

Source: U.S. Department of Labor. *Employment of Selected Hospital Occupations, 2000 and Projected 2010.* Washington, DC: Bureau of Labor Statistics; 2000.

workforce shortage will only increase. The aging population, increased demand for health care, technological and clinical advances, and a more educated patient population will be key drivers of this problem. Combined with a projected increased demand on outpatient or ambulatory settings,[22] a growing uninsured population, and a greater need for multilingual staff, the recruitment challenge for public health organizations and their HR staffs cannot be overstated. Public health settings and their HR professionals have attempted to solve this growing problem in several notable ways: engaging communities and educational institutions, studying best practices, searching worldwide, offering language instruction, establishing career paths, using more assertive personnel, and restructuring the care delivery process. Additionally, using independent contractor employees where permitted by the Internal Revenue Service (IRS), contract employees who are separate from independent contractor status, grant-funded salary structures, evidence-based bonus systems, and rigorous salary and wage data have all proven effective in attracting and retaining staff.

Gathering market data that use comparable statistics (i.e., average actual pay), compare job duties as well as job titles, are current, and are based on an appropriate geographic recruitment area is an important first step in this process. It helps create fair and competitive pay practices, without which recruitment difficulties are amplified. According to ASTHO, states are considering numerous strategies to ensure adequate staffing of public health agencies:[19]

- Increasing pay and benefits
- Offering flexible work schedules and telecommuting
- Providing professional training
- Training future public leaders
- Marketing public health careers at high schools and colleges
- Partnering with educational institutions
- Using information technology and the Internet for recruitment

While these strategies are important and likely to have some impact, they are essentially the same as those employed by most industries experiencing a labor shortage. In that sense, they do not give public health a competitive advantage or highlight its distinctive attributes. Public health settings offer unique opportunities and practice environments that attract a special group of providers. For these people, their values, life experiences, professional needs, and goals find their best match in these kinds of environments.[23] In addition, the work environment and scheduling in public health clinics are often more attractive than those in acute care settings. These characteristics can and should be used to attract job applicants and to market these careers. Also, linking with grant-funded programs and other sources of operating revenue can be an effective way to create funds and interest for staffing and attracting staff. Finally, engaging communities in diverse, multi-institutional, community-led collaborations to address this problem is essential and has proven to be very effective.[24] After all, this is not a public health "industry" problem; it is a public problem!

At the national level, the Health Resources and Services Administration (HRSA) commissioned a report entitled *The Public Health Workforce: An Agenda for the 21st Century*, which made several strategic recommendations to deal with healthcare workforce shortages.[25] Table 5-2 lists these suggestions. Their primary emphasis is the creation of a

Table 5-2 HRSA Public Health Workforce Recommendations

- Continued national oversight and planning for development of a public workforce capable of delivering essential public health services across the nation
- Establishment of mechanisms to support workforce planning and training in all states and local jurisdictions
- Greater use of a standard taxonomy to identify the size and distribution of the public health workforce in official agencies and private and voluntary organizations
- Refinement and validation of public health practice competencies associated with each of the various professions that make up the workforce to improve basic, advanced, and continuing education curricula for the public health workforce and strategies to certify competencies among practitioners
- Strengthening of distance-learning strategies and technologies

Source: U.S. Department Health and Human Services, Core Functions Steering Committee. *The Public Health Workforce: An Agenda for the 21st Century.* Washington, DC: DHHS-PHS; 1997.

national, "systemic" approach to public health workforce development. Getting a clear idea of need and, therefore, a quantifiable sense of the problem, standardizing practice competencies, organizing and increasing resources, and, most importantly, establishing policies and a national priority for public health workforce development are the key components of this systems approach. In addition, creating increased capacity in our current education and training delivery methods, including schools via technology, going to students versus having them commute, modifying curricula, and creatively engaging communities, are alternatives for addressing this "throughput" problem. Although these recommendations are intended for national action, many of the ideas contained in the report could be implemented at the local community level.

EMPLOYEE SAFETY

Although most federal law applies to public health settings, one area of federal regulation that does not typically apply to public health employers is the Occupational Safety and Health Act (OSHA).[23] While employees are thus not protected under the federal OSHA guidelines, local jurisdictions often mandate a comparable program. Also, regardless of requirements, it is advisable—for reasons of prudent management and constructive employee relations—to design and implement a safety and work-related injury documentation, follow-up, and compensation system. Such a system can aid in recruitment, retention, operations improvement, and public perception.

Although workplace safety and security functions are not always directly managed by HR professionals, they are highly interdependent. Employee relations, training, and benefits are some HR functions that are impacted by and impact employee safety and security. Human resources leaders should help develop work site safety audits, identify roles in employee safety and security, participate in crisis management teams, develop programs that help injured employees return to work, write policies for and plans in response to workplace violence, provide and/or coordinate employee safety training programs, and be involved in prevention and security plans in relation to terrorism. Given the diverse and very open environments of public health organizations, this is a complex and increasingly critical HR and organizational issue.

COMPENSATION AND BENEFITS

As mentioned in the previous section, public health units are often subsumed under a municipal umbrella on matters of safety. This is equally true in the area of pay and benefits. This "umbrella" usually takes the form of universal pay policies, practices, benefit programs, and pay and benefits administrative functions that are intended for all public employees within a jurisdiction. When a pay structure is established, jobs are evaluated for placement within this pay structure, and, when hiring offers are made, a centralized HR function for municipalities often dictates what kinds of offers are extended.

Pay delivery in the public sector is often less than in the private sector. While this difference does not create an insurmountable obstacle, it does require a certain amount of "creative commitment" on the part of HR professionals. Being able to invent solutions, understanding the range of opportunity in each policy, and adding diverse people and processes to develop alternatives are methods for adding divergent thinking while living within the "letter of the law." (As an aside, it should be noted that all federal pay provisions such as the Fair Labor Standards Act apply to public health settings.)

Benefits for public sector employees do not appear to be a competitive advantage when compared to the benefits offered by private employers.

According to ASTHO, many states are considering improving their benefits programs to bring them in line with those of private employers. Trends in benefits development and administration in all sectors of the healthcare industry include choice, flexibility, spending accounts, pay in lieu of benefits, benefits designed to increase with seniority, and greater attention given to retirement programs.

For example, one public health system has designed a retirement program that increases employer matching contributions based on an employee's age and length of service. This program is intended to retain employees as they get older and to attract older job applicants who would otherwise start over with regard to retirement benefits. These new, older employees get greater employer matching contributions than new, younger employees. Retaining and attracting older employees is critical not only because these workers bring an increased level of experience and expertise, but also helps address the labor shortage mentioned earlier in this chapter. Being able to attract older job applicants, who would otherwise lose retirement seniority, and retaining employees by increasing matching contributions in light of an aging workforce are value-added HR strategies. Additionally, rehiring employees who have already retired is an increasingly common practice. A majority of states are considering ways to do this.[19]

Among other issues that this trend presents is the need to create flexibility in and alternatives for state or locally mandated retirement plans. Given the increasing government oversight of retirement plans in general and the need to very carefully manage departure from retirement guidelines, adoption of such a plan will require thoughtful work by HR professionals.

The design and administration of benefits programs in public health settings, like other aspects of HRM, are carried out by government agencies and municipalities and, therefore, are intended to cover a broader workforce than just healthcare workers. In this sense, it is incumbent on HR professionals who work in public health settings to be advocates for their staff's special needs and to use creativity in administering their benefit programs.

EMPLOYEE RELATIONS

Legal Framework

As mentioned earlier, many complex federal laws govern the relationship between employee and employer. Laws such as the Americans with

Disabilities Act (ADA), Fair Labor Standards Act (FLSA), and Equal Employment Opportunity Act are intended to ensure that employees are treated fairly and consistently with respect to policies, procedures, and practices that govern day-to-day occurrences in the workplace. Additionally, in public health settings, employee relations policies and practices are frequently informed by state, local, and contractual relationships between employer and employee. For HR professionals in public health, this multiplicity of jurisdictions creates complex operational challenges. For example, while the FLSA provides federal guidance on pay practices, one local public health clinic was able to modify its overtime pay practices based on local interpretation of shift work needs and demands on staff by the public. Another example of operational complexity is worker's compensation. While federal regulations inform the management of worker injuries for most employers, chiefly through OSHA, states are largely responsible for worker's compensation provisions and insurance programs. Some states permit employers to opt out of state-sponsored worker's compensation programs entirely.

While public health organizations may be exempt from some of these provisions, HR professionals in these settings must be aware of the implications that these various regulations have for them. There are several perspectives on this issue:

- Employee relations perspective: Do employees believe that management is concerned about their safety and well-being?
- Labor market perspective: Do prospective job applicants understand that they will be treated fairly in the event of a job-related injury, particularly when other employers have programs in place to do this?
- Public perspective: Citizens want to make sure that their governments treat public employees fairly.
- Statutory/regulatory perspective: The complexity of requirements must be adequately addressed. Being aware of federal mandates that affect employee safety, state provisions for employee safety, and local government requirements for all public employees in this area increases the need for well-thought-out HR policies and practices.

Because of this complexity, it is often useful for HR professionals to seek advice to determine how much flexibility they have in managing to the intent of these policies while maximizing the utility for their operating units. One jurisdiction has done so by establishing "implementing procedures" that allow for a relevant and business-related application of overarching policies.[26] For example, to help public health organizations be more competitive in a tight labor market, an expedited hiring process might eliminate approval layers while staying within the framework of a hiring policy.

Policies and procedures that relate to employee discipline take on particular significance in public health arenas because of the legally mandated attention to due process. Public employees generally have a greater right to due process than do employees in the private sector. It is critical to have a well-developed "progressive discipline" process that lays out several levels of sanction for employees to go through before or if involuntary termination is considered. This process should also include a well-developed, clearly communicated grievance process.

Because public employees may be more directly connected to the political process, and because elected officials are often members of governing boards of public health providers and thus can make or influence HR policy and procedures, HR professionals need to manage these relationships and be aware of the impact of their policy decisions and actions in this light. It is not uncommon for employees who believe they have been treated unfairly or who dislike an HR policy to contact a public official for help and/or some level of intervention!

Managing Relationships and Employee Relations Programs

Establishing a constructive, high-quality work life is fundamental to employee relations. Effective supervision, growth, affirmation, autonomy, communication, and job design are some important variables to consider in creation of a productive work environment. Public health settings offer unique opportunities for implementation of these strategies. Public health organizations tend to have a much lower turnover rate than the healthcare industry as a whole: Average turnover for the healthcare industry as a whole is about 20%,[27] whereas turnover rates for public health environments are 10–14%.[19] Given this stability, there are ample opportunities to develop sustainable, constructive relationships with staff.

An axiom in managing employee relations is that, to the extent effective relationships are developed with employees, there will be a decrease in the need for a "legalistic environment." Put another way, if employers focus on developing a positive relationship with staff, they are less likely to need to rely on policies or laws to govern their actions. Establishing employee-valued methods for communication, seeking staff input on key decisions, providing opportunities for job-related autonomy, assisting leaders to develop the capacity for establishing a constructive employee relations environment, providing growth and affirmation programs and systems for employees, and being fair (not necessarily consistent!) in the treatment of staff are only a few ways to achieve this environment.[28]

In the public health setting, there is also a unique opportunity to match the value systems that many staff bring to their work in the form of goal congruence.[1] The values espoused by these employees tend to be altruism, social justice, care for the underserved, and public service. Public health organizations can identify and communicate organizational goals and cultural values and offer opportunities for staff to experience these values in their work. Given the typical diversity of public health settings, highly differentiated methods are often available that could be used to achieve this employee relations goal. In other words, one size does not fit all employees and work sites. The HR professional should develop several approaches and methods, geared toward the particular staff composition and work site characteristics, to achieve this constructive relationship.

Training and Education

While the standards found in the Joint Commission on Accreditation of Healthcare Organizations (JCAHO) do not apply to any of the HR functions found in public health settings, including training and education, several public and private auditing agencies do review these organizations' performance. In addition, HRSA has developed a set of "core competencies" for public health professionals (discussed later in this section).[4]

State health departments, local review boards, and grant funding agencies set their own standards and, in the case of grant funders, often have HR requirements that differ from and conflict with state and local HR requirements. This multitude of perspectives adds to the complexity of HR management. Human resources record keeping, work rules, pay structures, and employment relationships are a few of the challenges that these differing requirements bring.[23]

Also, while JCAHO has explicit requirements and standards regarding staff development and training, state and local review agencies and grant sources have their own educational regulations. While JCAHO might provide "one-stop shopping" for private sector healthcare employers with regard to education requirements, these requirements in public health settings often derive from diverse, sometimes conflicting sources and require

HR departments to establish multiple tracking systems, documentation processes, and delivery methods.

This complexity is usually coupled with the challenges associated with having a geographically dispersed staff. The wide distribution of employees creates difficulty in training delivery, securing staff time for training, documenting training, and measuring training effectiveness. It has required that training be done more frequently, via computer-based technologies, self-guided learning methods, "just-in-time" training, and training delivered by peers.

Core Competencies for Public Health Professionals

Of the more than 450,000 public health workers in the United States, only a fraction receive formal public health training.[29] Most professionals who do earn public health degrees receive their education from schools of public health and, to a lesser extent, from public health degree programs. Unlike members of virtually all other health professional groups, graduates of these programs are not certified as to their competencies.

In recent years, interesting and useful work has focused on the development of core competencies for public health professionals.[30] For example, public health practitioners and academics who participated in a Public Health Faculty/Agency Forum developed the list of suggested core competencies shown in Table 5-3. They can be organized under two categories: technical skills and intrapersonal/interpersonal skills.

The technical core includes problem solving, data analysis, research design, policy development, program and financial planning, and basic health science skills. While no one best method for developing this set has been identified, it lends itself more to a didactic teaching/learning style. This might involve a lecture, rule-driven approach for novices and case studies for more proficient learners. These technical skills could also be embedded in academic curricula and reinforced by employers through their training resources or outsourced to local academic institutions.

The intrapersonal/interpersonal core includes communication, group effectiveness, creating participative environments, cultural competence, managing people, and applying basic "people" skills. This set of skills lends itself to team- or organization-based experiential methods that should be facilitated by content experts and focus on real issues within an organization. Ideally, an organization's leadership will play a central role in this process. Leaders should set learning priorities, participate in the

Table 5-3 Universal Competencies for Public Health Professionals

- Defining a problem
- Determining appropriate use of data
- Understanding basic research designs used in public health
- Communicating effectively
- Leading and participating in groups
- Soliciting input from individuals and organizations
- Policy development and program planning
- Cultural competence
- Basic public health sciences skills
- Financial planning and management skills
- Managing personnel
- Applying basic human relations skills

Source: Public Health's Infrastructure. A status report prepared by the Centers for Disease Control and Prevention, 2000.

design of major training events, participate in the set of training activities, and be interested in follow-up.

Human resources professionals often have skills in many, if not all of, these areas and can serve as in-house consultants to the process. Obtaining this set of skills is important for all levels of staff. Educational methods include self-appraisal, values clarification, role-plays, instrumentation that provides individual or group feedback, and dialogue. It is important to link all forms of skill development to outcomes. Answering questions such as "What will be different after we undertake this training?" or "How does this training help us meet our goals?" keeps it relevant and value added.

Interestingly, the issue of credentialing for public health professionals appears to be unresolved. Although it is viewed as important, the American Public Health Association is still considering this topic.[10] In keeping with a key dimension of job satisfaction, many states are considering incentives designed to advance the competencies of their public health workforce, such as scholarship and school loan repayment programs, work-study arrangements, professional training, and distance-learning opportunities. By partnering with educational institutions, many states are beginning to educate all health professionals about public health skills and are developing basic public health curriculum units that can be integrated within formal degree programs. This trend is consistent with the theme of developing and implementing core competencies for public health professionals, whether they be caregivers or others.

Of particular importance in public health settings is the development of management talent. The success of any organized health program depends on effective management, but unfortunately health systems worldwide face a lack of competent management at all levels.[31] Management development, particularly at the first-line level in public health, should be given a high priority by senior leaders, funding agencies, and political leaders. Human resources leaders should have the capacity to facilitate this process and consult in the development of management education systems that demonstrate a positive outcome for their agencies and, ideally, show a return on investment. One problem that lack of management capability fosters is development of "vertical" health programs that are narrowly targeted and centrally planned. This practice discourages decentralization, program integration, local participation, and initiative. In other words, weak management is the enemy of fundamental public health values.[31] A useful place to start management development is to ask the question, "What does it take to be successful as a manager in our organization?" Explicitly linking management education to organizational goals, strategies, values, and mission in an evidenced-based way is another excellent starting point. Training managers on the job and with the team has proven to be the most useful approach for delivery of education.[32]

The American Public Human Services Association (APHSA) has taken a very active approach toward defining leadership roles and competencies.[33] APHSA, founded in 1930, is a nonprofit, bipartisan organization that brings together individuals and agencies concerned with human services. Members include all state human services agencies, more than 150 local agencies, and several thousand individuals who work in human services programs, including public health. APHSA has as its central role the education of members of Congress, the media, and the broader public on what is happening in the states around welfare, child welfare, healthcare reform, and other issues involving families and the elderly.[33] It offers HR professionals a valuable resource when thinking about training and education for their own organizations. The APHSA leadership and practice department currently offers the following services:

- Unique leadership development programs
- Leadership for high-performance training

- A leadership "train the trainer" program
- Personal mastery training
- Leading major organizational change
- Executive team development
- Executive coaching

The intent is to focus on the special characteristics and dynamics of public health environments as the key element in this education and development activity.

STRATEGIC PLANNING

Public health organizations offer ample opportunities for strategic thinking and acting in the HR arena. The desire to contribute to the achievement of organizational goals is an important starting point for HR strategizing. Table 5-4 lists some challenges that have been identified by leaders in the public health arena. How can HR practices help address these challenges in a strategic way? Mintzberg defines strategy as an intuitive, creative thinking process that involves both emergent and deliberative strategizing.[34] In this sense, it comprises both analysis and synthesis. To the greatest extent possible, HR actions must be invented that can demonstrate a relationship to organizational outcomes, further goal

---

Table 5-4 Selected Public Health Challenges

- Growth of managed care
- Privatization
- Welfare reform
- Steering versus rowing
- Invisibility of public health
- Government and health department reorganization
- Emergence of new diseases and reemergence of old diseases
- Changing demographics
- Enhance role of prevention
- Growing number of uninsured
- Shifting public expectations

Source: Rowitz L. *Leadership for the 21st Century. Public Health Leadership.* Gaithersburg, MD: Aspen Publishing; 2001.

achievement, and use valid and reliable metrics. Starting with an end or outcome in mind and a measurement method is critical. For example, Table 5-4 indicates that one challenge is the "growth of managed care." A likely result from this growth is reduced revenue when compared to charges. Human resources might help meet this challenge by developing creative ways to reduce overhead costs through restructuring, increasing the use of technology, redistributing HR roles, focusing or refocusing compensation and benefit plans, and making HR practices (e.g., hiring) more effective and efficient. As Mintzberg indicates, following this path requires creative, intuitive thinking and acting. Additionally, HR professionals need to show how these actions will, in fact, help reduce costs.

Additional strategic challenges in public health include addressing the labor shortage, changes in patient populations, growing uninsured populations, increased diversity, and changes in the regulatory environment. In short, they require anticipating and creating the future! In addition, HR professionals need to stay aware of and anticipate changes in the HR field itself. In this sense, it is important to have systems or methods in place to support this need. Certainly being connected to HR organizations such as the American Society for Healthcare Human Resources Administration is important. Likewise, being linked to experts in the benefits, compensation, employment/labor law, HR technology, and training areas is particularly useful in staying current and getting a sense of future trends. One organization has responded to this problem by getting on e-mail distribution lists of consultants and experts in these areas. This was done at no charge and resulted in frequent updates regarding changes and "pending" changes. To the extent possible, it is most useful for HR professionals to fully partner with their organization's leadership in this effort. Human resources strategizing is most effectively done through cocreation with and support of senior leaders.

Having listed all of these strategic opportunities for human resources in public health, it is important to emphasize the limited shelf life of plans in turbulent environments such as health care. Specific plans tend to have minimal value in this context. More useful strategically is what some describe as having a management philosophy designed to provide the organization with a long-term collective purpose and direction.[35] Having a strategic "stance" rather than a hard-and-test "plan" might be more appropriate in public health organizations. Having a clear, compelling vision, understanding how an organization intends to relate to its employees, making sense of the external and internal environment, emphasizing core competencies, and being able to act spontaneously using this information as a grounding are the essence of strategy in fast-changing environments. Conversely, there is no "either/or" equation in public health. Having specific actions for each of the major HR functions that is connected to an overall vision or stance is likely to be most productive.

CONCLUSION

Public health professionals provide a wide variety of services in an environment that is both rewarding and demanding. The growing public awareness of what was once an "invisible" part of the nation's infrastructure is creating both opportunities and challenges. In addition, threats such as terrorism, the need for greater coordination between public health providers, and the increasing sophistication required of public health professionals create a critical and rich setting in which human resources can add value. Being aware of what distinguishes the management of human resources in a public health context is an essential starting point.

Understanding the unique employment/legal environment and being able to creatively manage within it requires strategically addressing the current and increasing public health labor shortage; playing a key role in helping staff acquire additional skills, including the move to core skills; aligning compensation and benefits programs with public health organization needs and goals; and, perhaps most importantly, being sensitive to and skillful in establishing employee relations policies, programs, and actions that amplify and reaffirm the values, interests, and professional goals of those people who enter the field of public health. This chapter offered suggestions, guidance, and overall approaches that HR professionals and public health organizations can use to add value and achieve success in these areas.

REFERENCES

1. Franco LM. Health sector reform and public sector health worker motivation: a conceptual framework. *Social Science and Medicine.* 2002; 54:1255–1266.
2. Ulrich D. A new mandate for human resources. *Harvard Business Review.* 1998; Jan–Feb:124–134.
3. Center for Health Policy at the Columbia University School of Nursing. Public health work force declining in numbers. *Nation's Health.* 2001; 31:1–2.

4. Health Resources and Services Administration. The health professions workforce. *Health Workforce Link.* 1999.
5. Turnock B. Public Health: *What It Is and How It Works.* Gaithersburg, MD: Aspen Publishing; 2001.
6. U.S. Department of Health and Human Services. Available at: www.hhs.gov. Accessed June 10, 2005.
7. Welch N. In the hot seat of public health. *The Virginia Pilot.* February 18, 2005:8.
8. Austin City Connection. Available at: www.ci.austin.tx.us/health. Accessed May 15, 2005.
9. Robbins S, Rakich J. Hospital personnel management in the late 1980s. *Hospital and Health Services Administration.* 1986; July/August:18–33.
10. Rowitz L. *Leadership for the 21st Century: Public Health Leadership.* Gaithersburg, MD: Aspen Publishing; 2001.
11. Center for Health Policy at the Columbia University School of Nursing. Public health workforce declining in numbers. *Nation's Health.* 2001; 31:1–2.
12. U.S. Merit System Protection Board. *Federal Personnel Officers: A Time for Change?* Washington, DC: U.S. Merit System Protection Board; 1993.
13. Lengnick-Hall M. *Human Resource Management in the Knowledge Economy.* San Francisco: Berret-Koehler; 2003.
14. Ban C. The changing role of the human resource officer. *Handbook of Human Resource Management in Government.* 2nd ed. San Francisco: Jossey-Bass; 2004.
15. Burns L. *Polarity Management: The Key Challenge for Integrated Health Systems.* Report prepared for the Physician/Hospital Institute of the Illinois Hospital and HealthSystems Association. 1997; December:1–13.
16. Susser P. *State and Local Government Employment Law and Practices Handbook.* Austin: Sheshunoff Publishers; 2004.
17. Community Care Services Department. Austin–Travis County, Austin, TX. Interview notes, April 2005.
18. Buerhaus PI. Implications of an aging registered nurse workforce. *Journal of the American Medical Association.* 2002; 283:54–58.
19. Association of State and Territorial Health Officials. *State Public Health Employee Worker Shortage Report: A Civil Service Recruitment and Retention Crisis.* Washington, DC: 2004.
20. U.S. Department of Labor. *Employment of Selected Hospital Occupations, 2000 and Projected 2010.* Washington, DC: Bureau of Labor Statistics; 2000.
21. American Hospital Association. Vacancies Rampant Beyond Nursing. Available at: www.aha.org. Accessed August 30, 2001.
22. American Hospital Association. *Workforce Facts and Trends at a Glance.* Prepared by the Center for Health Workforce Studies, University at Albany, State University of New York, 2003.
23. Gertz F. Austin/Travis County Health and Human Services, Human Resources Unit. Austin, TX. Interview notes, April 2005.

24. Greene L. Engaging communities in workforce development. *Pulse: Journal of the American Society for Healthcare Human Resources Administration.* 2003; Winter.

25. U.S. Department of Health and Human Services, Core Functions Steering Committee. *The Public Health Workforce: An Agenda for the 21st Century.* Washington, DC: DHHS-PHS; 1997.

26. Leasure T. Austin/Travis County Emergency Medial Services, Human Resources Unit. Austin, TX. Interview notes, April 2005.

27. Bureau of National Affairs. *Report on Job Absence and Turnover.* Washington, DC: 2001.

28. Herzberg F. One more time how do you motivate employees? *Harvard Business Review.* 1968; January–February.

29. Institute of Medicine of the National Academies. *Who Will Keep the Public Healthy? Educating Public Health Professionals for the 21st Century.* A report from the Institute of Medicine of the National Academies. Washington, DC: National Academy of Science; 2002.

30. Sorenson A, Bialek RG. *The Public Health Faculty/Agency Forum.* Gainesville, FL: University of Florida Press; 1992.

31. Filerman GL. Closing the management competence gap. *Human Resources for Health.* 2003; 1:7.

32. Mintzberg H. *Managers Not MBAs.* San Francisco: Berrett-Koehler Publishers; 2004.

33. American Public Human Services Association. Available at: www.aphsa.org. Accessed June 10, 2005.

34. Mintzberg H. The fall and rise of strategic planning. *Harvard Business Review.* 1994; Jan–Feb:107–114.

35. Zallocco R, Joseph B, Furey B. Do hospitals practice strategic planning? An empirical study. *Healthcare Strategic Management.* 1984; 2:16–20.

CHAPTER 6

Managing Human Resources in an Integrated Healthcare System

Kanak Gautam

VIGNETTE

In 2000, Mount Carmel Health Systems had a human resources crisis on hand. Employees were unhappy and leaving their jobs. Overall, staff turnover at the central Ohio health system was 24%. The nursing vacancy rate was at 12%. Only 47% of staff rated Mount Carmel a great place to work.

To reinvigorate employee morale, Mount Carmel initiated a cultural transformation program dubbed "Higher Ground." The program aimed to reconnect people with the reasons they came into health care. More than 700 managers went on week-long retreats where facilitators helped them discuss the benefits of leading subordinates by inspiration and a call to service. The Higher Ground program helped unite Mount Carmel employees around a shared commitment to service. Over time, staff turnover came down to 12%, and nursing vacancies decreased to 3%.[1]

High turnover and cultural disenchantment have been common problems in many integrated health systems. Integrated health systems were often created from an amalgam of organizations that were very different in terms of their community served, size, mission, and culture. Forging a common purpose among such disparate entities remains one of the foremost challenges facing human resources managers in health systems today.

INTRODUCTION

Integrated health systems (IHSs) like Mount Carmel Health Systems emerged in the 1990s in response to declining reimbursement and managed care; they represented an attempt to improve the negotiating power of healthcare providers, control costs, and expand revenues. An IHS is an entity formed through acquisition or merger that provides a coordinated continuum of care to a defined population. Organizations that form the care continuum generally include physician practices, hospitals, long-term care, and home health. Three features distinguish IHSs. Unlike stand-alone facilities, they provide coordinated patient care across a care continuum in an attempt to provide comprehensive care to patients. Second, IHSs rely on primary care physicians (PCPs) to control costs by acting as gatekeepers to manage illness and monitor specialist care. Many IHSs acquired physician practices for precisely this purpose. Third, IHSs assume responsibility for delivering high-quality patient care within a fixed dollar limit set by payers. They contract with managed care organizations at the system level, using their network of physicians and facilities as negotiating leverage.

According to the American College of Healthcare Executives, there are 324 integrated healthcare systems in the United States. Some of the largest IHSs are well-known names in the healthcare field—for example, Intermountain Healthcare, Providence Health System, Advocate Healthcare, Henry Ford Health System, Presbyterian Healthcare Services, Sentara Healthcare, and BJC Health System. The number of hospitals that are part of health systems has remained stable over the past several years due to slowing of merger and acquisition activities since the late 1990s. This slowdown reflected the mixed results achieved by early mergers. While many IHSs of the 1990s were able to improve their financial and clinical performance through integration, others faced resistance to change from constituent hospitals and physicians. Another problem was the excessive prices paid to acquire physician practices, which caused financial distress and led to a wave of "de-integration."

Despite the recent slowdown in IHS formation, today's healthcare markets are more concentrated because of IHSs. According to one study, in 2000, the average market shares for the top four health firms in urban markets was 99% for markets of 250,000 and less; 93% for markets between 250,000 and 1 million; and 73% for markets of more than 1 million. Today's IHSs have survived the de-integration phase and are the market leaders in most urban healthcare markets. This chapter provides an overview of human resources practices within IHSs. After introducing the IHS setting, the chapter focuses on such human resources issues as the formation of HR, strategic planning, recruitment, selection, retention, training and education, performance management, compensation, ben-efits, unionization, and concludes by highlighting areas HR must strengthen.

OVERVIEW OF THE SETTING

IHSs enjoy several strategic advantages over stand-alone entities:

- They enjoy economies of scale because they can spread their fixed costs over a large patient base. They can also lower their overhead costs by centralizing several departments across operating units such as finance, legal, and laundry services, and by consolidating expensive clinical services such as open-heart surgery, thereby reducing duplication of services.
- Their large patient base and wide geographic distribution of hospitals and physician practices gives them power in negotiating rates with managed care organizations.
- Their continuum of care allows patients (e.g., at a physician's office) to use downstream services as needed (e.g., hospital services), thus ensuring them revenue for multiple services provided to the same patient.
- They generally have strong system boards that are involved in strategic planning and resource allocation and that are able to pool system resources and maximize revenues across the system. System boards,

by acting centrally, are also more successful in clinically integrating services across the system and instituting quality standards.

Not all IHSs have realized these advantages. Indeed, IHSs have had to fulfill several strategic requirements to be successful:

- *Centralized strategic planning.* Achieving agreement among diverse operating units of IHSs, such as hospitals, physician practices, and long-term care facilities, is difficult. It is important that all operating units back a centralized system-level mission, vision, and strategic plan.

- *Functional integration.* Departments such as finance, human resources, purchasing, and quality, if maintained in each facility, are duplicative. Several functional activities need to be centralized and coordinated to control overhead.

- *Clinical integration.* Coordination of care between different operating units is essential. There should be consolidation of services, emphasis on continuity of care, good communication among caregivers, and smooth transfer of patients and patient information. This is essential for reducing clinical costs and improving patient care outcomes system-wide.

- *Physician integration.* All clinical initiatives, whether related to quality improvement or continuity of care, require physician support. Physicians must be involved in making key decisions, and physician leaders must be identified and developed within the system. Physician compensation must also be aligned with system goals.

- *Integrated information systems.* Disconnected information systems in operating units must be replaced with integrated information systems to provide centralized financial, clinical, and human resources (HR) information to implement system plans.

- *Cost cutting.* Given reduced reimbursement, IHSs must reduce their labor, supply, and clinical costs to survive in a managed care environment.

- *Effective staffing.* Due to rampant worker shortages, creative recruitment and selection programs must be instituted system-wide.

- *Supportive organizational culture.* Diverse organizational cultures in different operating units make integration difficult. A strong system-wide culture is needed to unite employees from diverse operating units.

- *Managing change.* Widespread change is critical for system formation. IHSs must educate employees about change, minimize their resistance to that change, and provide ongoing support for required fiscal and clinical changes.[2]

The Human Resources Function in an IHS

The HR function is important for healthcare organizations in general, because healthcare organizations are labor-intensive and depend on effective recruitment, training, and motivation of qualified personnel to take care of patients. In IHSs, the HR function plays an additional role that is critical in meeting strategic goals, such as centralized planning; clinical, financial, and physician integration; cost cutting; managing change; and fostering a unified culture. At the outset, a distinction must be drawn between corporate HR within an IHS and the HR offices in various operating units, such as individual hospitals, physician practices, and skilled nursing facilities. Corporate HR operates at the system level by formulating and implementing policies for the entire IHS (see Figure 6-1).

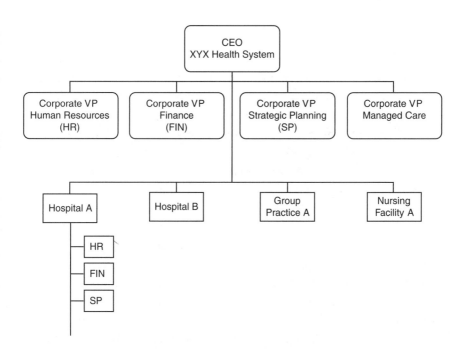

FIGURE 6-1 Organizational Chart of an Integrated Health System

Because this chapter focuses on HR in IHSs and not stand-alone hospitals or physician practices, it will examine the activities of corporate HR.

The following sections discuss corporate HR activities, starting from the time at which a health system is formed to its functions in the later stages of system consolidation and growth. During system formation, the corporate HR department is established, along with other corporate departments such as finance, contracting, and physician relations. In this phase, corporate HR must help recruit system executives and deal with other birthing pains experienced by the health system. This formative phase of corporate HR is characterized by challenge and uncertainty. Only after this phase is completed can corporate HR get down to the business of developing and implementing corporate-level HR policies that will apply to operating units across the system. These policies relate to fundamental HR activities such as planning, recruiting, training, evaluation, and compensation that are critical to effectively managing the system's human resources.

The Role of Corporate HR During IHS Formation

In the early stage of IHS formation, a corporate office is created with separate departments such as planning, finance, HR, and managed care contracting. The first major challenge faced by the corporate HR department is to hire senior vice-presidents and other system-level executives. Corporate-level managers require different qualifications from managers in operating units: They must combine "big picture" thinking with interpersonal and coordination skills for implementing and monitoring corporate policies. To achieve this goal, internal talent within various operating units must be assessed, and development of system executives must be planned. It is common to recruit many executives from within the system, as they are likely to be familiar with the IHS's internal realities and better able to negotiate change processes. At Barnes Jewish Christian (BJC) Health System in St. Louis, for example, recruiting and developing system executives was a high-priority project when this IHS was formed. The corporate HR department identified core competencies needed by system leaders and compared available management talent with business plans. A decision was made to recruit most system executives internally. A continuity plan was prepared that outlined the bench strength of BJC's management and recommended planned assignments to strengthen and develop internal managers.[3]

Another challenge encountered early on in IHS formation is helping the health system deal with dislocations and changes caused by the merging of functions and changing employee roles and work conditions. During this period of turmoil, strong employee communication is needed to maintain morale and commitment. Corporate HR must conduct employee surveys to assess and promote employee understanding of the rationale for the IHS and its goals. Surveys often reveal that employees understand IHS goals but question the need for an IHS. Corporate HR must explain the state of managed care development in the region and the need for integration to compete effectively. In light of changes in employee roles, organizational development staff should teach managers and staff how to manage personnel change, assist their subordinates to deal with such change, and maintain and/or improve productivity. At Albert Einstein Health Network (AEHN), for example, the HR department used the term "surround communication" to explain the need for forming an integrated health network. Bulletin boards were filled with stories of unexpected closures and consolidations, all of which reminded employees that such events could happen there. Bulletin board banners asked employees if they were prepared for change and had the skills for future growth. Newsletters featured stories of employees who had successfully retooled their skills to meet new challenges. Workshops on "survival tactics in times of change" were offered to employees at all levels.[4]

Another major issue is dealing with facility closures and layoffs. These events can be demoralizing for employees, and how they are handled may be critical in keeping operating units and their employees committed to the new system. When Minnesota-based Health One closed the Metropolitan–Mount Sinai Medical Center (MMSC), an inner-city hospital in its newly formed IHS, this move could have caused 2,000 layoffs. Instead, the system's leadership, in concert with corporate HR, implemented an HR strategy instituting a hiring freeze at all units to provide job openings for displaced MMSC employees. An off-site placement center was used to match displaced employees with job offers throughout the Health One system. In addition, the center was used to provide appropriate job training to workers. Ultimately, most laid-off employees were absorbed within Health One's multiple facilities.[5]

Naturally, employees in a newly formed IHS tend to be anxious about changes in compensation, benefits, and other HR practices. Many organizations delay addressing HR issues until late in the process. This tactic can have a negative effect on productivity and creativity by bringing out the staff's worst fears about their jobs, pay, and working conditions. While detailed HR policies cannot be provided immediately, the timelines for making HR decisions should be shared with employees. A broad framework for dealing with anticipated changes in other HR practices should be provided. To allow staff to give their full attention to their jobs, decisions about jobs, benefits, and other HR issues should be addressed on a priority basis at this stage.

Beyond System Formation: Formulating and Implementing Corporate HR Policies

After negotiating this early, uncertain phase, corporate HR can begin formulating corporate-level policies that are applicable across the system. The remainder of this chapter deals with these corporate HR policies. Note that this discussion of corporate HR policies includes a large number of examples related to nursing. Although healthcare organizations have a wide variety of professional and nonprofessional personnel, nurses spend the most time with patients and act as central coordinators of clinical services at the point of care that are provided by other employees, such as therapists, technicians, and aides. Not surprisingly, within the professionally diverse workforce in hospitals, nurses are most closely identified with patient care. In this labor-intensive area, nurses are also the largest employee group and account for the largest proportion of the labor budget. Due to their centrality, the shortage of nurses is the most pressing staffing problem facing hospitals and healthcare systems today, and creating effective HR policies relative to nurses is a crucial concern. Also, more has been written about nurse-related HR problems than about HR problems for any other set of caregivers. This lack of HR examples for other types of caregivers is another reason for focusing on nurses in this chapter.

STRATEGIC PLANNING

Before discussing corporate HR policies, a word of caution for senior vice-presidents of corporate HR is in order. It is imperative that HR and other functions in different operating units of an IHS be involved at an early stage in developing corporate-level HR policies—policies must not be formulated by the corporate office alone. This is important, as corporate policies can preempt powers of local operating units. Corporate policies address several key issues related to operating units: For example, which corporate guidelines for recruiting and selection should govern operating units? Which exceptions should be allowed, keeping in mind the local market conditions? To what extent will the compensation structure of operating units be retained or replaced? To obtain buy-in of operating units on such issues, a representative task force is needed to discuss the nature and scope of corporate HR policies. Fairview Hospital and Healthcare Services in Minneapolis appointed a 20-member employee task force representing various Fairview organizations for this purpose. Representatives included middle managers, supervisors, team leaders, and front-line employees to help formulate corporate HR policies.[2] A participative process is essential, because unilateral changes imposed by corporate HR can cause widespread dissatisfaction.

Policies Related to Strategic HR Planning and Information Systems

After addressing early formation-related challenges, corporate HR must turn its attention to the foundation of other HR policies—that is, the HR planning process. Strategic HR planning is essential for systematically addressing the HR needs of the system. The senior vice-president of HR should be involved in the health system's strategic planning process and align HR planning with the overall system's strategic plan. IHS goals typically include building a continuum of care, achieving cost-efficiency, creating profitable service lines, and instituting system-wide quality standards. HR planners must establish strategic priorities based on these goals. For example, based on system projections related to revenue growth and service-line expansion, what is the demand for personnel system-wide? What is the internal availability of personnel and the extent of external recruitment needed? What is the system-wide staff turnover rate, and what kinds of retention policies are required? What skills, competencies, and abilities are available and needed by system employees? What training and development programs are needed to address areas of deficit?

If corporate HR's strategic plan is not properly aligned with the system strategies, this discrepancy can thwart efforts to implement the system's strategies. For example, building profitable service lines across the system requires time-intensive recruitment of service-line managers with appropriate clinical and financial expertise. Instituting quality standards requires provision of adequate numbers of trainers and equipment in the right time and place. Sometimes IHSs do not sufficiently involve the head of corporate HR in their strategic planning process. Another common mistake is allowing the finance and managed care functions to dominate planning. Given the importance of having trained and motivated caregivers for providing cost-efficient, high-quality care, this exclusive focus on bottom-line issues can be very short-sighted.

HR planning at the system level also requires a well-integrated HR information system (HRIS). Systems without an integrated HRIS find the planning process challenging. With different systems for payroll, recruiting, and training functions, or different software platforms for different operating units, managers may receive multiple reports that must be combined manually to analyze system-level statistics. Similarly, staff must be trained on several systems to extract different types of information. Implementing a single information platform eliminates those problems and makes it easier to export company-wide HR data to various operating units and departments. For example, training departments at the corporate and local levels can get a single expert file regarding new hires, allowing them to plan and coordinate training schedules.[6]

An integrated HRIS also facilitates HR planning. For example, caregiver training based on Joint Commission Accreditation of Healthcare Organizations (JCAHO) standards is a key activity for health systems. Catholic Healthcare West uses its HRIS to plan and monitor its training activities. The HRIS keeps track of employee certifications, licenses, and required training courses for employees throughout the organization; it also tracks employees' expertise. HRIS software can track the inventory of skills people have—for example, what type of patient care training registered nurses have received and who in finance is a certified public accountant.[7] This capability helps the organization figure out which areas need development. Similarly, recruiters can search the database to find candidates for job openings, and software exists to set up "what if" scenarios to help determine how buying a new piece of equipment would affect staffing levels.

RECRUITMENT

Corporate recruitment and selection policies must resolve system-wide staff shortages by attracting external candidates with appropriate skills and values, accessing the internal pool of candidates, and controlling recruitment and selection costs through resource sharing among operating units. Some organizations, such as Inova Health System, have centralized the recruiting function by instituting strong corporate recruitment and employment policies, including policies related to internal transfers and employee reassignments.[8] Most health systems, however, extend significant discretion to operating units, allowing them to adapt central recruitment policies to their unique needs.

In the current environment, most operating units within IHSs are emphasizing creativity in recruitment programs so that they can survive in a highly competitive labor market. For example, there is a significant demand–supply gap for nurses across the United States. Fewer people are entering the nursing profession, and those who are in the market can be extremely choosy when looking for jobs. IHSs are implementing a variety of traditional and creative recruitment policies to address this problem. Organizations such as Tenet Health System and Massachusetts General Hospital are targeting nurses with sign-on bonuses of between $1,000 and $7,500, with the exact amount depending on experience and specialty.[9] Some health systems are paying bonuses or finder's fees to their own employees who refer a nurse; the logic is that bonuses for joining the organization encourage job hopping by candidates. Other sign-on incentives include assistance in acquiring necessities such as car loans, housing loans, and payment of relocation expenses for the right candidate.

Systems are also offering experienced nurse candidates preferential allocation of day shifts. Some hospitals are offering a "season plan" to contract nurses: They may work 12 weeks in a position and then opt to accept a full-time position in the hospital. Systems are also offering career-oriented incentives. For example, students are being invited to open houses, lunch with nursing managers, and "shadow a nurse" programs. The goal is to give them worthwhile work experience and organizational exposure, thereby motivating them to join the sponsoring organization. Some systems are offering nursing students tuition reimbursement and scholarships if they agree to join the organization following their graduation. Experienced nurses are also being offered fellowship programs involving advanced training. For example, Baylor Health System in Dallas offers 6- to 11-month advanced training programs for experienced nurses who join the organization.[10]

Systems are also hosting open houses for regular nurses and promoting their facilities and equipment to them. Some systems are taking a long-term view by targeting junior high schools, where students are told about the benefits of a nursing career before they have decided which career to pursue. Students are told about the promising employment prospects in the healthcare industry and the subjects they need to take to pursue a nursing or allied health career. Some systems are targeting area nursing schools and building good relationships with them to attract nursing interns who may one day join the organization. Baylor Health System, for example, gave the nursing program at University of Texas at Arlington a grant of $430,000 in 2002 to hire additional faculty and increase student enrollment. Most of the program's students go on to join Baylor or other Dallas-based health systems.

IHSs are focusing on their internal pool of candidates as well. Cincinnati-based Sister of Charity Health System's (SCHS) corporate office arranges for facilities to collaborate on in-house operating room training that helps hospitals fill vacancies in the operating room with their own staff. SCHS also encourages employees who want to leave the system to apply at other operating units within the system. Employees receive credit for benefits such as health insurance and retirement benefits if they leave one operating unit and join another within the system. In addition, SCHS has developed explicit policies that facilitate transfers among operating units without much red tape. Clearly, internal recruiting has emerged as an important tool to tackle staff shortages.

As a result of the ongoing staff shortages, recruiting costs have been rising in health care. Many IHSs have encouraged their operating units to share recruitment costs in an effort to reduce recruiting expenditures while improving selection quality. At SCHS, instead of each facility within the system sending recruiters to national conferences, schools, or job fairs, the system now sends a few representatives to recruit on behalf of several units. Similarly, SCHS's member hospitals in Colorado have been sponsoring a single hospitality suite at the annual conference of the American Physical Therapy Association for recruitment purposes, instead of each hospital recruiting separately.[11]

SELECTION

While recruitment enhances the quality and quantity of the candidate pool, candidates' cultural fit with the IHS is a critical consideration during selection. Corporate HR must emphasize alignment between the cultural values of the system and the cultural values of selected candidates. Post-merger, IHSs must build a common culture around their core values (e.g., initiative, teamwork, mission orientation) and must hire candidates who are compatible with that system culture. For example, Sentara Healthcare redesigned its selection process to identify potential employees with the appropriate service orientation. Recruited employees were shown a movie regarding Sentara's cultural values and administered a screening tool to ascertain whether they fit the cultural profile required. Interviews investigated each candidate's value orientation in great depth.

Some IHSs have trained managers to do value-based selection. For example, Eastern Mercy Health System (EMHS) offers managers an educational course on recruitment and selection, where they are taught how to select candidates based on their institutional culture.[4] In the course, managers discuss their organization's history and mission and the competencies needed for leadership success at EMHS. In addition, managers review appropriate interview procedures and discuss open-ended questions to ask candidates.[12] Albert Einstein Health Network's (AEHN) "Hiring the Best" program requires assessment of applicants' core values by means of "situational interviewing," in which candidates are asked what action they would take in a hypothetical situation. AEHN's training program for managers has been a great success. In fact, several new hires at AEHN indicated they were influenced in their decisions to join in part by the clear organizational values communicated during the situational interviewing process.[4]

Selection involves other activities as well, such as use of tests and use of structured and unstructured interviewing. SSM Healthcare in Saint Louis utilizes a uniform psychological test to recruit healthcare managers in its system. This IHS has identified management as a system-level resource. Managers are expected to rotate across system facilities and, therefore, are selected based on "system-wide" requirements (in contrast, selection of nurses and other clinical caregivers differs across facilities within SSM).

RETENTION

Employee turnover in health care is higher than the turnover rates found in most industries. Turnover translates into lower productivity, because employees deciding to leave the organization typically have reduced productivity in the months prior to their exit. Additionally, new hires take several months to achieve the normal productivity of their predecessor. Other costs accrue as well, such as use of agency nurses until a new employee is hired. It is estimated that turnover costs the organization 50–100% of an employee's annual salary—a cost systems can ill afford. Accordingly, employee retention is a key HR priority.[13]

Systems are implementing several strategies for retaining nurses. Retention bonuses are offered to newly recruited employees. For example, they may receive bonuses of 8%, 10%, and 12%, respectively, at the completion of their first, second, and third years within the organization. Organizations are also helping repay student loans and paying nursing license fees for new recruits. New employees are being introduced in special ceremonies and made to feel more welcome within the organization.

Scheduling is now often tailored to the life-stage of nursing employees. Older nurses may be offered shorter shifts of 8 hours instead of 12; calmer work environments, such as duty in clinics instead of in medical or surgical units; and fewer weekend shifts, to allow them greater leisure. Married nurses with family responsibilities may be offered flexible schedules and fewer night shifts, to accommodate their needs. Nurses are being helped in developing their careers through tuition reimbursement and mentoring programs. In addition, they are being educated on the latest equipment and new drugs, to improve their self-efficacy and sense of growth within the organization.

Poor relations between nurses and their managers are a major cause of nursing turnover. Therefore, systems are now holding nursing managers accountable for what happens in their units. They are linking the merit increases obtained by nurse managers to the turnover rates in their units. The goal is to motivate nurse managers to establish healthy relations with their nursing subordinates, monitor the employee climate within their units, and act to reduce employee turnover.

On another front, retention of agency nurses is being stressed. HR must contract with staffing agencies to supply agency nurses in times of shortage due to staff turnover. Often, concerns exist regarding the competence and quality of care provided by agency nurses. At the same time, organizations need to offer a suitable work climate for agency nurses. Several health systems are taking steps to assess and orient agency nurses to enable them to perform better. Assessment is based on compiling data on agency nurses to identify patterns and trends related to undesirable behavior, and developing and administering skills assessment programs for agency nurses. Orientation programs for agency nurses include organizational nursing philosophy, care standards, and quality assurance/

improvement programs. Policies related to infection control, fall precautions, restraint use, skin care, patient rights, documentation, informed consent, and other matters are discussed as well. A point person, such as a clinical coordinator, is available for agency nurses who need assistance.

It is HR's responsibility to monitor employee dissatisfaction and formulate appropriate retention strategies. This monitoring should not be limited to employee opinion surveys, however. In an era of chronic shortages of clinical personnel, HR must periodically conduct interviews and focus groups among key clinical employee groups to learn about areas of concern. Inova Health System had serious turnover problems with its finance division, which was losing employees to higher-paying "dot.com" companies. Divisional leadership joined with the corporate HR office to interview employees of the finance division to identify the causes of this high turnover rate. Interviews revealed that employees' primary concerns were lack of adequate rewards, absence of career planning opportunities, and unrealistic performance expectations. Accordingly, the division instituted a salary adjustment based on market value. Retention bonuses were added that were paid in quarterly increments. These measures dramatically improved Inova's employee retention.[13]

Besides higher pay, creating a culture of empowerment is necessary for retaining employees. For example, while nurses are always interested in higher pay and better working conditions, many joined the profession to serve patients as care advocates. Restructuring of care, increased inpatient acuity (as many former inpatient services are now performed on an ambulatory basis), and multiskilling programs have increased nurses' workload and reduced their autonomy. Retaining nurses requires involving them in strategic decisions and in care planning, listening to their concerns, recognizing their patient advocacy role, and providing developmental training for career advancement. HR should pay adequate attention to these kinds of "softer" issues related to retention.

TRAINING AND EDUCATION

Education should be a strategic tool in IHSs' business planning process. Training and development, when integrated with other HR processes, is likely to ensure employee competence needed for the future and development of managers and physician executives to handle appropriate system responsibilities. In contrast to this idealized view, training budgets are always under pressure in IHSs and among the first to be cut in times of financial scarcity. This tendency in part reflects the lack of evidence regarding the effectiveness of training programs. Another issue is the dominance of JCAHO-mandated training programs in healthcare organizations related to preventing workplace violence, promoting patient and employee safety, and continuing in-service programs. Mandated training programs often leave inadequate time and money for other training activities.

From a systems perspective, development of system-level managers should be a strategic priority of the training and development department. Systems need system leaders who are proactive, strategic thinkers and who have a good understanding of finance and the ability to deal with complex changes. At St. Louis–based BJC Health System, leadership development is handled as a partnership between the organization and its managers. Within the partnership, BJC provides managers leadership development and other educational workshops, on-the-job training, and work experiences that expand managerial skills and abilities. Eleven management competencies provide a benchmark for an annual career development discussion between every BJC manager and his or her boss; this evaluation leads to an individual development plan (IDP) that guides development aimed at improving the manager's leadership skills. The IDP also plays a key role in BJC's succession planning process.[3]

Another priority for IHSs is identifying and developing physician leadership that can help facilitate strategic changes in clinical areas. The continuation of BJC's success relies on its ability to partner with its physicians in both leadership and practice roles. For example, the organization must identify and develop physician leaders to assume administrative positions in BJC hospitals and corporate offices. A physician executive leadership program has been developed jointly between BJC, the Washington University School of Health Administration, and the Washington University School of Medicine Continuing Medical Education Office for developing physician management knowledge and skills. This program delivers a certificate-level curriculum designed to fill the gap between short, two-day management courses and a complete MHA/MBA degree program.[3]

Another priority is clinical training. Clinically, care for the patient across the continuum of care requires a vast array of expertise in a number of settings. At BJC Health System, a task force of critical care educators and nurse specialists designed and implemented a comprehensive critical care curriculum consisting of introductory, basic, and advanced critical care courses; this program was offered monthly at rotating sites at no cost to BJC employees.

Given today's omnipresent staff shortages, another problem that IHSs face is census fluctuation in different units. For example, Trihealth System in Cincinnati, Ohio, faced census fluctuations in perinatal units in its three hospitals, leading to increased overtime and rotation of agency nurses to the units in times of high demand. Nursing leaders in the three system hospitals conducted cross-training programs in which perinatal nurses from each hospital learned to work in perinatal units of other hospitals, in essence becoming a single team. The result was reduced overtime and use of agency nurses, reduction in rotation of untrained staff to perinatal nursing units, improved morale, and reduced turnover.[3]

As mentioned earlier, mandatory training is a large part of the training and development conducted in health care. The JCAHO standards focus on staff training and ongoing and continuous efforts of assuring staff competency through orientation, training and development, and encouragement of self-development. JCAHO requires that data on competence patterns be monitored to identify trends and respond to employees' learning needs. It also requires organizations to monitor patient care and safety incidents to determine employee-learning needs and to provide remedial training as necessary. Because violation of JCAHO standards can reflect adversely on the accreditation of facilities, corporate HR must ensure that adequate training staff and equipment are available at each operating unit for staff training, competence assessment, and remedial training. Given the scarcity of training dollars, meeting these needs is always a difficult problem. However, patient safety is a key priority, and corporate HR must ensure that JCAHO training standards are met in each facility.

In some organizations, training and development is being used as a powerful way to transform the culture of organizations. In the early 1990s, Albert Einstein Health Network (AEHN) undertook to transform its organizational culture and to change itself from a stable organization to an active, change-hardy, integrated health network. AEHN's CEO unilaterally established a set of core values for the organization. During the early years of this effort, embedding and sustaining these core values became the central HR initiative. For a year, AEHN's 14 top executives spent time clarifying and debating the core values, developing an understanding of living out core values, and enacting plans to disseminate those values throughout the organization. Core values were woven throughout the employee communication process in video and audio tapes, scripts, print pieces, and e-mail messages. Managers, supervisors, and trainers were coached on the content, meaning, and application of the core values. Managerial estimates indicated that approximately 70% of exempt and 50% of nonexempt employees truly understood, shared, and consciously lived the core AEHN values on a day-to-day basis on the job. The training was effective in transforming the culture of the organization.[4]

Among the many management skills, managing change is a meta-skill that employees of health systems need. Integrated health systems must constantly change so as to adapt to their environments, and managing such change is a key skill that needs to be taught system-wide. At BJC, organizational development staff teach managers and staff how to manage personnel change through anticipation, cognitive reorientation, and active communication. Employees are also taught to assist subordinates to understand and deal with change. Finally, an important component of the program focuses on how to maintain and even improve productivity in the midst of change.[3]

Employee orientation also serves to introduce new employees to the system culture, values, and expectations. For example, at AEHN in Long Island, a half-day session was added to the standard new employee orientation process to explain and demonstrate the meaning of the system's core values and to stress the importance of living them every day. At New Samaritan Health System, when employees start work, they have to be oriented to the entire system, not just their facility. They are taught the rationale of the system and the values of teamwork and service required by the organization.[14]

The most effective training programs have also learned to cope with shrinking budgets and increasing training needs with creativity. For example, more front-line training and "train the trainer" programs are being used to deliver training programs at the work site instead of the classroom. Front-line training involves job training for new employees that occurs on site by supervisors or co-workers. This strategy avoids classroom training, which can be expensive and can mean that the skills taught are less transferable to the work situation. "Train the trainer" programs involve classroom training of selected individuals, who in turn train various employees on the job—a process that saves both time and money. Another challenge for training programs is lack of time and motivation among trainees to attend class sessions. Creative methods are being utilized to deal with this problem. At SSM Healthcare in St. Louis, for example, certain training content related to patient safety was posted in restrooms as a way of reinforcing important lessons for employees.

PERFORMANCE MANAGEMENT

Performance management (PM) refers to a continuous and development-oriented performance evaluation system. It differs from the more traditional performance appraisal (PA) system in that it avoids some of the problems identified with PA (although many argue that PM includes all elements of PA but is simply more result focused). For example, PM is prospective—not retrospective—in orientation. It emphasizes frequent meetings between employees and managers to identify incipient performance problems, discuss developmental needs and barriers faced by the employee, and candidly explain performance implications for pay, so as to avoid surprises later on. Given the need to rein in labor costs and improve employee productivity, many health systems are instituting PM systems. For example, many IHSs have traditionally had PA systems that allow automatic pay increases every year. Such a system can be a liability for organizations that operate in highly competitive markets, so some organizations are trying to change to a system that discourages automatic increases. At the same time, increases in patient acuity and personnel shortages are causing organizations to stress teamwork, and other organizations are redesigning their PM systems to be more team based, rather than individual based.

The choice of a PM system depends on the organization's particular environment and culture. Good Samaritan Health System in Phoenix, Arizona, and SSM Healthcare in St. Louis, Missouri, demonstrate two ways in which PM systems can be redesigned to instill divergent but relevant performance cultures in an organization.

At Good Samaritan, a seven-hospital IHS, the PA system was revamped to emphasize the importance of individual accountability and performance. Earlier, Good Samaritan employees had been assured minimum increases every year. Because the IHS operated in the Phoenix market, which was characterized by high provider competition and high managed care penetration (70%), cutting staffing costs and improving employee productivity became essential for survival. Accordingly, the PA ratings were changed. Jobs were broken down into functional competencies (technical skills needed to perform assigned tasks) and core competencies. Functional and core competencies were emphasized in hiring, orientation, training, and development. Based on these competencies, employees were rated as "developing," "competent," or "master." The biggest raises (e.g., 6%) went to the master performers, the lowest (e.g., 3%) to those in the developing zone. Although not everyone welcomed the revised PA system, it led to a dramatic change in the work culture in the organization.[14]

At SSM Healthcare, the PM process for all 90 staff members in the corporate office, including the system president and senior executives, is team based. Employees share responsibility for developing their own goals and soliciting and analyzing feedback from people they work with as team members or co-workers. The PM system rewards teamwork and eliminates pay raises based on individual performance. It is geared toward promoting values of SSM Healthcare in the behavior of corporate employees—for example, acting with justice and fairness, giving primary importance to patients, and providing caring service. Feedback forms sent by corporate employees to co-workers ask the recipients to discuss how the sender's behaviors support SSM's values. Feedback forms are returned to employees only and are not seen by their supervisors. Each employee incorporates the substance of the feedback into his or her self-developed performance plan, which is then discussed with the supervisor in a coaching session.[15] Regarding compensation, the organization believes that teamwork is discouraged by rewarding individual performance. Accordingly, employees who have not contributed as actively as others to the organization receive only a market adjustment, while those who have contributed actively (the majority of employees) receive a market adjustment as well as a "contribution increase." SSM does not offer bonuses or incentives linked to performance, consistent with its desire to deemphasize hierarchical structures and its commitment to team building.[15]

These two cases demonstrate how PM systems are integral to defining performance in an IHS. At the same time, the type of PM system selected depends on the type of work culture the system desires. While some systems emphasize individual accountability, others stress teamwork and team accountability. Regardless of the type of culture involved, the PM system is integral to an IHS's work culture and values.

COMPENSATION

Health care is a service industry in which labor accounts for 50–60% of total costs, and payrolls increase every year to keep up with inflation. Controlling compensation costs is critical for overall cost-efficiency. At the same time, increasing pay is essential for recruiting and retaining employees.

While most healthcare organizations maintain a traditional compensation program with substantial base salaries, the growth of base pay has begun to slow, while more dollars are being put into strategies that reward performance. Performance is no longer judged by financial results, but rather by quality outcomes, patient satisfaction, and market share. This shift in emphasis is seen most clearly in the growth of incentive programs. With the exception of government hospitals, more than half of all hospitals now have annual incentive-based plans in place that extend eligibility far beyond executive suites. This is significant because hospitals have traditionally lagged behind other fields in the use of incentives.

Within health care, incentives are more popular in IHSs than in free-standing hospitals. A survey by Hay,[16] the healthcare consulting company, revealed that, of more than 100 healthcare systems, 79% made use of annual incentive programs. Other pay-for-performance programs that are growing in popularity include gain sharing, pay for competencies and skills, team-based pay, broad-banding, and key contributor plans. While incentive/bonus plans have found slow acceptance at the clinical and professional levels, integrated systems have instituted incentive plans linked to performance measures, including nonfinancial measures such as quality and customer satisfaction.[16]

As discussed earlier, Good Samaritan Health System established a pay system linked to performance so that it could survive in the competitive managed care market in Phoenix, Arizona. Good Samaritan's old pay system ratcheted up salaries automatically. At the same time, managed care payers and government were pressing reimbursements down, even as admissions and length of stay were declining. Good Samaritan felt it needed a flatter organization with fewer job titles, so it developed a system that

aligned pay and performance. Under the new scheme, annual performance evaluations rather than automatic increases determined raises.
Supervisors rated whether their people were "developing," "competent,"
or "masters" at their jobs. The biggest raises (6%) went to master performers; the lowest raises amounted to 3% of pay. Some employees could
get no raise at all. Not everyone welcomed the new compensation system.
At Desert Samaritan Medical Center, there was dissatisfaction in the nursing area. At the same time, people knew that this system would affect
their pay if they didn't excel on relevant performance criteria.[14]

The use of gain-sharing arrangements has also increased. Gain sharing
is an incentive program focused on improving operating results, typically
implemented at the group or organizational level. Such a program also
tends to be an organizational development technique designed to generate a major cultural change. Typical gain-sharing programs provide some
methods for employees to suggest ways to increase productivity and cut
costs, and some mechanisms for sharing the increased earnings or cost
savings with employees. For example, at one Florida hospital, a gain-
sharing plan for hourly staff helped reduce patient stays by half a day,
which saved the hospital about $2.3 million annually. Time to get lab re-
sults was reduced from an average of 2 hours and 37 minutes to 48 minutes. By implementing a gain-sharing plan for nurses and lab technicians,
the hospital had aggregate savings of 248 hours of labor on every shift.

Scanlon plans are the best known of gain-sharing techniques, where
employees serve on incentive design committees during the planning
stage and vote on the plan. Scanlon plans typically require an 80–90%
positive vote to be installed. Employees also serve on governing committees for administering the ongoing program.

A number of gain-sharing programs based on suggestion systems have
been very successful—for example, those at Baylor Health Systems,
Henry Ford Health System, Franciscan Health System, and Sutter Health
System. Sutter Health System has been a pioneer in gain sharing through
its SutterShare program, which is designed for all employees of the healthcare network.[17] Measurements in SutterShare compare system productivity against nationally published standards for income over budget and
departmental quality. The plan measures performance every two months
and provides timely and repeated feedback. It incorporates a formal suggestion system and gives special recognition to those employees who make
four or more suggestions per quarter. The greatest achievement of the

plan is the improvements made in areas of customer responsiveness by employees and profitability. It has also achieved a high level of employee involvement.[17]

Several organizations looking to introduce pay-for-performance policies are contemplating broad banding. In broad banding, jobs and roles are grouped into fewer but wider pay ranges to encourage initiatives such as management development, career ladders, and skill- and competency-based pay. Such a system reduces the number of job titles and accompanying salary scales. As a consequence, it avoids the problem of employees "topping out" at the highest point of the scale because they were hired at higher salaries or because they have high productivity, as such employees cannot be paid in excess of the pay range ceiling.

At AEHN, where work was redesigned, a broad-banding exercise sought to simplify the compensation system and make it consistent with job redesign. Earlier, the pay had been job based, with pay levels pegged to midpoint of the market and pay increases determined by a combination of ability to pay, cost-of-living adjustments, and merit. Now, from time to time, a few positions are reevaluated to reflect sustained changes in work redesign, and sometimes pay levels of a few high-performing individuals with rare technical skills are significantly adjusted by pegging their rates to the 75th rather than 50th percentile of the market.[4]

In light of the nursing shortage, many systems are trying to redress pay compression issues related to nurses and other clinical personnel.[18] Pay compression occurs when new employees in an organization are hired at much higher starting pay than old-timers, resulting in newcomers overtaking old-timers in terms of compensation, or being paid much higher salaries relative to their experience and contributions. A significant problem is the growing gap between the salaries of nurse managers, who have traditionally been paid more than staff nurses, and newly hired registered nurses, who are hired at market rates that pay them more on an absolute or relative basis than nurse managers who have been in the organization for many years. Many organizations are introducing new approaches to tackle this problem, such as giving across-the-board increases to all nurse managers to bridge the gap, engaging in individual negotiations with nurse managers, and establishing a fixed proportional difference between staff nurses and nurse managers, with the lowest-paid nurse manager being paid at a higher rate than the highest-paid staff.[18]

PHYSICIAN COMPENSATION

IHSs acquire physician practices or contract with physicians for primary and specialist care services so as to extend their geographic reach and ensure patient referrals to their hospitals and post-acute facilities. Physicians employed by IHSs must have a compensation structure that is aligned with system objectives in terms of enhancing revenues, improving clinical outcomes and customer service, and controlling costs.

During their formation, however, many IHSs did not devote sufficient effort toward incentive alignment. A typical assumption was that if a hospital was profitable earlier and the medical group at least broke even earlier, the IHS would at least be as profitable as the hospital was prior to integration. Typical compensation flaws included multiyear guaranteed salaries that led to drops in physician productivity, lack of individual productivity incentives, productivity incentives unrelated to staffing and other support costs, lack of compensation linkage to IHS performance, and allowing physicians to "cherry pick" payer classes.

Physician compensation in IHSs should be based on certain underlying principles:[19]

1. Compensation should be market based, but also sensitive to market realities on a specialty basis as well as type of practice setting.
2. Some portion of physician compensation should depend on the overall performance of the IHS. This helps physician compensation align strategically with the system.
3. Some portions of physician compensation should be linked to productivity.
4. Compensation should not be solely linked to productivity in terms of patient volume, but must also account for staffing and other support costs. Enhanced revenues from higher patient volume accompanied by higher staffing and support costs are not likely to make a net positive contribution to the system's bottom line.
5. Physicians should participate in development of the compensation plan and be accountable for administration of the plan. Frequently, compensation plans for physicians fail because no physician buy-in exists, and plans are designed solely or mostly by administrators.
6. The full cost of a primary care strategy should not be placed on the backs of all physicians. For example, a PCP in a rural site may not

be able to recover full costs from his practice, yet he is strategically valuable to the IHS.

In the mid-1990s, Meridia Health System of Cleveland, Ohio, acquired several PCP practices to form the core of an integrated delivery system.[18] All physicians received two- to three-year guaranteed salary and benefits packages based on a review of each physician's current salary level and years of experience. Unfortunately, Meridia's physician compensation plan lowered productivity among physicians and increased Meridia's losses to more than $100,000 per physician per year. Many physicians spent less time in the office, saw fewer patients, and provided fewer services than they had before their practices were acquired. Also, billing was contracted out and inadequately managed. Eventually, Meridia placed a moratorium on physician recruitment and appointed a task force composed of all physician group presidents, additional physician representatives, and representatives from Meridia's practice management, human resources, and finance and accounting departments. This task force developed a new compensation plan that based pay on the application of an estimated collection rate percentage to each physician's gross fee-for-service billings to arrive at estimated collections per physician, then applied an overhead rate to gross fee-for-service billings to arrive at an overhead amount. The difference between gross billings and overhead was the physician's total budgeted salary for the next six months. While not perfect, the new compensation plan helped Meridia and its physicians achieve their mutual goals of high-quality care, reasonable productivity, and operating efficiency. The success of the compensation plan is, in great measure, due to the willingness of physicians to work with other administrators in designing their compensation system.[20]

Another issue is linking physician compensation to specific behaviors required by managed care organizations related to efficiency, prevention, and customer service. Several systems have implemented bonus systems for physicians that are linked to cost-efficiency (e.g., based on the percentage of patients referred to specialists, adjusted for acuity), prevention activities (e.g., the percentage of diabetics given semiannual $Hb1_{ac}$ tests, Pap smears for women over age 40), and customer service (based on patient satisfaction surveys). Often, a portion of the total compensation (e.g., 5%) is placed "at risk" to motivate physicians to be efficient and provide customer service and preventive activities. A key consideration here is to allow physician participation in the design of such incentive systems.

BENEFITS

Reducing benefits costs and providing desired benefits to recruit and retain employees are twin challenges for IHSs. Because benefits are not performance related, they are similar to a fixed cost that must be adjusted every year for inflation. A major challenge is reducing the cost of health benefits in the system, given the increase in healthcare benefits costs of 10–30% annually nationwide, and the higher frequency of use of healthcare benefits by healthcare employees. More systems are increasing copayments for drugs and office visits, introducing coinsurance for drugs and procedures, and increasing deductibles. Annual premium increases of 15–30% are common. Also, companies are reducing pharmacy benefits, behavioral health, and vision care and hearing care benefits. Several organizations are eliminating fee-for-service and PPO options for employees. Some are introducing health management programs. Responding to the facts that 10% of employees generate one-third of costs for chronic care, 5% of employees drive 50% of acute care costs, and 60% of costs are due to modifiable lifestyle conditions, integrated programs are being put in place for providing the right intervention to the right people at the right time. IHSs are also becoming interested in consumer-directed healthcare plans, which are characterized by high deductibles and low-cost insurance products for catastrophic care, medical savings accounts designed to create financial incentives for prudent purchase of health care, and access to health information to help consumers choose providers, drugs, and other services intelligently.[20]

Some healthcare systems that own HMOs are asking employees to join the system HMO and motivating them to make this switch with lower rates and higher benefits. For example, BJC Healthcare System offered membership in its HMO to its 15,000 employees, along with other HMO, PPO, and fee-for-service options.[3] More than two-thirds of employees chose the HMO product that BJC partially owns. Sometimes this is a win-win situation for both sides: The system gains additional enrollees who can actually add to its bottom line, while employees enjoy lower rates. The danger is that healthcare employees tend to utilize healthcare services more than the average person, and this higher utilization rate can prove detrimental to system HMOs, especially those with a small enrollee base that lacks the numbers to compensate for increased utilization from the employee group.[3]

An increasing number of IHSs have revamped their retirement benefits by moving to defined-contribution programs.[21] Earlier defined-benefits plans (traditional pension plans) promised participants specific monthly benefits at retirement, based on a formula related to pre-retirement salary, length of service, and cost-of-living adjustments. Benefits were post-retirement annuities (fixed annual amount). Employees generally didn't have to contribute to the plan, and benefits did not depend on partici-pants' ability to save. Although they offered guaranteed retirement in-comes for employees with little investment risk, these defined-benefits plans were difficult to understand, limited upside gains for employees from profitable investments, and shifted investment risk to employers. By contrast, defined-contribution plans [e.g., 401(k) plans, 403(b) plans] provide individual accounts for each employee to invest in certain options (e.g., stock funds, bond funds), require contributions from both employer and employee, and yield variable benefits that depend on investment in-come. The advantages of this system are its low investment risk for em-ployers, unlimited upside payout for employees willing to take calculated risks, and employee incentive to save. The disadvantage is the unlimited downside investment risks for employees, which may be partly addressed by offering only conservative and moderate-risk options to employees in the retirement accounts and holding retirement planning seminars.

Given that health care is a round-the-clock profession that takes a toll on employees' home lives, many systems have tried to retain employees by providing family-friendly benefits that help reduce work-related pressures on their family lives.[22] Foremost among these benefits are flexible working hours, generous maternity leaves, career break schemes (e.g., to look after dependents), temporary and part-time work as a phased return to full-time work, and compressed work weeks to allow employees to fit their work lives to their personal needs. Many hospitals offer work-site childcare cen-ters with hours that parallel the work hours of employees both night and day. Moreover, many centers have a higher than average ratio of caregivers to children, and children are offered loving, responsible care and helped to develop social skills, motor skills, preliteracy competencies, and beginning concepts in math and science to help employees feeltheir children are well looked after. Other benefits help employees complete various personal and family-related chores at work, such as laundry drop-off and dry-cleaning services, grocery shopping services and on-site stores, and fitness centers.

UNIONIZATION

Since the 1990s, reduced reimbursement from payers has led hospitals and health systems to cut costs through layoffs, reengineering, lower staffing ratios, and subcontracting services. Many healthcare workers remain convinced that organizations are putting profits ahead of patient care and putting workers in positions that compromise both their own health and safety and that of patients. This dissatisfaction has led to increased unionization in the last decade, especially among nurses. IHSs must recognize unionization trends nationwide and develop appropriate labor relations policies.

Most unionization efforts focus on individual facilities, rather than entire IHSs. Because the law recognizes separate bargaining units for unionization within a hospital (e.g., physicians, clinical workers, technicians), unions tend to organize along these lines rather than trying to organize an entire hospital or health system. Nevertheless, many unions have begun issue-based regional campaigns against several multihospital systems (e.g., Tenet) and IHSs (e.g., Sutter Health System) related to overpricing of services or degradation of staffing ratios. For this reason, the labor relations policies discussed in this section emphasize monitoring union trends and internal labor practices, but do not deal with contract negotiations, which are the responsibility of individual health facilities within a system.

There are several leading causes of unionization in health care today. First, providers in states with high rates of managed care (such as California) have been forced to decrease nurse staffing ratios to survive capitation rates. Conversely, nursing unions, such as the California Nursing Association (CNA), have begun to bargain for higher staffing ratios, better wages, and repeal of mandatory overtime in these states.[23] IHSs in states with increased managed care need to be aware of such trends and monitor their staffing and overtime policies. Second, for-profit hospital chains, such as Tenet and Columbia, have been targeted by Service Employee International Union for overpricing of services and low staffing ratios. For-profit IHSs need to be particularly careful, along with IHSs accused of any unethical practices. Third, cost pressures in health care and resultant problems for employees and patients have increased interest in unionization in health care by national unions, such as the Teamsters, Steelworkers, and United Auto Workers.

To avoid unionization within their system, HR personnel should monitor key measures related to unionization, such as staffing ratios, mandatory overtime, no-layoff guarantees, subcontracting of services, and pay increases. Other issues, such as pricing of healthcare services, including for the uninsured, should be watched carefully as well. IHSs should also monitor the union environment in local facilities and in nearby states and regions.

At the top of this list of key concerns is an increase in staffing ratios. In California, the CNA was able to force legislation on minimum staffing ratios in the state, and staffing ratios are a staple item in many union contracts.

Mandatory overtime is another key criterion. Hospitals have imposed mandatory overtime to work around nursing shortages, but this move has been resisted by nurses on grounds of poor patient care resulting from overworked nurses. Recently, CNA had the mandatory overtime clause repealed in its negotiations with Kaiser.

Nursing unions are also looking for "no layoff" guarantees to get protection from downsizing by providers.[23] Although absolute guarantees have been rare, unions have won limited guarantees for very senior workers in the organization. Restrictions on subcontracting of services have also been resisted, though the maximum restriction imposed on providers is limiting intimidation of workers prior to subcontracting work.

Which preventive policies should IHSs pursue? In general, they should provide factual information to workers to persuade them against joining the union. Unfair labor practices, such as intimidating workers, offering monetary inducements, or making other promises to workers to vote against the union, should be avoided at all costs. Not only are they against the law, but such attempts are likely to backfire and result in considerable negative publicity for the organization, as happened at Columbia-HCA in the mid-1990s. An administrative law judge assigned by the National Labor Relations Board found Columbia's number two executive, David Vandewater, guilty of intimidation of nurse managers.

What should an IHS do if one or more of its facilities are unionized? Experts suggest being positive, being aware of and dealing with stumbling blocks, and building a good rapport with union officials. In the first months after a labor agreement is reached, organizational leaders should create a climate of engagement and dialogue by meeting with the union leadership right away, clarifying priorities, and committing to positive language by assuring the union it won't be disparaged by management. Leadership should also be aware of potential stumbling blocks. If some practice, such as a staffing or management practice, angers employees at a unit, it should be put on the table for discussion, even if it cannot be altered immediately due to fairness or other reasons. If a manager is very confrontational or insensitive, this behavior is likely to create a bad context for union relations, and the manager may have to be reassigned. For most organizations, issues that are important to employees surface in the year prior to contract negotiations (e.g., overtime, scheduling, workload, acuity assignment, and pay and benefits). Leaders need to be aware of employees' emotional commitment to specific issues and approach them sensitively. Any ambiguity related to interpretation or application of the contract should also be clarified. Finally, it is essential to build a good rapport—by arranging for the nurse executive and management team to meet with union leaders at least once a month, involving union leaders in strategy and planning, and providing visible programs of management training in union and staff relationship building.[24]

CONCLUSION

The corporate HR function within IHSs faces major challenges in present times. Strategically, IHSs face internal resistance to attempts at functional and clinical integration. Operationally, reimbursement continues to decrease for IHSs even as costs of patient care increase, at the same time as shortages are making it difficult to adequately staff facilities. Corporate HR departments must strengthen their strategic planning by linking it with the health system's strategic plan. These departments must find creative ways of recruiting and retaining workers to keep the health system fully operational. They must train and develop managers, physician leaders, and employees on a limited budget while simultaneously meeting JCAHO training standards in the system. They must control compensation and benefit expenditures in the face of inflation while providing nonmonetary benefits and rewards to attract and retain employees during staff shortages.

They must design an appropriate compensation structure for physicians to enhance their productivity and efficiency without alienating them, and give physicians a dominant role in designing this system. Finally, they must deal with the possibility of unionization at healthcare facilities at a time when patient care restructuring, layoffs, and inadequate staffing ratios have made unions more popular. The corporate HR department is critical to the survival and success of integrated healthcare systems today.

REFERENCES

1. Dalton A. Happy workers. *Hospitals and Health Networks.* 2004; November: 26–27.
2. Satinsky M. *The Foundations of Integrated Care.* Chicago: American Hospital Publishing; 1998.
3. Lerner W. *Anatomy of a Merger.* Chicago: Health Administration Press; 1997.
4. Shafer R, Dyer L, Killy J, Amos J, Ericksen J. Crafting a human resource strategy to foster organizational agility: a case study. *Human Resource Management.* 2001; 40:197–212.
5. Matthes K. The pink slip turns into something rosier. *Management Review.* 1992; 4:5.
6. Cross M. Software becomes a strategic tool for human resources departments. *Health Data Management.* 1997; July:1–5.
7. Morrissey J. CHW plans IT initiative. *Modern Healthcare.* 2004; 8:16.
8. Savill P. HR at Inova reengineers recruitment process. *Personnel Management.* 1995; 6:109–111.
9. Deslodge R. Tenet, St. John's offer bonuses, tuition payments to lure nurses. *St. Louis Business Journal.* 2002; 10:9.
10. Perotin-Star M. Fort Worth–Dallas hospitals step up efforts to recruit nurses. *Knight Ridder Tribune Business News.* Sept. 29, 2003: 1.
11. Fordyce M. Regionalization of human resources. SCHS facilities collaborate to head off labor shortages. *Health Progress.* 1992; 7:41–43.
12. Fritsch S. Skills for selecting valued leaders: Eastern Mercy takes a nine-step approach to choosing managers. *Health Progress.* 1992; 7:36–40.
13. McDonald L. Raising the bar on recruitment and retention. *Healthcare Financial Management.* 2000; 6:58–61.
14. Moore D. Samaritan's revolution. *Modern Healthcare.* 1996; 26:31.
15. Cassidy J. Teamwork rewarded. *Health Progress.* 1995; 76:43–45.
16. Pagoaga J, Williams J. Hay survey: Reform spurs shift in compensation strategies. *Trustee.* 1993; 11:12–15.
17. Markham S, Scott KD, Little B, Berman S. Gainsharing experiments in healthcare. *Compensation and Benefits Review.* March–April: 1992; 57–68.

18. Brennan M. Salary compression of nursing managers. *Nursing Management.* 1993; 4:46–49.
19. Zismer D. *Physician Compensation Arrangements.* Gaithersburg: Aspen Publishers; 1999.
20. Miller J. Quality progress. *Managed Healthcare Executive.* 2003; 6:28.
21. Norris R. Detroit hospital mulls freezing pension contributions for 11,000 workers. *Knight Ridder Tribune Business News.* Feb. 13, 2003: 1.
22. Keeshan, B. Hospitals serve as pioneers in family-friendly benefits. *Modern Healthcare.* 1994; 51:40.
23. Wolkinson B, Hames D, Lundy C. Nurse staffing issues: from conflict to collaboration. *Journal of Collective Negotiations in the Public Sector.* 2003; 2:135–147.
24. Porter-O'Grady T. Collective bargaining: the union as partner. *Nursing Management.* 2001; June: 30–32.

CHAPTER 7

Human Resources Issues in Managed Care Settings

Marie L. Kotter and Karen S. Burnett

VIGNETTE

Sara Hunter is the Director of Human Resources for a well-integrated managed care organization that includes more than 20 hospitals, employed physicians, and a health plan. Sara faces unique challenges every day. It is getting tougher to keep the care provider at the patient's bedside. Turnover at the hospitals is increasing as the bedside caregiver moves into nontraditional nursing roles within the integrated system. The nurse vacancy rate is a growing concern among the physicians, and they want Sara to develop appropriate incentives to keep the nurses at the bedside. The piece-rate compensation package for claims processors at the health plan needs to be updated, and the five-year strategic plan for human resources is due in three days.

OVERVIEW OF THE SETTING

For most of the twentieth century, the U.S. healthcare system was financed through traditional indemnity health insurance plans that paid doctors, hospitals, and other healthcare providers on a fee-for-service basis. With economic prosperity and comparatively low costs of health care, the ample funding resulted in the widespread provision of ever more advanced care.

Table 7-1 Comparisons Demonstrating the Increase in the Amount of Healthcare Spending in the United States and the Sources of Funds That Have Shifted to Third-Party Payers

	1929	1965	2002
Total health spending ($ millions)	3,656	41,012	1,545,900
Adjusted for inflation (2002 $ millions)	32,400	192,300	1,545,900
Per capita (adjusted) ($)	305	962	5,427
As a percentage of GDP	3.5%	5.7%	14.7%
Percentage Paid by			
Self (out-of-pocket)	81%	44%	15%
Third parties	19%	56%	85%
Government	13%	25%	45%
Private insurance	<1%	25%	35%
Philanthropy, other	6%	6%	5%

Source: Getzen T. *Health Economics Fundamentals and Flow of Funds.* 2nd ed. New York: Wiley & Sons; 2004. Reprinted with permission of John Wiley & Sons, Inc.

In 1965, as seen in Table 7-1,[1] 44% of the U.S. population personally paid for their health care. By 2002, only 15% of the population were paying for their care, and 85% of the costs were covered by third-party payers. This shift in the source of funds made the end user immune to the cost of health care, and accessing all of the technological advances became very desirable. In addition, the aging of the U.S. population, coupled with the fact that people are no longer dying from acute, short-term diseases, has resulted in an increase in healthcare system treatment of chronic diseases that were once considered hopeless. Finally, there has been a shift in the recipients of expenditures—from doctors to institutions such as hospitals and nursing homes. All of these factors resulted in a bill for healthcare spending in 2002 that amounted to $1.58 trillion, which was 15% of the gross domestic product (GDP), and a healthcare workforce that includes 1 out of every 12 people in the U.S. labor force.[1]

All of these reasons combined to produce a very rapid escalation in premium increases in the 1980s. The value of healthcare benefits provided by U.S. industry was equal to 36% of after-tax profits in 1970, 43% in 1980, and 108% in 1990.[1] Industry countered the skyrocketing costs with widespread adoption of managed care approaches by employer-sponsored health plans.

The fundamental difference between traditional reimbursement in fee-for-service or indemnity models and managed care is a *manager* who monitors and controls the transactions between healthcare providers and the patient. Because the managed care organization has financial responsibility for medical care, it has an incentive to provide efficient, quality care and to control costs. Of course, the potential configurations of managed care are very diverse and should be viewed on a continuum ranging from unmanaged to tightly managed. The most loosely organized managed plans are preferred provider organizations (PPO) or point-of-service (POS) operations.

Variations of the managed care approaches used in employer-sponsored health plans were adopted in Medicaid and Medicare programs. By the mid-1990s, this widespread acceptance of managed care plans had substantially reduced the growth rate of healthcare expenditures, and the need for large premium increases declined (see Figure 7-1).[2]

All published studies show that health maintenance organizations (HMOs) and other managed care plans have delivered health care of

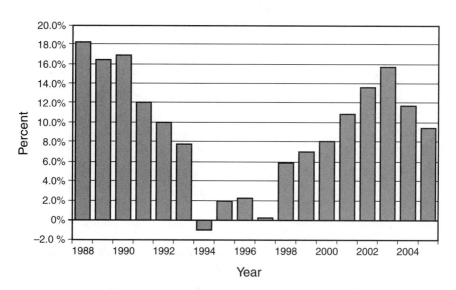

Source: Managed Care National Statistics, MCOL, 2005. Available at: http://www.mcareol.com/factshts/factnati.htm. Accessed July 20, 2005. Reprinted with permission of the publisher of Managed Care National Statistics, MCOL, 2005.

FIGURE 7-1 Premium Increase Comparisons Demonstrating the Decrease in Premiums from 1990 to 1997, When Premiums Began to Increase

equal or better quality than traditional indemnity insurance plans, and at a lower cost.[3] In 1995, a Pew Commission report[4] projected major changes in healthcare structure and delivery based on increased managed care market penetration and a spillover effect to the structure and function of the total healthcare system. However, in the late 1990s, concerns about overall costs lessened, and the public and physicians became less willing to accept restrictions on choice of physician and treatment. National HMO enrollment began to decline in 2002 (see Figure 7-2).[2] As a result of this backlash, the healthcare industry is reworking the structure of its managed care products. In some areas of the country, managed care has moved into third-generation models. Many HMOs, such as Kaiser (the largest HMO in the United States), began as nonprofit organizations with closed staff models. Today, many for-profit corporations use corporate business models, and Kaiser's 10 million enrollees represent only 10% of the market.[1] Employer-sponsored health plans are following three trends. First, they are using plan deductibles, copayments, and premium costs to shift more of the financial burden from employers to employees. Second, they are making employees more accountable for their healthcare cost decisions. Third, they are moving toward PPOs and away from

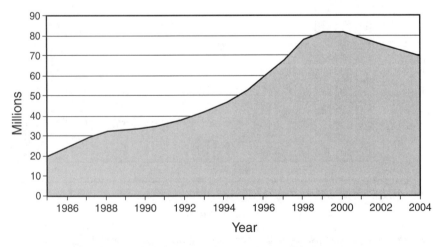

Source: Managed Care National Statistics, MCOL, 2005. Available at: http://www.mcareol.com/factshts/factnati.htm. Accessed July 20, 2005. Reprinted with permission of the publisher of Managed Care National Statistics, MCOL, 2005.

FIGURE 7-2 HMO Enrollment in the United States, 1985–2004 (in millions)

HMOS. These trends reflect efforts to control overall healthcare benefit costs and provide employees with more choice.

Organized delivery systems are a newer development that are composed of hospitals, physicians, and insurers in various forms of ownership and alliances designed to provide more cost-effective care to defined populations by achieving desired levels of functional, physician system, and clinical integration. Evidence suggests that, compared to less integrated delivery forms, these organized delivery systems provide more accessible coordinated care across the continuum, and appear to be associated with higher levels of inpatient productivity, greater total system revenue, greater total system cash flow, and greater total system operating margin. To optimize these gains, several key factors have been identified—namely, organizational culture, information systems, internal incentives, total quality management, physician leadership, and the growth of group practices.[5] These systems should be viewed as an additional step along the managed care continuum.

Today, healthcare costs are rising once again. Tables 7-2 and 7-3 and Figure 7-3[1] illustrate the current health insurance coverage of the U.S. population, the distribution of types of insurance, and the percentage of workers insured, based on size of employer. The United States is spending significantly more per capita on health care than are other developed

Table 7-2 Health Care Insurance Coverage of the U.S. Population for Non-elderly and Elderly Groups

	Non-elderly	Elderly
Total people	250 million	35 million
With insurance	74.2%	99.3%
Employment	34.9%	34.1%
Employment (dependent)	33.5%	N.A.
Other private insurance	5.7%	27.9%
Military	2.8%	4.3%
Medicare	2.2%	96.9%
Medicaid	10.4%	10.1%
Uninsured	15.5%	0.7%

Note: Percentages add to more than 100% because many people have multiple coverage.
Source: Getzen T. *Health Economics Fundamentals and Flow of Funds.* 2nd ed. New York: Wiley & Sons; 2004. Reprinted with permission of John Wiley & Sons, Inc.

Table 7-3 Annual Premiums for Employee Health Insurance Coverage, 2002

	HMO	PPO	POS	Indemnity	Average
Single					
Total premium	$2,764	$3,109	$3,175	$3,582	$3,060
Employee pays	$455	$432	$527	$426	$454
Family					
Total premium	$7,541	$8,037	$8,173	$8,479	$7,954
Employee pays	$1,960	$2,152	$2,186	$1,630	$2,084
Percentage of all insured employees	26%	51%	18%	5%	100%

Source: Getzen T. *Health Economics Fundamentals and Flow of Funds.* 2nd ed. New York: Wiley & Sons; 2004. Reprinted with permission of John Wiley & Sons, Inc.

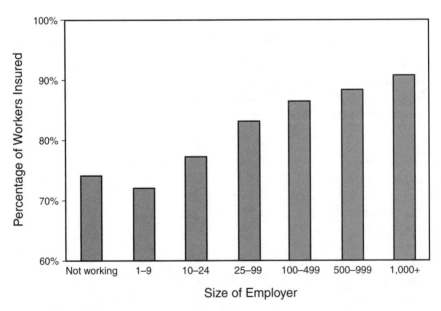

Source: Getzen T. *Health Economics Fundamentals and Flow of Funds.* 2nd ed. New York: Wiley & Sons; 2004. Reprinted with permission of John Wiley & Sons, Inc.

FIGURE 7-3 Percentage of Insured Workers by Size of Employer

countries, with no demonstrable improvement in health outcomes. Estimates suggest that, in the next 30 years, healthcare costs will again rise at a rate faster than that of the economy as a whole. Further, rising costs will reflect the impact of the aging population, with more than 20% of the U.S. population being 65 or older by 2030.[5] These market forces are coinciding with shortages in various health professions, such as nursing, pharmacy, and clinical laboratory sciences, which will make human resources management (HRM) a key issue for all healthcare delivery systems, including managed care organizations.

This chapter focuses on the differences and similarities between HRM in the healthcare industry in general and managed care organizations in particular. The chapter is divided into several sections, which coincide with general HR functions, such as staffing, employee development, compensation, and governance.

STRATEGIC PLANNING

Human resources' leadership role in health care is more important than ever due to the changing dynamics in the industry. The continued growth of managed care as a system for healthcare delivery provides both challenges and opportunities for HR managers. Proactive management of HR strategy can help a managed care organization gain or keep a competitive advantage in the industry. The HR department in a managed care organization must formally contribute to the overall organizational strategic planning process. Many of the issues facing managed care today are important workforce, staffing, and work flow design issues.

Successful strategic HRM in a managed care organization requires the entire HR department to become a strategic business partner with the rest of the organization. The HR staff must participate in business strategic planning; they must know how HR systems and decisions affect the organization; and they must be viewed as experts in their field if they are to become a integral part of the strategic planning process.

Planning and Implementing HR Strategy in Managed Care Settings

Strategic workforce planning within a managed care organization brings unique challenges. While the healthcare industry in general is facing nationwide workforce shortages, managed care organizations face stiff competition in the business world for competent employees. In today's world, a greater variety of jobs are available outside of managed care for the traditional managed care employee, requiring managed care organizations to plan their HR strategy carefully.

Many production facilities are employing RNs in their operating plants to design wellness programs and review worker's compensation injuries. RNs are also being recruited by attorneys for case review positions. Technicians who historically were employed by the managed care organization are being heavily recruited by privately owned, niche providers in the area of radiology, heart services, women's services, and other specialties. Additionally, the health plan clerical employee has a number of career opportunities outside of the managed care organization. Given all of these available opportunities, the HR strategies for the organization are clearly very important.

Managed care organizations not only employ the traditional bedside nurses, but now must also employ claims processors, actuaries, case managers, and benefits review specialists, just to name a few. In addition to these specialized clerical and professional jobs, many nontraditional roles for nursing staff are available. Many managed care organizations stress the importance of wellness, prevention, and early intervention with the patient. The managed care nurse's role may include development of wellness programs, disease management programs, and patient safety initiatives. As a result, the managed care nurse of today must not only understand direct patient care, but also possess highly developed critical thinking skills to be able to understand and advocate for the entire patient experience.

Because a managed care organization's workforce can be highly dependent on the workforce to which its customers belong, planning the appropriate size of the healthcare workforce can be especially challenging. Ensuring the right amount of staff at the right time is a skill that managed care leaders must carefully develop. Because of the stiff competition they face, managed care organizations must be diligent in providing employees with a stable work environment so as to increase their retention rates.

Additionally, advanced technology plays a role in HR strategy in the managed care organization. This technology has forced the managed care workforce to be more technologically skilled and to adapt to changing dynamics quickly. Advances in technology promise to allow customers access to even more information about their care, their medical records, and their caregivers in the future.

For all these reasons, HR strategic planning in all managed care organizations, regardless of their size, is critical. Failure to plan proactively will result in an HR culture that is reactive and not able to respond quickly to the changing demands in the industry.

Managing the Flow of Work in Managed Care Settings

Like its counterparts in many nonhealthcare industries, the managed care organization must have a continuous improvement process. Administrative expenses must be kept to a minimum if the organization is to achieve financial success. Successful managed care organizations not only focus on patient safety and outcomes, but also on the financial impact of claims management. They continually update their processes, review claims administration processes, and reduce administrative costs. The work process must be continually improved to eliminate waste, redundancy, and unnecessary steps.

Typically, organizations have relied upon senior management to evaluate work flow processes and make necessary changes. A successful managed care organization will seek input from front-line staff members about work flow and process improvement. Successful work flow and process improvement must begin with the people who are doing the actual work, who can identify barriers and recommend improvements. It is short-sighted to exclude the front-line staff member from important work flow and process improvement decisions.

Understanding Equal Opportunity and the Legal Environment in Managed Care Settings

The expectation of equal opportunity and the legal environment are no different in a managed care organization than in any healthcare organization. Ensuring equal opportunity and fair treatment in the workplace is the responsibility of every leader, whether in a managed care setting or a non-managed care environment. Human resources staff members must ensure that the organization's culture is characterized by fairness and equal opportunity. Any deviation from fairness or equal opportunity must be addressed quickly and aggressively, regardless of the type of healthcare organization.

RECRUITMENT AND SELECTION

The healthcare system in the United States continues to face severe workforce shortages. In July 2002, the U.S. Department of Health and Human Services, Health Resources and Services Administration, Bureau of Health Professions, and the National Center for Health Workforce Analysis distributed a report titled "Projected Supply, Demand and Shortages of Registered Nurses: 2000–2020." This report focuses on the challenges the healthcare industry will face over the next two decades with recruiting and retention. The report data indicate that a national shortage of registered nurses, once expected to begin around 2007, was already evident in 2000.[6]

In 2000, the national supply of registered nurses was estimated at 1.89 million, while the demand was estimated at 2 million, a shortage of approximately 6%. Based on trends in the supply of RNs and the anticipated demands, this shortage is expected to grow to 29% by 2020. This projected shortage will result from a projected 40% increase in demand between 2000 and 2020, compared to a 6% growth in supply.

Factors driving the growth of demand for healthcare workers include growth in the U.S. population, a larger proportion of elderly persons, and medical advances that heighten the need for healthcare providers. In contrast, the declining supply of RNs can be attributed to a declining number of nursing school graduates, the aging of the RN workforce, decreases in nurses' relative earnings, and the emergence of alternative job opportunities.[6]

The managed care organization will face an even greater staffing challenge. While the healthcare industry struggles to recruit and retain bedside RNs, managed care organizations need a consistent supply of not only bedside nurses, but also registered nurses who function as case managers, patient educators, triage nurses, utilization reviewers, risk managers, and provider liaisons. All of these positions require a licensed RN, but they also require that the RN be removed as the primary care provider for the patient.

Physician recruiting represents another challenge. In a study of primary care physicians, the majority of HMO-affiliated physicians joined HMOs to avoid a perceived penalty associated with lack of affiliation, rather than for positive reasons. The data also suggest that physicians with managed care experience affiliate with an HMO more often for "quality of life" reasons.[7]

The number of physicians who are choosing to become employed and salaried is increasing rapidly. For those physicians who are newly out of residency and saddled with large medical school debt, accepting a salaried position is a wise decision. For managed care to continue to be successful, a fully committed and engaged physician workforce is imperative. Benefits of becoming an employed physician include the ability to achieve work–life balance, a predictable minimum income level, and reduced administrative activities.[7]

A successful managed care organization must be staffed to match the size of the community it serves. If staffing levels are not appropriate, physician income and professional satisfaction may be at risk. It is important for the organization to formulate a physician recruitment plan as part of its long-term strategy. In developing this plan, the managed care organization must assess its mission and vision, the priority healthcare needs in the community, the organization's current ability to meet the needs of the community, and the projected growth and development of the community. The managed care organization must also carefully assess its current physician workforce and plans for future employment. After the physician recruitment plan has been developed, the medical staff leadership must partner with HR personnel to develop a successful recruiting strategy.[8]

Clearly, recruiting and retention strategies are increasingly important in maintaining an engaged and energized workforce in a managed care organization. Recruiting methods for managed care systems generally include Internet recruiting, internal recruiting, and external recruiting.

Competition for well-qualified healthcare providers is also strong. Managed care systems must compete in this marketplace not only on the basis of cost and quality of care, but also as part of their effort to attract and retain a competent workforce. Prior to beginning any recruiting, the managed care organization must define the competencies necessary for specific positions. Managed care employees are unique because they must be technically sophisticated and experienced people who also have a clinical background.

Internet Recruiting

Today, the Internet has become the primary source through which many healthcare employers search for qualified candidates and many applicants search for jobs. In the United States, it is estimated that 74% of those with Internet access use the World Wide Web as a component of their job searches. HR professionals are using the Internet as well. When questioned, recruiters report that 77% of their new hires responded to openings posted on the Internet, compared with 17.5% who responded to newspaper advertisements.[6]

Today's Internet recruiting includes not only generic career Web sites, but also Web sites dedicated solely to healthcare recruiting. There are even managed care recruiting and managed care nursing certification Web sites (www.abmcn.org). In the managed care setting, nurses have moved away from their traditional roles, so the recruiting must follow suit and move away from its traditional methods.

Internal Recruiting

Oftentimes, the best sources for qualified candidates come from within the healthcare facility. A popular method of internal recruiting includes job posting and bidding. Some managed care systems maintain an applicant tracking system that includes a computerized internal database of skills.

One of the most reliable sources of qualified candidates is referrals by current employees. Current employees can discuss with potential candidates the advantages of a job with the company and encourage them to apply.[6] Some employers pay employees incentives for referring individuals with experience or specialized skills that are hard to recruit.

External Recruiting

In an era of many workforce shortages, Internet and internal recruiting sources often do not produce the required number of qualified candidates. As a consequence, managed care HR professionals often turn to schools, colleges, and universities for additional candidates. Due to the unique aspects of educational preparatory requirements for most clinical degrees, many healthcare employers already have a flow of candidates through the educational system.

Clinical rotations are required for such fields as nursing, pharmacy, and medical technologies. A clinical rotation program requires students to have hands-on educational experiences. These rotations generally occur in a hospital or related healthcare setting. Many employers use this clinical rotation as an opportunity to recruit qualified candidates.[9]

Additionally, many graduate degree programs in healthcare administration, public health, and health planning include postgraduate fellowship programs. These fellowships place qualified candidates in high-level support positions to executives, administrators, and CEOs of managed care systems. Some of the fellowships result in opportunities for the candidate to move into middle- or upper-management positions at the completion of the fellowship.[9]

Managing Workforce Diversity in Managed Care Settings

Both non-managed care and managed care organizations desire inclusiveness in their workforces. Likewise, both strive to ensure that the organization's culture supports and encourages inclusiveness. In addition to the professional clinical staff found in all healthcare organizations, managed care organizations have a large workforce of hourly, clerical employees to process claims and answer members' questions. Organizational commitment to diversity and job satisfaction of a diverse workforce are requirements for any managed care organization to be successful. Indeed, celebrating and valuing cultural diversity within a managed care organization are important not only for workforce satisfaction, but also for a better understanding of the patient's experience, which leads to greater patient satisfaction.

Many cultures view the healthcare experience differently and have unique and distinct customs regarding healthcare decisions and the roles that family members play in making those decisions. A comforting gesture by a patient care provider from one culture might be perceived as an insult to a patient of another culture. Many cultures require that the elder male member of the family take responsibility for medical decisions for family members. If the patient care provider is not aware of this cultural expectation, the entire experience for the patient and the family can be negatively affected if the expectation is not met. Cultural sensitivity is imperative with an inclusive workforce and customer base.

Both non-managed care and managed care organizations must make a strong effort to seek out a diverse workforce and must shape their recruiting and retention strategies around the goal of a multicultural workforce. Customers in the managed care environment include patients, physicians, and health plan members. To provide the excellent customer service required for a managed care organization's success, the workforce must mirror the diversity of the customers. Additionally, the workforce must be educated to the needs and expectations of a culturally diverse customer base.

Selection

Selection entails more than just choosing a person to fill a job. It is important to have the right person in the right position. The selection process can best be defined as a matching process: It seeks to match what the organization needs with what the candidate needs from the organization. Such a "fit" is critical to ensure a successful placement. In today's managed care environment, if the candidate has the necessary minimum qualifications, then employers are often willing to hire for "fit" and train for any additional skills. During the selection process, to help determine whether an employee will be an appropriate "fit," past behavior is the best predictor of future behavior. As a result, the selection process should include a measure of past behavioral events. For instance, behavioral event–based interview questions require employees to give specific examples of how they have handled a specific problem in the past, what they learned from the experience, and what they might do differently in the future. The candidate's answer can give important insight into how he or she might handle a similar situation in the future.

Orienting the Workforce

New employee orientation can be especially challenging in a managed care setting. New employees must be oriented to JCAHO standards, their specific jobs, and the overall organization mission, vision, and values; they must also receive any special, technical orientation required to do their jobs. Their initial competence must be assessed, and then unit/job-specific orientation must be tailored to their needs. Additionally, many managed care organizations orient new employees to critical thinking skills.

In today's managed care environment, great emphasis is placed on customer service skills. Oftentimes, the only thing that separates one organization from another is the level of customer service provided. As a result, service excellence training and education must be an integral part of orienting the managed care workforce. Employees should be educated on how to resolve customer issues and concerns in a timely fashion.

Confidentiality is another important component of managed care employee orientation. Managed care employees must commit to maintaining the confidentiality of employee and patient information, including sensitive medical record information. They must understand their legal obligations as managed care employees with access to such confidential information.

RETENTION

Retention of valued employees is a significant concern for the managed care organization. Organizational performance is improved in any industry when there is continuity of employees who are experienced in their jobs and who understand the organization and its culture. Successful managed care organizations intuitively understand the link between retention and overall patient satisfaction. Increased demands placed on managed care employees to provide patient care for more patients while managing costs can lead to higher turnover rates. Turnover costs not only include the actual cost of recruiting a replacement, but also the cost of the experience level of the incumbent who left. As a result, retention of valued staff members is critically important to the successful managed care organization.

Employees consider several factors when choosing whether to stay with their employer or to leave for another employer. For example, they consider organizational factors, including what the mission and culture of the organization are, how well managed the organization is, and whether the organization provides job security. Career opportunities, competitive pay and benefits, and the organization's reward system are other factors that the employee assesses. In addition, a number of personal factors must be considered, including job autonomy, work–life balance, and supervisory support.

One advantage of an integrated managed healthcare organization is the availability of many different opportunities and different work environments within the same organization. For the long-tenured nurse who is looking to leave the bedside, opportunities in utilization review, case management, and employee health—to name only a few—exist within the same organization. Overall organizational retention increases when greater opportunities are available. A successful integrated managed care organization has the ability to offer greater flexibility in scheduling, a culture that allows autonomy in decision making, and the ability for staff members to be involved in the patient experience at all levels.[9]

Managing Separations and Outplacements

Both non-managed care and managed care organizations must manage separations and outplacements in a legally appropriate and ethical manner. Successful management of employee separations includes a well-defined corrective action policy that addresses expectations as well as consequences. It also provides an understanding of wrongful discharge and the importance of documentation.

To reduce employee separations, organizations should develop standards of behavior, or organizational values, to identify what the organization expects from the employee and what the employee can expect from the organization. It is imperative that these values be incorporated into the organizational culture and practiced at every level in the organization. If expectations are made clear and employees are held accountable to these expectations in a fair and consistent manner, then employee separations can be reduced. The result will be a culture where employees feel valued and choose to stay with an employer and meet that employer's expectations. Reducing the number of employee separations will reduce employment liability and risk to the organization.

PERFORMANCE MANAGEMENT

Because more than half of the expenses of a healthcare organization are related to compensation, compensation strategies, including performance appraisals, must be aligned with the organization's business strategies and goals.[8] Managed care organizations usually support more job classifications than are found in a traditional healthcare setting. These range from physicians and hospitalists to nurse case managers and patient educators, in addition to the traditional hospital employees. This diversity of positions requires a rethinking of the traditional appraisal methods.

For example, in a study by Duberman[10] that assessed the critical behavioral competencies of outstanding managed care primary care physicians within a network-model HMO, six performance measures were used: (1) member satisfaction, (2) utilization, (3) patient complaints, (4) emergency room referrals, (5) out-of-network referrals, and (6) medical record completeness. Physicians performing above the mean on all of these measures were classified as outstanding and then participated in a behavioral event interview and a picture story exercise. Outstanding physicians demonstrated higher achievement orientation, concern for personal influence, empathic caregiving, and empowerment scores. They were also more competent in building team effectiveness and reaching interpersonal understanding when compared with the control group of typical primary care physicians. Duberman's data suggest that primary care physicians' performance is the product of measurable competencies that can be targeted for improvement. Using competency assessment methods of appraisal combined with a good development program can benefit organizational efficiency and increase both physician and patient satisfaction.

In a 2001 American Society of Health-System Pharmacists (ASHP) survey[11] of ambulatory care responsibilities of pharmacists in managed care and integrated health systems, the 24 performance functions used were related to five "enabling" factors: (1) pharmacists on interdisciplinary care teams, (2) automated dispensing systems, (3) integrated electronic medical records, (4) very supportive medical staff, and (5) very supportive senior managements. These enabling factors speak to the support needed in the managed care environment for the pharmacists to perform well. (These factors may also be required for pharmacists to perform well in more traditional healthcare settings.) Ambulatory care pharmacists' functions expanded into new areas and decreased in more traditional areas, such as negotiating pharmaceutical contracts, immunization screening, and administration. These changes in responsibility may reflect the current pharmacist shortage and the increase in the number of prescriptions and patients. This study supports the idea that performance measures must be continually updated to match the current environment and business strategies of the organization.

Garcia, Safriet, and Russell[12] argue that, as pay-for-performance compensation plans become more prevalent, these programs will require the selection of appropriate performance criteria, accurate assessment of their financial impact, development of an effective means of communication between the health plan and physicians, and gradual implementation of the plan. If such compensation programs are implemented correctly, they will allow health plans and physicians to balance economic incentives and operational outcomes, which in turn will encourage improved performance and benefit providers, payers, and patients alike.

A well-defined pay-for-performance plan is built on a solid foundation: By rewarding employees and providers for quality outcomes, significant improvement in the quality of service and care will result. In a typical plan, incentives are calculated using a series of clinical and service indicators that measure results. A successful plan relies heavily on data collection and new information technology that is only now emerging.

It is important that a pay-for-performance program contain incentives and measures that actually motivate the stakeholder to improve the quality of care or service. The outcomes should be measurable, specific, and consistent. The outcome measures must also be flexible and adapt to a quickly changing healthcare environment.[12]

Examples of outcome measures for physicians include clinical process measures, patient grievance rates, and transfer rates. Outcome measures for health plan employees could include report accuracy, complaint resolutions, and satisfaction of members' employers.[12] It is important to remember that pay-for-performance plans must be built and adopted gradually. Successful plans require education, trust in the data, and sustained achievements.

In summary, appraising and managing performance in a managed care setting requires that appropriate, continually updated appraisal criteria be used in conjunction with required "enabling" support. For employees who are lacking in performance, action plans should be developed and training provided, if necessary, to empower employees to improve their performance.

TRAINING AND EDUCATION

Although "training" is a term often used in conjunction with "development," the two are not synonymous. Training typically seeks to provide employees with specific skills or help employees correct deficiencies in their performance. In contrast, development provides employees with the abilities the organization will need in the future. These two types of activities are important in all healthcare organizations, but they are essential in managed care organizations, which are continually trying to improve their quality and service while controlling costs. Indeed, in the current environment of double-digit cost escalations and healthcare employee shortages, these programs are crucial.

Salaried employment among primary care physicians is becoming the rule rather than the exception. This trend has forced managed care organizations to focus on the consequences of physician employment, types of practice revenues, and overall career satisfaction.

A 2003 study of physicians employed in a nonprofit HMO, which used interviews, observations, and archival data over a five-year period, revealed that the "form and substance of individual physician adaptation to organizational life is dependent upon social exchanges over time with the HMO."[13] This study suggests that, in a managed care environment characterized by structural diversity and constant change, individual physician adaptation is an emergent, evolutionary process and may be slow and delayed, particularly if the change makes physicians more dependent on their employing organization. This process appears to be more amenable to nontraditional career development methods than the traditional training programs the healthcare industry has used in the past. In managed care organizations, career development must be seen as a key business strategy that will improve the quality of employees' work lives, prevent job burnout, meet diversity goals, improve retention, and meet organizational needs that require adaptation to constant change.

COMPENSATION AND BENEFITS

Developing compensation strategies in a managed care organization can be a very complex process. Managed care is designed to be a cost-effective way to deliver quality healthcare. Managed care organizations must focus on providing a full spectrum of quality healthcare services while remaining cost-effective. However, the nontraditional roles found in many managed care organizations bring a unique and complex challenge to HR professionals, who are accountable for developing a compensation strategy that not only is aligned with business needs, but also meets the needs of the workforce.

More than half of a healthcare organization's expenditures are related to compensation.[8] Healthcare HR professionals are accountable for directing the development and administration of the organization's compensation system, including its base pay systems, pay structures, and organizational compensation policies and procedures. An effective compensation management system should include four objectives:

- Legal compliance with all appropriate laws and regulations
- Cost-effectiveness for the organization
- Internal, external, and individual equity for employees
- Performance enhancement for the organization[9]

Managing Compensation and Rewarding Performance in Managed Care Settings

To recruit and retain a highly qualified, highly engaged workforce, managed care organizations are competing not just with non-managed care organizations, but with the business industry as well. Managed care systems that include hospitals, employed physicians, and a health plan business deal with a wide variety of compensation needs and must be creative when developing their compensation plans. While much of the traditional clinical workforce is compensated based on market-driven factors, the nontraditional healthcare workforce may be compensated much differently. In particular, health plan employees may be compensated at a lower base rate, with their total compensation being supplemented by incentives. Incentives, which are normally paid in production or assembly work, are effective for health plan employees as well. For example, piece-rate incentives may be paid for the number of calls received by a telephone service representative at the health plan or for the number of claims processed by a health plans claims processor. Many of these positions are clerical in nature, but they still require basic clinical knowledge to be able to answer questions appropriately and process claims correctly. Managed care organizational systems that include a health plan business will employ a sales staff to market and sell the health plan, so incentives may be paid to these employees, including sales commissions.

These examples illustrate the unique challenges facing HR professionals in managed care organizations. These organizations are forced to be creative and often move away from traditional compensation approaches. Many managed care organizations might wish to be the leader in their market with their compensation scheme, but face significant pressures to control costs and may have to redefine this compensation strategy.

While the employee's base rate of pay should be based on market conditions, adjustments to the employee's compensation should reflect his or her individual performance and contributions to the organization's goals.[8] Resources for compensation can be limited, based on the managed care organization's desire to reduce overall costs. Compensation must reflect this reality.

Scoggins,[14] in a study measuring the effect of practitioner compensation on HMO consumer satisfaction, found that consumer satisfaction with HMOs was negatively correlated with the percentage of practitioners on a capitated-fee basis and positively correlated with the percentage compensated with a fee-withholding incentive. Fee-withholding programs hold back a fraction of the fees paid until specific quality and cost-control goals are reached. This study implies that the compensation method for practitioners in managed health plans can affect participant satisfaction.

In a study on trends in the nurse labor market, Buerhaus and Staiger discuss the differences in employment and wage growth in low-enrollment and high-enrollment HMO states.[15] In low-enrollment states, the employment growth of RNs between 1983 and 1997 increased, compared to high-enrollment states. However, the wage growth during this same time span was higher in high-enrollment states. (See Figures 7-4 and 7-5.) This

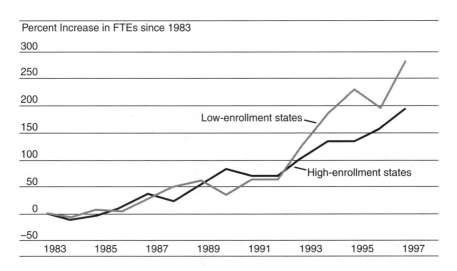

Source: Buerhaus P, Staiger D. Trouble in the nurse labor market? Recent trends and future outlook. *Health Affairs.* 1999; 18.1:218. Reprinted with permission of *Health Affairs.* Online (Project Hope).

FIGURE 7-4 The Higher Employment Growth of RNs in Low-HMO-Enrollment States, 1983–1997

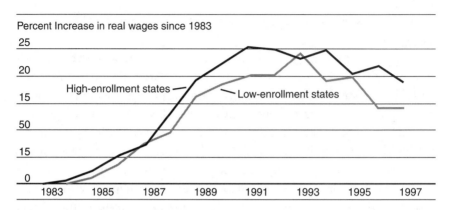

Percent Increase in real wages since 1983

Source: Buerhaus P, Staiger D. Trouble in the nurse labor market? Recent trends and future outlook. *Health Affairs.* 1999; 18.1:219. Reprinted with permission of *Health Affairs.* Online (Project Hope).

FIGURE 7-5   Higher Wage Growth of RNs in High-HMO-Enrollment States, 1983–1997

study demonstrates that the number of RNs hired may have been less in high-enrollment states, but wage growth was higher. This probably reflects the increased responsibilities of the RN workforce in HMO organizations and the emphasis on cost controls, which decreased RN full-time equivalent (FTE) growth.

Compensation decisions must be viewed strategically. Because the organization dedicates such a large percentage of its funds to compensation and related activities, it is extremely important that compensation decisions be closely aligned with business strategies and goals. To have a successful compensation program, an organization should consider what its pay philosophy is, how the organization will react to market fluctuations, and what approach it will take regarding compensation.[9]

Designing and Administering Benefits in Managed Care Settings

Within the total compensation package, healthcare organizations provide benefits to their employees for being part of the organization. Benefits are forms of indirect compensation that may include retirement benefits, paid time off, health insurance, educational and professional development assistance, and many other programs.[9] Designing and administering benefits in a managed care setting is similar to that in the non-managed care setting, with a few differences.

In a managed care setting, HR professionals are responsible for designing and administering benefits programs that meet the needs of the organization. Time off for employees must be structured to satisfy business needs, as many parts of the organization operate on a 24 hour per day, 7 day per week schedule. A distinct advantage for managed care systems is that they are part of a system, yet are a single employer, so benefits offered to employees are the same throughout the organization.

Educating the managed care employee on the concept of total compensation is an important part of administering a successful benefits program. A comprehensive benefits program is costly to an employer, averaging 30% to 40% of payroll costs. Employees often think of their compensation as including only wages and salaries and fail to understand the value of their benefits package when considering total compensation.[9] Because a comprehensive benefits plan has significant implications for recruiting and retention, educating the managed care employee about total compensation is imperative.

Managed care systems often find themselves on both sides of the healthcare continuum. On the one hand, as employers, they must provide a competitive, comprehensive benefits package. On the other hand, they are also the healthcare provider and may be the health insurance provider. The managed care organization has to carefully plan and design benefits strategies so that it does not have competing objectives between its business units.

Managed care organizations must provide the same government-mandated benefits that non-managed care organizations provide. These include worker's compensation, Family and Medical Leave Act (FMLA), and unemployment compensation.

In today's competitive job market for managed care employees, organizations must carefully assess their benefits design strategy to improve both recruiting and retention. They must try to meet the needs of a changing workforce population, including generational differences and related benefits needs. Flexibility and choice are important aspects of any successful benefits program. The managed care organization must continue to focus on providing a quality, cost-effective healthcare product, while expending the appropriate amount of funding for benefits programs that will meet the needs of its workforce.

EMPLOYEE RELATIONS

Developing Positive Employee Relations and Communication in Managed Care Settings

Although developing positive employee relations and communication is the responsibility of all managers, effective employee relations require cooperation between managers and employee relations representatives in HR departments. Employee relations representatives are like internal business consultants who advise both supervisors and employees on policies, procedures, and problems. The effectiveness of this system is directly related to the quality of the healthcare organization's communications. This is particularly true of managed care organizations. Employee productiveness is also correlated with various enabling systems, such as electronic medical records, and various automated programs, such as dispensing systems in the pharmacy and automated standing orders derived from evidence-based medicine clinical protocols.

In addition to electronic communication, opportunities need to be available for two-way communication in formal and informal meetings between employees and managers. In managed care settings with large organizational or geographic barriers, this can be very challenging. Often, the employee relations representatives may be more accessible and can channel employee concerns properly, so that issues can be addressed appropriately.

Managing Discipline and Respecting Employee Rights in Managed Care Settings

There is a fine line between the rights of employees and the rights of management. In healthcare settings, issues such as random drug testing, electronic monitoring, and whistle blowing can cause problems. In addition to these difficult issues, managed care organizations must always balance cost, quality, and patient satisfaction concerns. In more traditional healthcare organizations, this balance may not be as prominent.

Courts have routinely protected employee rights in wrongful discharge cases and in statutory and contractual cases. Most healthcare organizations have discipline and discharge policies that they must follow to ensure due process rights for their employees. The *Potvin v. Metropolitan Life* case, which was settled in 2000 by the California Supreme Court, held that a physician provider, who is an independent contractor for a health insurer, may have a right to a fair procedure before being terminated if the insurer possesses power that will impair the provider's ability to practice medicine. Although this decision does not clarify whether this standard applies to other entities or decisions not involving termination or exclusion, it is a clear message to follow due process procedures regardless of the healthcare entity.[16] This message is particularly strong for managed care entities, which often have physician employees or service contracts with physicians.

So-called economic credentialing, which relies on economic criteria to determine an individual's qualifications for staff privileges, is a new method being used to protect hospitals from competition by medical staff members. For example, if a physician opens a separate outpatient surgery center that will be in direct competition with the hospital, the hospital can refuse to credential the physician, which will prevent him or her from admitting patients to the hospital. This type of credentialing can be used for a variety of healthcare providers, including physicians, nurse practitioners, and physician assistants. This method uses economic conflict-of-interest credentialing policies to ensure loyalty and maintain economic viability. Weeks[17] argues that hospitals should be able to implement these policies in ways that minimize liability in most jurisdictions. Because managed care organizations use many midlevel practitioners and physicians to achieve labor cost savings,[18] economic credentialing must be done carefully to ensure fair procedures.

UNIONIZATION

Due to the trends in healthcare financing and delivery described at the beginning of the chapter, there has been an increase in union membership among many types of healthcare providers, including physicians. This is particularly true in states with a significant percentage of patients in managed care plans. Scheffler[19] suggests that the union membership of physicians, which numbered 35,000–45,000 in 1998, will increase 5–6% per year.

Kaiser Permanente is a large managed care company, with 8.6 million enrollees in 18 states. In *Modern Healthcare* in 1997, one lead story was the Kaiser unions voting on a pact with the AFL-CIO. This pact covers 50,000 union workers.[20] This shift toward greater unionization in health care is occurring at a time when traditional union membership in the

United States is decreasing. Large unions, such as the AFL-CIO, are now concentrating on the new markets of health care and government.

Managers and HR employees are on the front line in dealing with employees on labor–management matters. When unions enter the picture, labor relations specialists are usually hired to resolve grievances, negotiate a labor contract, and advise top management on labor relations strategies. Because unionization is often found in areas with high penetrations of managed care plans, this is an important issue for managed care organizations.

When a company faces difficult labor relations, the most important strategic choice will be to accept or to avoid unions. If management decides to try to avoid unionization, union organizing may still continue, and companies have to be very careful to avoid engaging in unfair labor practices.

If a union is organized, then the next step is to negotiate a contract and then administer the contract, which usually includes a specific grievance procedure. In a managed care organization, with its emphasis on cost and healthcare quality, unionization will have a significant effect on the management of human resources. Human resources policies will have to reflect consideration for the preferences of workers, which usually include better wages and benefits, job security, the ability to express dissatisfaction with administrative actions, and having a voice in work rules that affect their jobs.[21]

Ensuring Workplace Safety and Health in a Managed Care Setting

Healthcare organizations must place a strong emphasis on workplace safety and health for employees and patients. Patient and employee safety are measured, tracked, and reported to the board of directors. JCAHO requires that all sentential events be reported to the board.

In addition to the traditional patient safety concerns, healthcare facilities must be sensitive to employee concerns, such as exposure to infectious organisms, violence in the workplace, smoking in the workplace, fetal protection, hazardous chemicals, and genetic testing. Human resources professionals often work on policies dealing with these issues, which have both legal and ethical concerns. Both managed care and non-managed care organizations must make a concerted effort to develop policies in these difficult areas to protect patient and employee safety.[21]

CONCLUSION

Three major human resources challenges arise in managed care settings: (1) meeting the shortage of licensed healthcare professionals, (2) managing quality with human resources, and (3) evaluating the HR system. Given the diversity of employee categories, unique compensation systems, and emphasis on cost control, these problems are particularly acute in managed care organizations. As a consequence, the HR system must be particularly effective and staffed with competent HR specialists. In addition, the HR office and other support offices must be evaluated for competence and quality, just as patient care centers are.

One method for accomplishing this goal is to do a regular HR audit. A typical audit should analyze the following issues: (1) turnover rates; (2) reasons employees are quitting; (3) compliance with government regulations; (4) effectiveness of recruiting, training, and compensation plans; (5) employee diversity; (6) managers' needs versus services provided; (7) employee needs versus services provided; and (8) HR policies and procedures' effectiveness in helping the managed care organization meet its goals.[21] Based on the results of these audits, changes in personnel, policies, and processes may be warranted.

REFERENCES

1. Getzen T. *Health Economics Fundamentals and Flow of Funds.* 2nd ed. New York: Wiley & Sons; 2004.
2. Managed Care National Statistics, MCOL, 2005. Available at: http://www.mcareol.com/factshts/factnati.htm. Accessed July 20, 2005.
3. Luke RT. Healthcare in the United States: current and future challenges. *Managed Care.* 2001; 10(suppl):2–6.
4. Pew Health Professions Commission. *Critical Challenges: Revitalizing the Health Professions for the Twenty-First Century.* San Francisco: University of California, San Francisco, Center for the Health Professions; 1995.
5. Shortell SM, Hull KE. The new organization of the healthcare delivery system. *Baxter Health Policy Review.* 1996; 2:101–148.
6. U.S. Department of Health and Human Services, Health Resources and Services Administration, Bureau of Health Professions, National Center for Health Workforce Analysis. Projected Supply, Demand and Shortages of Registered Nurses: 2000–2020. July 2002. Available at: http://bhpr.hrsa.gov/healthworkforce/reports/mproject/report.htm. Accessed February 21, 2005.

7. Schur CL, Mueller CD, Berk ML. Why primary care physicians join HMOs. *American Journal of Managed Care.* 1999; 5:429–434.

8. Griffith J, White K. Human resources system. In: Kenneth R. White (ed), *The Well-Managed Healthcare Organization.* 5th ed. Chicago: AUPHA Press; 2002: 279–325, 597–634.

9. Flynn W, Mathis R, Jackson J, Langan P. *Healthcare Human Resource Management.* Mason, OH: Thomson South-Western; 2004.

10. Duberman TL. Assessing the critical behavioral competencies of outstanding managed care primary care physicians. *Managed Care Interface.* 1999; 12:76–80.

11. Knapp KK, Blalock SJ, Black BL. ASHP survey of ambulatory care responsibilities of pharmacists in managed care and integrated health systems—2001. *American Journal Health System Phramacies.* 2001; 58:2151–2166.

12. Garcia LB, Safriet S, Russell DC. Pay-for-performance compensation: moving beyond capitation. *Healthcare Financial Management.* 1998; 52:52–57.

13. Hoff TJ. How physician-employees experience their work lives in a changing HMO. *Journal Health Sociological Behavior.* 2003; 44:75–96.

14. Scoggins JF. The effect of practitioner compensation on HMO consumer satisfaction. *Managed Care.* 2002; 11:49–52.

15. Buerhaus P, Staiger D. Trouble in the nurse labor market? Recent trends and future outlook. *Health Affairs.* 1999; 18.1:214–222.

16. Diaz DS, Ty MY. Termination of a physician contract: fair procedure under *Potvin v. Metropolitan Life. Managed Care Interface.* 2000; 13:77–79.

17. Weeks EA. The new economic credentialing: protecting hospitals from competition by medical staff members. *Journal of Health Law.* 2003; 36:247–300.

18. Roblin DH, Becker ER, Adams EK, Roberts MH. Use of midlevel practitioners to achieve labor cost savings in the primary care practice of an MCO. *Health Services Research.* 2004; 39:607–626.

19. Scheffler RM. Physician collective bargaining: a turning point in U.S. medicine. *Journal Health Politics, Policy, and Law.* 1999; 24:1071–1076.

20. Moore JD. Kaiser unions OK pact with AFL-CIO. *Modern Healthcare.* 1997; 127:30.1–30.3.

21. Gomez-Mejia LP, Balkin DB, Cardy RL. *Managing Human Resources.* 4th ed. Upper Saddle River, NJ: Pearson Prentice Hall; 2004.

CHAPTER 8

The Human Resources Function in Hospitals

Susan Sportsman

VIGNETTE

Paul Farmer is the newly hired Director of Human Resources (HR) at Mercy Hospital, a 400-bed, not-for-profit, acute care hospital in an urban area. He faces numerous challenges in this role. The hospital is preparing for a Joint Commission for the Accreditation of Healthcare Organizations accreditation visit in six months, and several human resources problems must be resolved before the visit. For example, physician credentialing files must be updated and the required education/training for clinical staff adequately documented. The average hospital-wide nurse vacancy rate is 18%, and the turnover rate is 23%. In addition, the hospital has been losing money for the last 18 months, and the administrative team is developing strategies to reduce labor costs without affecting the quality of care. Chapter 8 will provide Farmer—and other readers—with guidelines for dealing with such challenges in a hospital setting. Following an overview of the hospital setting, the chapter will address recruitment and selection, retention, hiring, competency validation and performance appraisal, work environment, training and education, employee relations, and unionization as related to hospitals.

OVERVIEW OF THE SETTING

In the last century, acute care hospitals have become, in many ways, the cornerstone of the U.S. healthcare delivery system. The majority of healthcare professionals work in hospitals, and a significant portion of the dollars spent on health care are generated there. As a result, the study of human resources in health care must include the unique challenges in acute care settings.

Acute care hospitals can be characterized in a number of ways: size/number of beds, function, ownership, location, mission, complexity, competitiveness, population served, endowment and financial situation, physical facilities, cost per patient day, or patient diagnostic category.[1] These categories help in making comparisons across the industry. Younis, in a comparison of the financial performance of urban and small rural hospitals,[2] found that for-profit hospitals were more profitable than nonprofit hospitals; teaching hospitals were less profitable than nonteaching hospitals; and hospitals with fewer than 50 or more than 400 beds were less profitable than hospitals having between 50 and 400 beds. In addition, hospitals in which the ratio of total Medicaid days to total days was higher were more profitable than those with a lower ratio, because hospitals with a higher proportion of Medicaid patients get additional money through the Medicaid disproportionate hospital share payments.[2]

Table 8-1 provides an overview of the most common hospital classifications. Hospitals may fit into more than one classification.

Regardless of the classification of an acute care hospital, patients in this setting require care and observation 24 hours per day for the length of their stay. A physician or designated extender must order admission to the hospital and necessary medical care related to diagnosis and treatment, including surgery or other invasive procedures to be provided. Nursing staff are accountable for coordinating patients' care during the hospital stay, but numerous other healthcare providers—including physical, occupational, and respiratory therapists; radiologic science professionals; pharmacists; lab technologists; dietitians; social workers; psychologists; chaplains; and support staff—give treatment to improve patients' condition and/or help them cope with limitations imposed by their illness. As patients' conditions improve and they require less monitoring, they are typically moved to a less intensive level of care, such as a long-term acute care hospital, rehabilitation center, or skilled nursing facility, or released to their home with or without support.

Table 8-1 Classifications of Acute Care Hospitals

Classification	Definition
Short-term	Patients have an ALOS of 30 days or less.
Long-term	Patient has an ALOS of more than 30 days.
Urban	Hospital located inside an MSA. An MSA is a territory containing a city with a population of at least 50,000 or an urban area with a population of at least 50,000 and a total metropolitan population of at least 100,000.
Rural	Hospital located outside an MSA.
Public	Hospital owned by federal, state, or local governmental agencies—usually a city or county governmental department or a free-standing governmental agency, such as a public health authority or district.
Federal	Hospital owned by the federal government, and designated for special populations (e.g., military, veterans).
Private	Hospital owned by a private entity, either nonprofit or for profit.
Nonprofit	Hospital that is not required to share profits with shareholders. Revenues in excess of expenses are returned to the organization as reserves or for future uses.
Profit/investor owned	Hospital that must share profits with shareholders.
Teaching	Hospital that has an affiliation with a medical school accredited by the Liaison Committee on Medical Education. These hospitals must sponsor or participate significantly in four approved, active residency programs, at least three of which must be medicine, surgery, obstetrics/gynecology, pediatrics, family practice, or psychiatric.

ALOS: average length of stay.
MSA: metropolitan statistical area.
Source: Kovner A, Jonas S. *Healthcare Delivery in the United States.* New York: Springer Publishing; 1999:162.

As the U.S. population has aged and technology has developed, there have been increasing employment opportunities in the acute care environment. For example, full-time equivalent (FTE) personnel in hospitals increased from approximately 3,420,000 to 3,911,400 between 1995 and 2000, despite a decrease in the number of community hospitals and beds per 1,000 population.[3] This expansion in employment opportunities has created multiple challenges for human resources personnel. The shortage of healthcare professionals and the increasing acuity of hospitalized patients have resulted in a stressful work environment. The need to reduce costs and the associated trend toward managed care have caused a shortened length of stay for most patients. The rapid turnover of patients has added to the stress of the work environment. Managed care has also reduced traditional fee-for-service reimbursement, placing many hospitals in financial jeopardy.

While all industries must address human resources challenges to stay competitive in the marketplace, inadequately managed human resources problems in acute care hospitals can have a profound effect on a facility's public relations. Negative publicity of any sort can increase the public's resistance to hospitalization at a facility. Of greater concern, however, is that numerous studies have shown poor working conditions in an acute care setting can affect employee job satisfaction as well as the outcomes of patient care. Because hospital care is "people driven," the human resources function plays a crucial role in ensuring high-quality care.

RECRUITMENT AND SELECTION

Recruitment and retention remain the most important human resources function in hospitals today because of the critical shortage of health professionals. The lack of available nurses, which has received widespread publicity, is the best-known marker of this shortage, because nursing is the United States' largest healthcare profession, and nurses represent the largest single component of hospital staff. The U.S. Bureau of Labor Statistics estimates that the rising complexity of acute care will see demand for RNs in hospitals climb by 36% by 2020.[4] According to the report *Acute Care Hospital Survey of RN Vacancy and Turnover Rates*, which was released in 2002 by the American Organization of Nurse Executives, the average RN turnover rate in acute care hospitals is 21.3%. The average hospital-wide nurse vacancy rate is 10.2%, with critical care units registering a 14.6% vacancy rate. Fifty-one percent of the nurse executives surveyed in this study indicated that staffing shortages contribute to emergency room overcrowding, and 25% blamed the nursing shortage for the need to close beds.[5]

Nursing is not the only discipline experiencing a shortage. The American Medical Association acknowledges a physician shortage in some specialties and in some areas of the country. The shortfalls are most striking in radiology and anesthesiology, but are also present in cardiology, dermatology, gastroenterology, general surgery, and surgical subspecialties. In November 2003, the government-approved Council on Graduate Medical Education, reversing a previous position, called for an expansion of medical school spaces and residency slots. Although it will not resolve the maldistribution of physicians, such an approach will increase the number of U.S. medical graduates to 3,000 per year by 2015, with a corresponding expansion in residency positions.[6]

The U.S. Department of Labor's Bureau of Labor Statistics predicts that the country will need 75,000 more radiographers in 2010 than it did in 2000, 16,000 more sonographers, 8,000 more nuclear medicine technologists, and 7,000 more radiation therapists.[7] *The Respiratory Therapist Human Resources Study—2000* of the American Association of Respiratory Care estimated that in 2000, 6,510 respiratory therapy positions were vacant, giving an overall vacancy rate of 5.69%. The Bureau of Labor Statistics expects employment of respiratory therapists to increase faster than the average for all occupations, increasing from 21% to 35% between 2000 and 2010.[8]

The shortage of all healthcare providers places a heavy burden on human resources professionals, who, in concert with administrators and clinical managers, must recruit and retain sufficient staff to deliver safe and effective care. In April 2002, the AHA Commission on Workforce for Hospitals and Health Systems recognized that, if left unresolved, the shortage of health professionals may result in a major healthcare crisis. The commission's report, titled *In Our Hands: How Hospital Leaders Can Build a Thriving Workforce,* included five major recommendations:

1. Broaden the base of healthcare workers by designing strategies that attract and retain a diverse workforce of men and women, racial and ethnic minorities and immigrants, and older workers.
2. Build societal support for public policies and resources needed to help hospitals hire and retain a qualified workforce.
3. Collaborate with hospitals, healthcare and professional associations, educational institutions, corporations, philanthropic organizations, and governments to attract applicants to the health professions.
4. Foster meaningful work by transforming hospitals into modern-day organizations where the work is designed around both patient and staff needs. The work environment must be structured so that workers can find meaning and be supported in their efforts to provide high-quality care.
5. Improve workplace partnerships by creating a culture in which hospital staff (clinical, support, and managerial) have ongoing input

into institutional policies and receive appropriate rewards and recognition.[9]

Recruitment strategies are classified into two categories: local and global. Human resources professionals in hospitals have greater control over recruitment at the local level. Competitive salaries are, of course, an important factor in recruitment and retention, even though most hospitals are struggling to break even financially. According to Hewitt and Associates, a compensation and benefits consulting firm, cash compensation for executive, managerial, and department director positions increased in the hospital industry by 6.7% in 2000, nearly double the average increase of the year before.[10] The wages of most hospital employees are market driven, and current wages and benefits packages can be determined through local, state, and national hospital or professional organizations. Table 8-2 outlines benefits that might be used either individually or in combination to recruit staff to a particular hospital or to encourage students to consider the health professions.

A popular local recruitment strategy in hospitals is flexible scheduling for staff providing 24 hour per day, 7 day per week care. For example, staff may choose a weekend option, working 24 hours every weekend, while being compensated for 36 hours, and receiving full-time benefits. Those who work Monday through Friday often work three 12-hour shifts with no weekends. They also receive full-time benefits. Examples of hospitals using this system include Summa Health System Nursing Service in Akron, Ohio, which reported a vacancy rate of 6%—below the national average for vacancies in nursing departments—after implementing flexible staffing.[11]

In an effort to deal with the widespread shortages in the health professions, numerous national recruitment initiatives have been implemented. Hospitals often benefit directly or indirectly from these programs, particularly when previously uninterested individuals are drawn to a career in one of the health professions. Some of these recruiting efforts include Johnson & Johnson's Campaign for Nursing's Future Initiative (www.discovernursing.org), Nursing for a Healthier Tomorrow (www.nursesource.org/nursing_careers.html), and a recruiting plan by the American Society of Radiologic Technologists (www.asrt.org). Federal legislation aimed at providing recruitment dollars includes the Nurse Reinvestment Act (www.bhpr.hrsa.gov/nursing/reinvestmentact.htm) and the Allied Health Reinvestment Act (www.asahp.org/billsummary.htm).

Table 8-2 Recruitment Strategies Used by Human Resources in Hospitals

Strategies to Recruit or Retain Professional Employees	Strategies to Encourage Entry into Healthcare Professions
Competitive salaries	Classroom visits in high school/junior high school by healthcare providers
Flexible staffing	
Scholarships for additional education	Job-shadowing experiences
Signing bonuses	Participating in "Bring Your Child to Work Day"
Tuition reimbursements for graduate education or degree completion programs	
	Volunteer opportunities for students and adults in healthcare settings
Tuition reimbursements for nonprofessional staff to become healthcare professionals	Student internships
	Part-time employment opportunities for students
Collaborative education programs between colleges/universities and hospitals at the hospital location	Visits to youth clubs and organizations (Boys and Girls Clubs, Boy and Girl Scouts, science clubs, 4-H Clubs)
New-graduate mentorship	Participating in community health fairs
Continuing education	Participating in "Adopt a Health Professions Student" program
Structured communication with management (e.g., newsletters, "CEOgrams")	
Staff recognition programs	Speaking to guidance counselors/home school organizations
Wellness programs	Summer or day camps for high school or junior high students to introduce them to the health professions
Career ladders (clinical)	
Rewarding experienced staff who serve as preceptors	Interaction with groups involved in counseling individuals looking for second careers
Leadership training	
Improving orientation	

Physician recruiting is another important human resources function, albeit one that often results in a financial burden for the hospital. In large hospitals, physicians in some specialties, such as emergency room physicians or hospitalists, may be employees. In such circumstances, the hospital must match the compensation the physician would receive in private practice. For example, the 2002 Medical Group Compensation and Productivity Survey listed the median income of physicians in emergency medicine as $204,921 and the median income of hospitalists as $146,551.[12] Even if physicians are in private practice, they may receive compensation from the hospital for administrative responsibilities, such as being director of a specialty medical service. Hospitals may also provide loans for office space or equipment to physicians who practice in proximity to the hospital and (as will be later discussed) may assist physicians with malpractice insurance.

Lack of Diversity in Healthcare Providers

The lack of diversity among healthcare providers creates another recruitment challenge in hospitals. The Sullivan Commission on Diversity in the Healthcare Workforce, in its report *Missing Persons: Minorities in the Health Professions,* indicates that, taken together, African Americans, Hispanic Americans, and Native Americans make up more than 25% of the U.S. population, but only 9% of the nation's nurses and 6% of its physicians. The study also pointed out the lower quality of health care and higher rates of illness, disability, and premature deaths among minority populations. These poorer health outcomes for minorities and the shortage of minority healthcare providers appear to be related.[13] Not only must hospital human resources professionals and administration focus on local and global recruitment, but they also must be cognizant of the need to recruit qualified professionals from minority populations.

RETENTION

Retention of hospital staff requires adequate compensation and flexible staffing. However, maintaining a positive work environment is equally important in retaining employees. A review of literature regarding job satisfaction of hospital employees—particularly nurses—consistently found eight influencing variables: professional autonomy, communication and interpersonal relationships, administrative aspects (e.g., the structure of the department and/or prevalent leadership style), recognition (both internal and external to the employment site), working conditions, professional practice, pay/benefits, and staffing/scheduling issues.[14] While these variables make a difference in all areas of health care, they are particularly important in acute care as an antidote to the stressful work environment. Often healthcare professionals—particularly nurses—leave the hospital seeking a less acute work environment. They report that such a move lets them implement the full scope of their professional role in a less stressful environment, which allows time for critical thinking and decision making. Ensuring that the previously mentioned variables have a positive presence in the acute care hospital may prevent nurses and other staff from resigning to work in less stressful work environments.

Recognizing that certain characteristics influence a positive work environment in hospitals is not new. In the early 1980s, during a previous nursing shortage, the American Academy of Nursing conducted research to identify organizational factors in hospitals that resulted in successful recruiting and retention of nurses. American Academy of Nursing Fellows nominated 165 U.S. hospitals with reputations for successfully attracting and retaining nurses and delivering high-quality nursing care. Ultimately, 41 hospitals were distinguished by their high nurse satisfaction, low job turnover, and low nurse vacancy rates, even while neighboring hospitals were experiencing nursing shortages. These hospitals were called "magnet" hospitals because of their successes in attracting and keeping nurses.[15] Table 8-3 identifies the core organizational attributes common to these "magnet" hospitals.

Ten years after the identification of the original magnet hospitals, the American Nurses Credentialing Center (ANCC) established a new magnet hospital designation process, similar to the accreditation scheme developed by the Joint Commission for the Accreditation of Healthcare Organizations (JCAHO). The process includes a self-appraisal using the *Scope and Standards for Nurse Administrators* published by the American Nurses Association (ANA), an assessment using ANA Quality Indicators, and a multiple-day site visit.[15] In the current competitive environment, receiving magnet status may serve as a recruiting and marketing tool for a hospital, attesting to its professional work environment and quality nursing care.

Since the early 1980s, significant research about magnet hospitals has provided empirical evidence that the organization of the nursing service in these hospitals has produced positive benefits for patients and staff alike. Hospitals that organize their nursing services around organizational

---

Table 8-3 Organizational Attributes Common to Magnet Hospitals

The chief nurse executive is a formal member of the highest decision-making body in the organization.

Nursing services have a flat organizational structure with limited supervisory personnel.

Decentralized decision making occurs at the unit level, giving staff nurses as much autonomy as possible in providing care.

The administrative structure supports nurses' decisions about patient care.

Good communication exists between nurses and physicians.

Source: Haven S, Aiken L. Shaping systems to promote desired outcomes: the magnet hospital model. *Journal of Nursing Administration.* 1999; 29:14–20.

factors supporting professional practice are associated with lower Medicare mortality rates, higher levels of patient and nurse satisfaction, lower levels of nurse emotional exhaustion, and fewer nurse-reported needle-stick injuries.[16] Table 8-4 outlines selected empirical studies that evaluated the nursing work environment in magnet hospitals.

Table 8-4 Selected Research on the Work Environment

Reference	Findings
Aiken LH, Smith H, Lake ET. Lower Medicare mortality among a set of hospitals known for good nursing care. *Medical Care.* 1994; 32:87.	After adjustment for patient severity, magnet hospitals demonstrated statistically superior ($p = 0.026$) outcomes, reflected by Medicare mortality rates. Magnet hospitals had slightly better RN-to-patient ratios and significantly richer nursing skill mixes. When differences in nursing staffing were controlled statistically, the lower mortality rate persisted.
Haven DS, Aiken LH. Shaping systems to promote desired outcomes: the magnet hospital model. *Journal of Nursing Administration.* 1999; 29:14–20.	Study explored empirical evidence associated with patient outcomes in magnet-designated hospitals and concluded that the evidence is significant that magnet organizations produce better patient and staff outcomes and so should be the model for re-configuring nursing services and delivery of patient care.
Havens DS. Comparing nursing infrastructure and outcomes: ANCC magnet and non-magnet hospitals. *Nursing Economics.* 2001; 19:258–266.	Survey was sent to the chief nursing officers that addressed recruitment difficulties, quality of care, and organizational structure. The characteristics of the hospitals were similar in terms of size and demographics. Findings included that magnet hospitals had higher JCAHO scores, had distinct departments of nursing, and were more likely to have a doctorally prepared nurse researcher on staff; also, the CNO received greater control of nursing practice, autonomy, and nurse–physician collaboration.
Kramer M, Schmalenberg C. Essentials of a magnetism. In: McClure M, Hinshaw A, Eds., *Magnet Hospitals Revisited: Attraction and Retention of Professional Nurses.* Kansas City, MO: American Nurses Publishing; 2002.	Staff nurses working in 14 magnet hospitals identified eight attributes as essential to quality care: • Support for education • Working with other nurses who are clinically competent • Positive nurse–physician relationships • Autonomous nursing practice • A culture that values concern for the patient • Control of and over nursing practice • Perceived adequacy of staffing • Nurse-manager support

Laschinger H, Shamian J, Thomson D. Impact of magnet hospital characteristics on nurses' perceptions of trust, burnout, quality of care, and work satisfaction. *Nursing Economics*. 2001; 19:209–219.	Staff nurses in magnet hospitals were surveyed using instruments that measured perceptions of autonomy, control, physician relationships, faith and confidence in peers, managers, emotional exhaustion, and job satisfaction. Findings suggested that perceived autonomy, control, and physician relationships influence trust, job satisfaction, and perceived quality of patient care. The authors suggest that practice models that address autonomy and control, while managing the flattening of organizational structures, could achieve positive staff perceptions.

Magnet hospital research has focused only on nursing services. As yet, there has been little or no research to evaluate the job satisfaction of other disciplines that work in these hospitals. However, it is logical to assume that the results of research on the effects of the work environment might be generalized to healthcare disciplines besides nursing.

Despite the results reported on magnet hospitals, there continues to be concern about the hospital work environment. In 2002, the Robert Wood Johnson Foundation published *Healthcare's Human Crisis: The American Nursing Shortage.* This report used nurse focus groups to explore the effect of the nursing shortage on the work environment. The report found:

> that nurses plan to stay in nursing but have concerns about workloads and the chaotic work environment, are confused by the financial issues surrounding healthcare, and feel powerless to change the work environment. Nurses believe that managers can make a difference in how nurses perceive their jobs, that the image of nursing is poor due to the poor work environment, and they see little commitment from nursing schools and employers for the development of nurses and themselves.[17]

One must assume that if other disciplines working in hospitals were interviewed, their responses would be similar to these.

THE HIRING PROCESS

Hospital Employees

Hiring employees in any setting involves entering into an implicit contract with the employee. The legal doctrine underlying contracts is the common-law "employment at will," which states that employment is at the will of either the employer or the employee and that either party may terminate employment at any time. An employer's right to terminate an employee can be limited by express agreement with the employee through a contract or a collective bargaining agreement. The major purpose of an employment contract is to specify legally enforceable agreements; therefore, the contract should outline various points of agreement between the employee and the employer, including the length of time the contract will remain in effect.[18 (p. 191)]

Over the years, the rights of employees have been expanded beyond the "employment at will" concept through federal and state regulations and judicial decisions based on verbal promises, historical practices of the employer, and documents such as employee handbooks and administrative policy and procedure manuals. For example, an employee might not be considered an "employee at will" if the employee handbook says that a nonprobationary employee can be discharged after written notice.[18 (p. 198)] In this circumstance, discharge would require written notice.

Each hospital, typically through its human resources department, develops its own policies and procedures for the employee selection process. Managers in the functional area of the hospital often will make the final choice of the employee, matching the candidate's credentials with those required by the job description. Other organizations utilize a two-tiered interview system for screening applicants. In such a system, an appropriately trained member of the human resources department will conduct the first interview, followed by an interview conducted by the supervisor of the service to which the applicant is applying.

Before licensed employees begin their assigned jobs, their licenses to practice must be verified. This confirmation may be done by the human resources department or through the service in which the employee works. To protect themselves and reduce the likelihood of nosocomial infections, employees must have certain immunizations, usually defined by state law, prior to beginning the job function. Criminal background checks may be required by state law or organization policy (www.jcaho.org). Documentation of immunizations and/or background checks is typically a human resources function.

Credentialing of Independent Practitioners

Independent practitioners provide a significant portion of the care offered in today's hospitals. Although they are not employees of the organization, the administration and governing body share responsibility for the care of their patients. Physicians are the primary independent practitioners in the hospital setting, although there are others, such as psychologists, physician extenders, and social workers. The role of an attending physician in the hospital environment is to ensure a comprehensive approach to patient care. At the same time, the hospital governing body bears ultimate responsibility for ensuring that other criteria are met:

- Medical care is supervised by a physician.
- A covering physician supervises the medical care of patients when the attending physician is unavailable.
- The physician reviews each patient's plan of care, including medications and treatments during each visit.
- Progress notes are current, signed, and dated.
- Physician orders are signed and dated.
- Patients are seen by a physician on a regular basis, as outlined by the organization's Medical Staff Bylaws.[18] (p. 103)

The governing body of the organization is legally responsible for the selection of medical staff members and determination of their ability to practice in the role they have requested (e.g., family practice physician, surgeon). The selection process, which should be spelled out in the hospital's Medical Staff Bylaws, is known as credentialing. Trustees have a duty to protect patients from physicians they know (or should know) are unqualified to practice medicine, particularly through actions that might result in the loss of the license to practice medicine. A state license to practice medicine may be revoked for the following reasons:

- Demonstration of a lack of good moral character
- Deliberate falsification of a medical record
- Intentional fraudulent advertising
- Gross incompetence
- Sexual misconduct
- Substance abuse
- Performance of unnecessary medical procedures
- Billing for services not performed
- Forged operative record[18] (p. 187)

The governing body and the medical staff delegate responsibility to investigate the application information submitted, including confirmation

of all references, to a credentialing specialist, typically from the human resources department. The National Practitioner Data Bank (NPDB)
(www.ama-assn.org/ama/pub/category/4543.htm) should be queried regarding any negative legal action taken against the applicant. Neglect of
either of these processes may result in the organization being held liable,
if this failure leads to injury of a patient.[18 (p. 188)] Table 8-5 outlines the

---

Table 8-5 Documentation Necessary to Screen a Hospital Medical
Staff Applicant

Written Documentation Provided by the Applicant	Questions That Should Be Asked During the Screening Process
Medical school, internship, residency	Are there any unaccounted-for gaps in education or employment?
Fellowships*	Is there any disciplinary action or misconduct investigation by any state licensure board?
State license to practice medicine	Has the applicant:
Board certifications*	• Had the license to practice medicine in any state denied, limited, suspended, or revoked?
Medical societies*	
Documentation of malpractice coverage (usually $1–3 million)	• Withdrawn an application or resigned from any medical staff to avoid disciplinary action?
Special skills and talents that are related to the practice of medicine	• Had any disciplinary proceedings at any healthcare facility?
Availability/willingness to provide on-call coverage as applicable	• Been named as a defendant in a lawsuit?
Availability/willingness to serve on appropriate hospital committees	• Been named as a defendant in a criminal proceeding?
	• Reviewed medical staff bylaws, rules, and regulations?
Medical staff appointments in other organizations	• Been restricted from participating in Medicare or Medicaid programs?
Disciplinary actions against applicant in the past	• Had malpractice insurance coverage terminated?
Unexplained gaps in the work history	• Been denied malpractice insurance coverage?
	• Had any settlements and/or judgments against him or her?
Previous limitations or relinquishment of staff privileges	Does the applicant have backup and cross-coverage?
	Does the applicant have any physical or mental impairment that could affect his or her practice ability?

---

*These are not legally acceptable criteria for determining eligibility for appointment.
Source: Pozgar GD. *Legal Aspects of Healthcare Administration.* Seventh Edition. Gaithersburg, MD: Aspen; 1999:194.

documented information that the credentialing specialist should prepare for the selection committee to review.

Medical staffs may be considered open or closed. They may accept all qualified practitioners (open) or they may limit medical staff, either temporarily or permanently (closed). For example, an organization may temporarily stop accepting applications because of an ongoing high inpatient census beyond available space. Other medical staffs may be permanently closed, usually related to the mission of the hospital, such as teaching or research, which requires a specific level of expertise that most practitioners do not have.

COMPETENCY VALIDATION AND PERFORMANCE APPRAISAL

Initial Competency Validation

Caring for patients in a hospital requires a variety of skills, depending on the scope of practice of the discipline. Healthcare professionals are accountable for practicing according to standards established by their state practice acts and national professional standards. However, JCAHO standards require hospitals to document competency on all employees at the time of hiring and, thereafter, on an annual basis. Most hospitals use checklists or computerized systems to document that employees (particularly clinical staff) have the necessary competencies required by their job description. These competencies typically contain a number of skills essential for safe functioning.

Granting Privileges to Independent Practitioners

Independent practitioners also have to demonstrate their competence in various patient care activities through a process known as privileging. The governing body must determine whether applicants are qualified to perform procedures that are part of the clinical privileges for their area of practice. Failure to properly screen an applicant's competence can lead to liability for injuries suffered by patients.[18 (p. 194)] The process for approval of privileges is spelled out in the Medical Staff Bylaws, and the credentialing specialist is responsible for collecting necessary information to allow the medical staff and governing body to make decisions regarding granting privileges for specific activities.

Ongoing Competency Validation

Annual competency validation required for clinical staff by JCAHO and other accrediting bodies and in-service training specific to the organization are often provided by clinical staff working in the human resources department, in collaboration with managers or educators assigned to specific clinical units. Some hospitals may hold "Competency Fairs" periodically throughout the year, as they represent an efficient approach to document staff competency. Booths may be set up to give employees the opportunity to demonstrate their competence in all skills that require annual renewal. The employee may be asked to do a self-evaluation of the skills and then have this assessment validated by a peer, supervisor, and/or staff development personnel. If the employee is unable to adequately perform a skill at the time of the validation, a specific remediation plan should be developed.

Performance Appraisal

Although competency validation is a part of the hospital employee's annual evaluation, other components of a performance appraisal must also be considered. Performance appraisals are designed to monitor work-related behaviors and stimulate individual growth and development through the identification of strengths and weaknesses. Marquis and Huston summarize management research in this area, suggesting that performance appraisals result in increased employee motivation and productivity if the following factors are in place:

- The employee must believe that the appraisal is based on a standard to which other employees in the same classification are held accountable.
- The standard should be clearly communicated to employees at the time they are hired.
- The employee should have some input into developing the standards or goals on which his or her performance is judged. This is vital for professional employees.
- The employee should know in advance what will happen if the expected performance standards are not met.
- The employee should know in advance how the information to be used in the evaluation, including sources and their relative weight, will be obtained.

- Appraisals tend to be more accurate if a variety of information sources are used.
- The employee must believe that the person doing the major portion of the review has actually observed his or her work.
- The performance appraisal is more likely to have a positive outcome if the appraiser is viewed with trust and professional respect.[19]

Most hospitals use performance appraisal forms, which are directly related to the job description of the employee. For example, if a responsibility of the nurse is to assess the condition of patients and provide appropriate nursing care, then the nurse's ability to perform these activities should be evaluated annually. Other related behaviors, such as attendance or collaboration with others, may also be included, as they may affect the employee's ability to meet the job expectations.

Performance appraisal forms usually require that the evaluator rate the employee's behavior according to a 2- to 5-level scale. Human resources policies should outline the frequency of the evaluation and the process by which it is accomplished. They should also detail the mechanisms for developing a plan to correct any deficiencies identified in the evaluation and the criteria for termination if the employee consistently does not meet the performance standard set.

Due Process

Human resources professionals and managers must be sure that due process is built into the performance appraisal process. Due process is based on the notion that the process/procedures for evaluation are fair, and that they allow an opportunity for the employee to present objections to a negative evaluation. While at-will employees have no property rights in continued employment, they do have the right to have negative decisions about their performance reviewed. The human resources department is usually responsible for developing procedures to provide this opportunity.

Defamation Liability

Human resources professionals must be aware of the hospital's liability related to defamation of character in the performance appraisal process. Defamation of character may be charged when an employee who has received a negative performance appraisal believes that the results have been shared with others inappropriately. This offense consists of a false oral or written communication to a third party that tends to hold a person's reputation up to scorn and ridicule in the eyes of a substantial number of respectable people in the community.[18 (p. 33)] Defamation includes both libel, resulting from the written word, and slander, resulting from the spoken word. Generally, the person being defamed must prove that defamation resulted in some damage. However, some statements may be so defamatory that the victim does not have to prove that the defamation harmed his or her reputation. Classic examples of this type of defamation include allegations of serious sexual misconduct, serious criminal misbehavior, or affliction with a loathsome disease.[18 (p. 33)]

Pozgar notes that two defenses to a defamation action are possible: truth and privilege.[18 (p. 37)] If the claim about a person's work performance can be proved to be true, this is protection against a finding of defamation. A privileged communication is one that might be defamatory in other circumstances, but is not defamatory because the person making the statement has a higher duty to another party. Under these circumstances, the person must make the statement in good faith, on the proper occasion, in the proper manner, and to people who have a legitimate reason to know.[18 (p. 37)] For example, the evaluator who shares a negative finding with a supervisor has a duty to the organization to discuss concerns that might prove harmful to patients or the organization as a whole.

Peer Review

Peer review is the method by which the quality of the practice of a healthcare professional (physician, nurse, or other allied health professional) is evaluated by a group from the same discipline. This process puts assessment of the quality of an individual's practice in the hands of the professional group rather than management. Implementation of a peer review process has the potential for increasing the discipline's performance and professional accountability and provides learning experiences for the peer reviewers as well as those whose practice is reviewed. On the downside, a peer review process takes a great deal of time and energy to accomplish.

Medical staff members (i.e., physicians, physician extenders, and psychologists) typically have the most formalized peer review process in hospitals. The criteria and procedures for this process should be documented in the Medical Staff Bylaws. The credentialing specialist typically manages this process. Other professional groups, if they are employees of the hospital, may or may not have such processes in place, particularly for routine annual performance evaluations. If peer review occurs within a discipline, the process is usually managed within the clinical department.

In some disciplines, such as nursing, peer review may be required by state regulations, such as when the competency of an individual nurse is questioned or when he or she is asked to do something that the nurse believes violates professional practice standards. In such circumstances, nurses may be placed in a situation where they must choose between refusing an employer's request and risking disciplinary action or agreeing to the request, which might result in disciplinary action by the Board of Nurse Examiners (BNE). In states that have peer review laws, nurses are protected from dismissal and action by the licensing board until a peer review panel evaluates the situation.

THE WORK ENVIRONMENT

Numerous reports have shown that an unsupportive work environment in hospitals may have a significant influence on the shortage of employees. A number of strategies have been suggested to create a "provider-friendly" environment, including changes in organizational structures, scheduling and staffing, and support of delegation rules required by licensing regulations. Each of these strategies supports professional practice, which most healthcare professionals find appealing in a work environment.

"Provider-Friendly" Organizational Structures

An organizational structure that supports participation in policymaking supports professional practice. Clinicians who are involved in patient care are in the best position to articulate the effects of a policy on patient outcomes. Not only does such an approach protect patients, but it may also reduce costs. Ashmos and colleagues measured hospital costs and performance benefits as they related to participation of clinical professionals and middle managers. Their study found that the more clinical professionals (in this case, physicians and nurses) were involved in strategic decision making, the more cost and performance benefits were realized.[20] Similarly, Erbin-Rosemann and Simms found that hospital nurses who felt that they had no influence over the work environment were more likely to experience a decrease in work excitement.[21]

Scheduling and Staffing

Hospitals must be staffed 24 hours a day, 7 days a week. Managed care, the nursing shortage, and the lack of trained auxiliary personnel make the establishment of standardized staffing patterns difficult.[22] Employees— particularly clinical staff—are required either to work a variety of shifts or to be on call in their off-hours. Both practices place a psychosocial burden on staff. Control of staffing patterns relative to the needs of the patients under their care—an important marker of professional practice—can reduce this burden.

Events within the nursing profession illustrate this point. Documentation of the number of nursing staff needed relative to the number and acuity of patients on a unit is a major challenge of staffing. In the last 20 years, patient classification systems (also called acuity systems) have been used to determine the number of nurses needed on a unit at any one time. Most patient classification systems are factor evaluation tools that use critical indicators of patient needs to categorize patient information. The resulting classifications suggest the number of staff needed to care for the patients. The daily workload of a specific unit, known as the workload index, is determined by the sum of the acuity values for each patient in the unit. The workload index provides a weighted census that considers the patients' nursing care requirements. Acuity systems then typically provide a staffing framework that addresses hours of care for each unit of work. These hours are identified as a range, within which the organization determines each unit's target.[23]

Patient classification systems, particularly with increased computerization and the ability to access the systems online, provide many benefits. In addition to determining acuity levels and workload for patient care units or specific clinical populations, they help managers determine how and where staff spend time; identify trends in patient population, staffing patterns, and workload and care practices; effectively allocate limited resources; and benchmark units to support financial decisions.[23]

After the trend of hospital downsizing in the 1990s, concerns arose regarding the number of patients assigned to each nurse. Organized nursing believed that the more registered nurses on a nursing unit at any one time, resulting in a lower patient-to-nurse ratio, the more effective care patients would receive. However, little empirical evidence was available to support this claim.

In 1995, the American Nurses Association commissioned research to identify common quality indicators associated with registered nurse involvement in patient care. The study identified 42 indicators in three classes: clinical outcomes (nosocomial infections, decubitus ulcers, postoperative pneumonia, shock, and urinary tract infections), structure (number of staff, type of staff, and hours per patient-day), and process (patient and nurse satisfaction).[24] Using these parameters, several studies, including one by Blegen and Goode, found that the total hours of care from all nursing personnel were associated directly with the rates of decubiti, patient complaints, and mortality. Further, as the RN proportion relative to the number of Licensed Practical/Vacational Nurses and unlicensed assistive personnel increased, adverse outcomes decreased.[25]

According to JCAHO, in 1,609 hospital reports of patient death or injury in 2002, low nursing staffing levels were a contributing factor in 24% of the cases.[26] Also in 2002, Aiken and colleagues found that patients who had common surgeries in hospitals with high patient-to-nurse ratios had as much as a 31% increased chance of dying.[27] Each additional patient in an average hospital nurse's workload increased the risk of death in surgical patients by 7%. The same researchers also identified a link between higher levels of nursing education and patient outcomes in surgical patients. In hospitals, a 10% increase in the proportion of nurses holding BSN degrees decreased the risk of patient death and failure to rescue by 5%.[27] These findings made it obvious that having an appropriate number of educated nurses available for care was a critical factor in delivering high-quality care.

Two approaches are used to determine the minimum number of nurses required in any given acute care unit: fixed staffing ratios and establishment of a hospital-specific written staffing plan. The latter technique typically uses computerized patient acuity systems as its basis. In 1999, California became the first state to pass comprehensive legislation requiring minimum patient-to-nurse ratios for RNs and LVNs in acute care, acute psychiatric, and specialty hospitals. The final version of the bill did not mandate ratios, however. Instead, the California Department of Health Services was charged with developing regulations, including the ratios. These regulations were released in January 2002. After two years of public comment and revision, they were implemented in January 2004.[28] Table 8-6 outlines the required California patient–nurse staffing ratios.

Table 8-6 California Staffing Ratios

Type of Nursing Unit	Nurse–Patient Ratio
Intensive/critical care	1:2
Neonatal intensive care	1:2
Operating room	1:1
Post-anesthesia recovery	1:2
Labor and delivery	1:2
Antepartum	1:4
Postpartum couples	1:4
Postpartum women only	1:6
Pediatrics	1:4
Emergency room	1:4
ICU patient in the ER	1:2
Trauma patients in the ER	1:1
Step-down initial	1:4
Step-down in 2008	1:3
Telemetry initial	1:5
Telemetry in 2008	1:4
Medical/surgical initial	1:6
Medical/surgical in 2005	1:5
Other specialty care initial	1:5
Other specialty care in 2008	1:4
Psychiatric	1:6

Source: California Nurses Association. RN Ratios Alert. Available at: www.calnurse.org.

When nursing resource requirements are defined by nursing hours per patient-day or as nurse-to-patient ratios, the underlying assumption is that all patients and patient-days are equal. In reality, the need for nursing care varies significantly among patients and over the length of each patient's stay in the hospital. As the intensity of patient care increases and length of stay decreases, hours per patient-day or the nurse–patient ratio may not adequately express the resources needed. "Prescribed minimums" often become the "maximum available," and the ability to make staffing changes relative to patient need is lost.

Establishment of a written staffing plan as a means of providing a structure to quantify needed nursing resources is another approach to assuring adequate staffing. Such a written plan should include the following critical factors:

- Establishing initial staffing levels that are recalculated at least annually or as necessary
- Setting staffing levels on a unit-by-unit basis
- Adjusting staffing levels from shift to shift based on the intensity of patient care
- Using outcomes and nurse-sensitive indicators to evaluate the adequacy of the plan

Written staffing plans should be developed by a hospital advisory committee composed of registered nurses, a significant portion of whom are involved in direct patient care at least part of the time. Some states, such as Kentucky, Virginia, Texas, and Oregon, have codified the need for a written staffing plan in legislation.[28]

Overtime

With the current shortage of health professionals in a hospital, which must provide care on a 24-hour basis, employees are encouraged and sometimes required to work overtime. Golden and Jorgensen looked at the cost of overtime to the general U.S. economy. While overtime helps to drive a healthy economy, it has some unhealthy associated social costs, especially if the overtime is involuntary. According to Golden and Jorgensen, accident rate begins to increase at the ninth hour of continuous work and to double that of the ninth hour after the twelfth hour of continuous work.[29] It is estimated that job stress from overwork is responsible for industry costs of $150 billion per year in absenteeism, health insurance premiums, diminished productivity, compensations claims, and direct medical costs.[29]

According to the National Sleep Foundation (NSF), a deficit of sleep is associated with decreased alertness, problems with task completion, problems with concentration, irritability, and unsafe action and decision making. These findings are consistent across studies.[30]

The fatigue factor has an effect on the quality of care delivered by health professionals. Gaba and Howard found that 41% of medical residents reported a fatigue-related error.[31] They also noted that being awake for 24 hours was equivalent to having a blood alcohol level of 0.10%. Jha and colleagues reviewed studies related to fatigue, sleepiness, and medical errors in a variety of medical personnel. Their results suggest that when adults, who typically require 6 to 10 hours of sleep, get less than 5 hours of sleep over a 24-hour period, their peak mental abilities decline.[32] After two nights without sleep, cognitive performance can fall to nearly 40% of baseline. Sleep debt is associated with slower response times, altered mood and motivation, and reduced morale and initiative.[32]

In a 2004 study, nurses were asked to keep log books for a month documenting the number of hours they worked each day, the amount of overtime they worked, and the errors, including "near-misses," they made.[33] The researchers found that the risk of making an error greatly increased when nurses had to work shifts that were longer than 12 hours, when they worked significant overtime hours, or when they worked more than 40 hours per week. The likelihood of making an error was three times greater when nurses worked shifts that lasted at least 12.5 hours. Working overtime also increased the odds of making at least one error, regardless of how long the shift was originally scheduled.[33] JCAHO has recognized problems associated with overtime and, in a 2002 white paper on the nursing shortage, stated that mandatory overtime should be used only in emergency situations.[26]

Hospital human resources professionals, along with administrators and clinical managers, must consider the risks associated with long shifts, overtime, or scheduling staff to work many days without a break. Despite the shortage of personnel and the need to provide adequate staffing on each unit, the research on overtime is clear. To allow—or, worse yet, force—staff to work long hours is to increase the likelihood of errors in patient care.

Delegation Rules

The practice of a number of hospital healthcare professionals is supported by employees with less education and training. Some of these employees have licenses or other credentials (e.g., licensed practical/vocational nurses, physical therapy assistants, pharmacy technicians). Others have been prepared through "on-the-job" training (e.g., unlicensed assistive personnel). For this support to be helpful, the health professional, the nonprofessional, and those who develop policies regarding patient care must recognize which activities can be delegated and which must be done by the licensed provider.

In most cases, the professional practice acts of the various disciplines determine delegation rules. For example, physicians cannot delegate diagnosis or prescribing of medications. A registered nurse may delegate some tasks, such as inserting a Foley catheter, but cannot delegate the related assessment. Policies and procedures that support this accountability support professional practice.

TRAINING AND EDUCATION

Clinical/functional area managers and the human resources department share the responsibility of providing education and training for hospital personnel. Human resources representatives are frequently responsible for staff orientation to the hospital, in which the new employee receives information about organizational structures, benefits, general policies and procedures, and safety training. Clinical/functional staff are typically responsible for determining specific topics to be included in the orientation for various disciplines, although the staff that actually deliver the clinical orientation may be employed by the human resources department.

Once new employees have been initially oriented to the hospital, they are frequently assigned to preceptors who have the same or similar job descriptions and who work in the same area of the hospital. The new employee and the preceptor work closely together while the employee learns the expectations and policies/procedures of the new unit. The role of a preceptor is critical to the successful integration of a new employee. Recognizing this fact, hospital education departments often spend considerable resources in preparing preceptors to effectively orient new employees. This role is so important that serving as a preceptor often is required for managerial promotion or clinical advancement.

Specific educational offerings related to the role of the employee are developed based on the initiation of a new standard of care or "best practice" or because quality management data highlight particular educational needs of staff. These programs are generally developed by specific clinical staff, although the education staff housed in the human resources department may also be involved. Finally, inadequate individual performance appraisals may cause managers to request that the educational staff work with employees on remediation plans.

Patient Safety

In 1999, the Institute of Medicine released a report called *To Err Is Human: Building a Safer Health System,* which documented the high rates of treatment-associated injury and mortality. The report set a goal of reducing fatalities associated with hospital-based care delivery by 50% within five years.[34] So began the intensive focus on patient safety in health care.

Although the target proposed in *To Err Is Human* has not been achieved, perhaps because of a lack of necessary federal funding,[35] the emphasis on safety continues in hospitals and in governmental and nonprofit agencies. The Agency for Healthcare Research and Quality (AHRQ) is the lead federal agency on quality-of-care research; its Web site, www.ahrq.gov, provides helpful information to hospital staff about patient safety.

Recent studies indicate that an average of 17 years is needed before new knowledge generated through research is widely incorporated into clinical practice, and physicians, nurses, and other caregivers report that the delivery of health care has become so complex that they can no longer devote the time necessary to assimilate the ever-expanding numbers of clinical studies and emerging treatment options.[36] In response to these concerns, AHRQ has examined the issues surrounding the adoption of improved clinical practice. Funding was provided for Stanford University– University of California at San Francisco Evidence-Based Practice Center to determine which strategies are more effective than others for introducing proven treatment methods. A visit to the AHRQ Web site (www.ahrq.gov) can provide hospital staff with important information about evidence-based practice designed to safeguard patients.

Reflecting the overall concern about patient safety, JCAHO also has established an initiative related to patient safety. Each year, the commission reviews safety goals for hospitals to use to foster a safer hospital practice. Table 8-7 outlines the 2005 patient safety goals proposed by JCAHO.[26]

AHRQ has also developed a set of quality indicators for hospitals, which reflect national hospital inpatient data. These data can be used to guide healthcare policy at the state and national levels. Likewise, they can be used to compare individual hospital performance with other organizations at the local, state, or national level. Reports using this approach are available at the AHRQ Quality Tools Web site (http://www.qualitytools.ahrq.gov). General questions about the AHRQ quality indicators can be found at http://www.qualityindicators.ahrq.gov/.

Because safety in hospitals depends on the actions of professionals and nonprofessionals in delivering care, human resources professionals and clinical managers must be involved in local patient safety initiatives. Injuries to patients from nursing-caused errors, for example, include

Table 8-7 JCAHO National Patient Safety Goals, 2005

Improve the accuracy of patient identification
Improve the effectiveness of communication among caregivers
Improve the safety of using medications
Eliminate wrong-site, wrong-patient, and wrong-procedure surgery
Improve the effectiveness of clinical alarm systems
Reduce the risk of healthcare-associated infections
Reduce the risk of patient harm resulting from falls
Reduce the risk of influenza and pneumococcal disease in older adults
Reduce the risk of surgical fires

Source: Joint Commission on the Accreditation of Healthcare Organizations. 2005 Joint Commission National Patient Safety Goals: Practical Strategies and Helpful Solutions for Meeting These Goals. Available at: http://www.jcrinc.com/subscribers/patientsafety. asp?durki=7916&site=22&return=154. Accessed January 9, 2006.

medication errors, knowledge errors, and procedural errors. Rarely do these errors result from the careless action of a single individual. Instead, most errors stem from a breakdown in the delivery system, often related to a fragmentation of care and a lack of communication between staff. Human resources professionals and clinical managers can do much to improve care delivery systems through critical analysis of processes and training of staff. Equally important is avoiding a "culture of blame." If staff members are encouraged to report errors so that the underlying factors can be identified, rather than being blamed or punished for mistakes, then they are more likely to report errors and become involved in finding solutions to systemic problems.

Technology and Patient Safety

Hospital care over the last 25 years has been characterized by the explosion of technology. Today, a particularly important emphasis for technology is to support patient safety initiatives. Examples of technology that provide support for multiple safe communications in a hospital include the following:

• Bar coding and other patient identifiers that reduce data input errors
• Decision support systems, such as personal data administrators (PDAs) that highlight adverse events before they happen, including drug interactions, inappropriate doses, and potential side effects

- Point-of-care technologies that allow providers to document interventions at the bedside, thereby streamlining work flow
- Computerized physician order entries that replace easily misinterpreted written orders[37]

Simpson suggests that although technology can facilitate the delivery of care and support the reduction of errors, most technology initiatives require four components for implementation

- A system that interacts with other technologies currently used
- A well-defined strategy for implementation
- A process design that remains focused on meeting the mission of the hospital
- Recognition that the change must be managed[37]

Malpractice

Despite efforts to enhance patient safety in the hospital, errors that could potentially harm a patient will always be a factor in the operation of a hospital. For this reason, malpractice insurance for the hospital and providers—particularly physicians—is necessary. An Economic and Budget Issue Brief from the Congressional Budget Office (CBO) defines *malpractice* as "the failure of someone providing professional services to exercise the degree of skill and learning commonly applied under all the circumstances in the community by the average prudent reputable member of the profession with the result of injury, loss, or damage to the recipient of those services or to those entitled to rely upon them."[38] The same reference defines *negligence* as a violation of a duty to meet an applicable standard of care.[38]

Pozgar describes three groups that are likely to purchase medical professional liability insurance:

- Individuals (physicians, nurses, dentists, and others)
- Healthcare institutions, such as hospitals
- Outpatient facilities and clinics where there are no regular bed or board facilities[39]

Insurance will provide for payment on behalf of the insured if an injury arises from either (1) malpractice, error, or mistake in rendering or failing to render professional services or (2) acts or omissions on the part of the insured. Although injury is not limited to bodily injury or property damage, it must result from malpractice, error, mistake, or failure to perform acts that should have been performed. The most common risks covered by medical professional liability insurance are negligence, assault and battery due to failure to obtain consent to a medical or surgical procedure, libel and slander, and invasion of privacy for betrayal of professional confidences.[39]

The cost of medical malpractice insurance for both physicians and hospitals continues to rise. For example, the CBO reports that premiums for physicians' medical malpractice insurance have climbed since 1999 for all physicians and, in some cases, insurers are not willing to cover certain physician groups. Recent analyses suggest that premiums have risen because insurance companies have faced increased costs to pay claims (from growth in malpractice awards), reduced income from their investments, and short-term factors in the insurance markets.[38–40] Kolodkin suggests that insurers are reluctant to insure certain medical specialists, such as obstetricians/gynecologists, pediatricians, internists, emergency physicians, anesthesiologists, and radiologists.[41] Some observers fear that rising malpractice premiums will cause physicians to stop practicing medicine, reducing the availability of health care in some parts of the country.[41] To alleviate this problem, some hospitals have begun to assume the physician's risk, by paying the insurance premiums.[42]

Medical malpractice insurance associations are also being formed in response to the malpractice crisis. The purpose of these associations is to provide coverage for institutions or physicians who are unable to obtain medical malpractice insurance at a reasonable price in the open market. Development of these associations was supported by legislation that required all insurance carriers engaged in writing personal liability insurance within a particular state to provide malpractice coverage through these associations.[39]

Some hospitals have also chosen to pursue self-insurance for their malpractice risk. In these circumstances, the hospital sets aside a certain amount of its own funds as a reserve against malpractice losses and expense. Generally, the hospital will retain the services of a self-insurance consulting firm and an actuary to determine the proper level of funding the institution should maintain.[39]

Accountability for Quality of Care

Although licensed professionals are responsible for ensuring that their own practice meets professional standards, the governing body bears the ultimate responsibility for the hospital's quality of care. From a practical point of view, this accountability is managed through the work of hospital committees. JCAHO requires that hospitals monitor, usually through committees, the following functions: quality management, pharmacy and therapeutics, safety, infection control, and medical records. Membership in these committees includes representative physicians and nurses and other disciplines involved in the particular function. The work of the committees is typically reported to the executive committee of the medical staff and, ultimately, to the governing body. Some other disciplines in the hospital, particularly nursing, have discipline-specific committees, similar to the medical staff, as a means of supporting shared governance between management and staff.

In the late 1980s, the concept of total quality management (TQM) or continuous quality improvement (CQI) began to be implemented as a way to improve processes within the hospital. In this approach to achieving quality, CQI teams representing staff involved in a particular process are appointed on an ad hoc basis to solve problems that affect efficiency or effectiveness. The results of this committee work are also typically reported to the medical executive committee and the hospital's board of trustees.

EMPLOYEE RELATIONS

Communication and Interpersonal Relationships

Effective communication among all members of the healthcare team is an important motivator for employees as well as a factor in ensuring patient safety. Improving communication between line staff and management and between physicians and other clinical staff currently seems to be a focal point for improving the work environment.

Numerous studies point to a flat organizational structure as a means of ensuring open communication throughout the chain of command.[20, 21, 43, 44] The need for physician support of nurses and other healthcare disciplines has also been documented.[45] In fact, the 2002 JCAHO report on the nursing shortage indicates that accountability for retention of nurses falls in part on physicians and states that the hospital administration should have zero tolerance for abusive behaviors by physicians and other health practitioners toward their colleagues.[26] In

2002, the Robert Wood Johnson Foundation sponsored nursing focus groups around the country to identify work environment concerns. Administrators who listened and addressed work environment concerns and those who provided respect and support that encourages physicians to treat nurses as colleagues were identified as important to improving the work environment.[17]

The importance of communication is illustrated in *Silence Kills: The Seven Crucial Conversations for Healthcare,* a 2005 study by the American Association of Critical-Care Nurses and VitalSmart.[46] Researchers conducted focus groups, interviews, and workplace observations and surveyed more that 17,000 nurses, physicians, clinical care staff, and administrators in rural, suburban, and urban hospitals throughout the United States during 2004. A few of their findings are especially notable:

- Eighty-four percent of physicians and 62% of nurses and other clinical care providers have seen co-workers taking shortcuts that could be dangerous to patients.
- Eighty-eight percent of physicians and 48% of nurses and other providers work with people who show poor clinical judgment.
- Fewer than 10% of physicians, nurses, and other clinical staff directly confront their colleagues about their concerns, and one in five physicians said they had seen harm come to patients as a result.
- The 10% of healthcare workers who raise these crucial concerns with their colleagues observe better patient outcomes, work harder, are more satisfied, and are more committed to staying in their job.[46]

The need for effective communication among healthcare workers in hospitals is great. Effective communication in "tough" situations leads to higher job satisfaction and reduces the potential for patient error. One way to improve such communication is through effective management of conflict.

Conflict Management

Traditionally, conflict has been viewed negatively as a power struggle, with the intent to neutralize, injure, or eliminate rivals.[47] However, in the 1960s, authorities began to suggest that properly managed conflict could actually facilitate organizational growth.[48] Conflict can have positive consequences if it is recognized and not ignored. Some types of conflicts—particularly those that deplete time or money resources, damage individuals, make cooperation difficult, or divert attention from established goals—are detrimental. Conversely, conflict that leads to constructive problem solving and a greater acceptance of change in general may support the growth and development of an organization.

People react in a variety of ways when faced with a conflict situation. Five specific strategies—avoiding, accommodating, compromise, competition, and collaboration—are typically used to manage the demands of one's self-interest and the interest of others. To be competent in managing conflict, a person must be able to effectively use multiple strategies, depending on the situation. Certain strategies may stimulate the use of other strategies, whereas other strategies tend to be incompatible. For example, when one party is unsuccessful in competing, that person may withdraw. Competition, however, is likely to preclude the use of collaboration.[47] Table 8-8 defines the five conflict management strategies.

The negative effects of conflict and poor communication on patient outcomes have been documented only recently. Most hospitals currently do not have specific training on constructive conflict management or strategies to handle difficult conversations. Despite the fact that there is no one right conflict management strategy to use or way to handle all conflict, given that circumstances dictate the appropriate approach, the increased complexity of the healthcare environment speaks to the need for better staff training in this area.

Table 8-8 Conflict Management Strategies

Strategy	Definition
Avoidance (denial, withdrawal	Choosing to do nothing that will enhance one's own interest; the interest of the opposing party is maximized
Accommodation (suppression, smoothing over)	Playing down differences, so the issues are not dealt with; neither self- nor other-interest is met
Competition	Using power to overcome the other party; the "winner's" interest is dominant
Compromise	Each side "giving a little" to come to a solution
Collaboration	Recognizing the interests of everyone, as a means of solving the problem so that all parties receive benefit

Source: Adapted from Wilmot W, Hocker J. *Interpersonal Conflict.* Sixth Edition. Boston: McGraw-Hill; 2001.

UNIONIZATION

Few issues in health care are more controversial than unionization of hospital employees, particularly professional staff. The controversy stems not only from the different perspectives of management and nonmanagement employees, but also from differences in professional and regional philosophies. These differences can best be managed by first understanding the legal implications of unionization and the process of collective bargaining.

Through the mid-1930s, union organizational activity in hospitals was minimal, and there was relatively slow growth in healthcare-related unions until the late 1950s. Since that time, however, unions in health care have grown as the opportunities for union expansion in other industries have diminished. In general, union activity in health care has been successful most often in those geographic areas in which unions have been active in other industries.[18] (p. 441)

O'Keefe describes collective bargaining in hospitals as a process by which employees have the right to join unions, designate representatives, and participate in negotiation and bargaining with management on a collective basis.[49] Collective bargaining is based on the principle that there is strength in numbers, with the goal "to equalize power between labor and management."[49]

The National Labor Relations Acts

The National Labor Relations Act (NLRA) was enacted in 1935 and modified by the Taft-Hartley amendments of 1947 and the Landrum-Griffin amendments of 1959. The main focus of this legislation is to define certain conduct of employers and employees as unfair labor practices and to provide for hearings when complaints arise that such practices have occurred. Both employers and employees have certain rights as defined by the legislation, which are balanced by certain responsibilities.[18] (p. 443) (See Table 8-9.)

The National Labor Relations Board (NLRB) is responsible for enforcement and administration of the NLRA. It is also responsible for investigation of claims of unfair practices submitted by the employer or the employee. The board reviews the claim, determines whether there have been unfair labor practices, and recommends a solution.[18] (p. 444)

Because patient care may be immediately affected during a labor dispute, some special problems must be considered during a labor–management

---

Table 8-9 Labor and Management Rights in Collective Bargaining Situations

Labor Rights: Employees May . . .	Management Rights: Supervisors May . . .
1. Organize and bargain as a group.	1. Receive notice of a strike at least 10 days before the event.
2. Distribute information when employees are *not* at work (i.e., mealtimes and coffee breaks).	2. Hire replacement workers.
3. Picket.	3. Keep union activity in a specified area and time to avoid interference with operations.
4. Strike (employees leaving work as a group as part of the negotiation).	4. Forbid union activity during work.
	5. Mandate that supervisors may not participate in activity.

Source: adapted from Pozgar GD. *Legal Aspects of Healthcare Administration.* Seventh Edition. Gaithersburg, MD: Aspen; 1999:443–454.

---

dispute in a hospital. This concern over patient safety resulted in an exemption for healthcare institutions in the original legislation in 1935. However, a 1974 amendment to the NLRA extended coverage to employees of nonprofit healthcare institutions that previously had been exempted, although the legislation designated procedures to limit strikes in healthcare institutions. These procedures ensure that the needs of the patients will be met during a strike. For example, a board of inquiry is created within 30 days after notification of either party's intention to terminate a contract if the dispute threatens to interrupt health care in the community. The board then has 15 days during which to investigate and report its findings and recommendations. Once the report is filed, both parties are expected to maintain the status quo for an additional 15 days.[18 (p. 451)]

Impact of Labor–Management Disputes in Hospitals

Hospitals are particularly concerned about the number of bargaining units that are allowed in any one institution. In 1989, the NLRB published rules and regulations that allowed up to eight collective bargaining units in healthcare organizations, as opposed to the three normally allowed in other types of organizations. Hospital workers may form separate bargaining units for physicians, registered nurses, technical employees, clerical employees, other nonprofessional employees, and security guards.[18 (pp. 444–455)]

Does the Act of Supervision Imply Management?

Many hospital employees for whom the collective bargaining process is intended are professionals who may have some supervisory responsibilities over less qualified employees. For example, staff registered nurses routinely delegate duties to unlicensed assistive personnel (UAPs) and supervise the work delegated. Supervisors are considered management and therefore cannot be a part of the collective bargaining process. However, many of these nurses do not hold formal management positions. To clarify whether these employees are supervisors, the NLRA provides a three-part test; each part must be met to determine whether a professional is a line employee or a supervisor. The professional must have the authority to hire, transfer, suspend, lay off, recall, promote, discharge, assign, and reward an employee. The judgment of the professional in this situation must be independent, not routine or clinical, and the decisions must be made for the benefit and interest of the employer, not the patient.[18 (pp. 444–455)] Under this definition, nurses who supervise specific care given by another employee, rather than the general performance of the employee, are eligible to join a union.

CONCLUSION

The effectiveness of the care delivered in a hospital is directly related to the competency of the healthcare providers who practice there. The goal of human resources professionals in hospitals must be to support multiple providers, so that the care delivered meets the needs of both patients and caregivers. The AHA report, *In Our Hands: How Hospital Leaders Can Build a Thriving Workforce*, states:

> Good hospital care is numerous caregivers in a variety of occupations providing services to patients on an individual, highly personalized basis. The provision of that care is made possible by workers in many fields who support the systems and resources that sustain both patients and caregivers. The work is demanding, but can and should be equally rewarding, because everyone in the hospital is helping to meet a vital human and community need.[9]

Care delivered in acute care hospitals in the future is likely to become even more complex. The shortage of healthcare professionals needed to provide this complex care will continue. Human resources professionals and management staff must work together in recruitment and retention, education and training, and assessment of competency to ensure that the care provided meets national standards. Successful management of these initiatives should improve the care delivered in all categories of hospitals in the United States. Fortunately, research suggests ways to insure a "provider-friendly" work environment that emphasizes patient safety. The future challenge is to implement such strategies in a cost-effective manner.

REFERENCES

1. Kovner A, Jonas S. *Healthcare Delivery in the United States.* New York: Springer Publishing; 1999:162.
2. Younis M. A comparison study of urban and small rural hospitals' financial and economic performance. *Online Journal of Rural Nursing and Healthcare.* Available at: http://www.mo.org/journal/issues/Vol-3/issue-1/Younis.htm. Accessed July 2005.
3. Bernstein AB, Hing E, Mass AJ, Allen KF, Siller AB, Tiggle RB. *Health Care in America: Trends in Utilization.* Hyattsville, MD: National Center for Health Statistics; 2003.
4. AACN. Nursing Fact Sheet. Media Background. February 2004. Available at: http://www.aacn.ncne.edu/Media/Backgrounders/nursfact.htm. Accessed July 2004.
5. HMS Group, Ltd. *Acute Care Hospital Survey of RN Vacancy and Turnover Rates in 2000.* Presented to the American Organization of Nurse Executives. January 2000. Available at: http://www.who.org.workForce/pdf/aone/surveyrnvacancy/pdf. Accessed July 2005.
6. Elliott VS. Physician shortage predicted to spread. *AMednews.com.* Available at: http://www.ama-assn.org/amednews/2004/01/05/pr/20105.htm. Accessed July 2004.
7. ASRT. The Personnel Crunch: A Crisis in the Radiologic Technologist Workforce. Available at: www.asrt.org. Accessed July 2004.
8. Dubbs B. Respiratory care workforce shortage. *American Medical Association.* Available at: http://www.ama-assn.org/ama/pub/category/9818.htm. Accessed July 2004.
9. AHA Commission on Workforce for Hospitals and Health Systems. *In Our Hands: How Hospital Leaders Can Build a Thriving Workforce.* Chicago: American Hospital Association; April 2002.
10. Moore JD. Healthcare compensations rises. *Modern Healthcare.* 2000; 30:29–30, 32, 34–36.
11. Santamour B. Staffing watch. Hospitals and healthcare network. *Health Forum.* 2003; 24. Available at: http://www.hhnmag.com. Accessed July 2004.
12. Medical Group Association. Median Compensation for Physicians in the Four Regions of the United States. 2002. Available at: www.amga.org. Accessed July 2005.

13. Sullivan Commission. Missing Persons: Minorities in the Health Professions: A Report of the Sullivan Commission on Diversity in the Healthcare Workforce. Available at: http://www.aacn.nche.edu/Media/pdf/SullivanReport.pdf. 2004. Accessed July 2004.
14. Kuhar P, Miller D, Spear B, Ulreich S, Mion L. The meaningful retention strategy inventory: a targeted approach to implementing retention strategies. *Journal of Nursing Administration.* 2004; 34:10–18.
15. Haven S, Aiken L. Shaping systems to promote desired outcomes: the magnet hospital model. *Journal of Nursing Administration.* 1999; 29:14–20.
16. Aiken L, Clarke S, Sloane D, Sochalski J, Silber JH. Hospital nurse staffing and patient mortality, nurse burnout and job dissatisfaction. *Journal of the American Medical Association.* 2002; 288(16):1987–1993.
17. Kimball B, O'Neil E. *Healthcare's Human Crisis: The American Nursing Shortage.* Princeton, NJ: Robert Wood Johnson Foundation; 2002.
18. Pozgar GD. *Legal Aspects of Healthcare Administration.* Seventh Edition. Gaithersburg, MD: Aspen; 1999.
19. Marquis B, Huston C. *Leadership Roles and Management Functions in Nursing: Theory and Application.* Third Edition. Philadelphia: Lippincott; 2000:416.
20. Ashmos D, Huonker J, McDaniel RR Jr. Participation as a complicating mechanism: the effect of clinical professional and middle manager participation on hospital performance. *Healthcare Management Review.* 1998; 23:7–28.
21. Erbin-Rosemann MA, Simms LM. Work locus of control: the intrinsic factor behind empowerment and work excitement. *Nursing Economics.* 1997; 15: 183–188.
22. Hader R, Claudio T. Seven methods to effectively manage patient care labor resources. *Journal of Nursing Administration.* 2002; 32:66–68.
23. Graf C, Millar S, Feilteau C, Coakley P, Erickson J. Patients' needs for nursing care. *Journal of Nursing Administration.* 2003; 33:76–81.
24. American Nurses Association. *Nursing Report Care for Acute Care Settings.* Washington, DC: American Nurses Association; 1995.
25. Blegen MA, Goode CJ. Nurse staffing and patient outcomes. *Nursing Research.* 1998; 47:43–50.
26. Joint Commission on Accreditation of Healthcare Organizations. *Health Care at the Crossroads: Strategies for Addressing the Evolving Nursing Shortage.* Chicago, IL: JACHO; 2002.
27. Aiken L, Clark S, Cheung R, Sloane D, Siber I. Educational levels of hospital nurses and surgical patient mortality. *Journal of the American Medical Association.* 2003; 291:1617–1623.
28. Spetz J. California's minimum nurse-to-patient ratios: where are we, how did we get here, and where do we go next? *California Health Workforce Studies.* San Francisco: Center for Health Professions, University of California, San Francisco; 2004. Available at: www.futurehealth.ucsf.edu/cchws/ratios.html. Accessed July 2004.
29. Golden L, Jorgensen H. *Time After Time.* Washington, DC: Economic Policy Institute; 2002.

30. Tabone S. Nurse fatigue: the human factor. *Texas Nursing.* 2004; 78(5):8–10.
31. Gaba DM, Howard SK. Fatigue among clinicians and the safety of patients. *New England Journal of Medicine.* 2002; 347:1249–1255.
32. Jha A, Duncan B, Bates D. Fatigue, sleepiness and medical errors. Evidence Report/Technology Assessment No. 43. *Making Healthcare Safer: A Critical Analysis of Patient Safety Practice.* 2002. Available at: http://www.ahcpr.gove/clinic/ptsafety/index.html. Accessed August 2004.
33. Rogers AE, Hwang WT, Scott LD, Aiken LH, Dinges DF. The working hours of hospital staff nurses and patient safety. *Health Affairs.* 2004; 23:202.
34. Kohn LT, Corrigan JM, Donaldson MS. *To Err Is Human: Building a Safer Health System.* Washington, DC: National Academic Press; 1999.
35. Young D. Five years after the IOM report, experts gauge progress of patient safety. *American Journal of Health-Systems Pharmacy.* 2005; 62:12, 14, 20.
36. AHRQ Fact Sheet. Closing the Quality Gap: A Critical Analysis of Quality Improvement Strategies. 2004. Available at: http://www.ahrq.gov/clinic/epc/qgapfact.htm. Accessed July 2005.
37. Simpson R. Patient and nurse safety: how information technology makes a difference. *Nursing Administration Quarterly.* 2005; 29:97–101.
38. Congressional Budget Office. *Limiting Tort Liability of Medical Malpractice.* Economic & Budget Issue Brief. January 8, 2004.
39. Pozgar G, Santucci N. *Legal Aspects of Healthcare Administration.* Eighth Edition. Gaithersburg, MD: Aspen; 2002:434.
40. United States General Accounting Office. *Medical Malpractice Insurance: Multiple Factors Have Contributed to Increased Premium Rates.* GAO-03-702. June 2003.
41. Kolodkin C. Expert Commentary: Medical Malpractice Insurance Trend? Chaos! 2001. Available at: http://www.irmi.com/irmicom/expert/articles/2001/kolodkin09.aspx. Accessed July 2005.
42. Borbjerg R, Bartow A. Understanding Pennsylvania's Medical Malpractice Crisis. The Project on Medical Liability in Pennsylvania. June 2003. Available at: http://www.medliability.pa.org/research/report0603. Accessed July 2005.
43. Kangas S, Kee, C, McKee-Waddle R. Organizational factors, nurses' job satisfaction and patient satisfaction with nursing care. *Journal of Nursing Administration.* 1998; 29:32–34.
44. Laschinger H, Shamian J, Thomason D. Impact of magnet hospital characteristics on nurses' perceptions of trust, burnout, quality of care, and work satisfaction. *Nursing Economics.* 2001; 19:258–266.
45. Havens D. Comparing nursing infrastructure and outcomes: ACCN magnet and non-magnet hospitals. *Nursing Economics.* 2001; 19:258–266.
46. Maxfield D, Grenny J, McMilan R, Patterson K, Switzler A. *Silence Kills: The Seven Crucial Conversations for Healthcare.* American Association of Critical-Care Nurses & VitalSmart; 2005. Available at: www.rxforbettercare.org. Accessed July 2005.

47. Wilmot W, Hocker J. *Interpersonal Conflict.* Sixth Edition. Boston: McGraw-Hill; 2001.

48. Valentine P. Management of conflict: do nurses/women handle it differently? *Journal of Advanced Nursing.* 1995; 22:142–149.

49. O'Keefe M. *Nursing Practice and the Law: Avoiding Malpractice and Other Legal Risks.* Philadelphia: F. A. Davis; 2001:255–288, 533.

CHAPTER 9

Human Resources Management Along the Continuum of Care
Donna L. Gellatly

VIGNETTE

Another day, another resignation. It seemed that the cycle would never end. The turnover rate for nurse aides was more than 100%. Salaries in this inner-city Medicaid-predominant nursing home could not even keep up with the pay rates offered by the local fast-food restaurants. Indeed, the restaurants offered better benefits. If it wasn't the pay rates, the legal rules and regulations governing long-term care personnel added to the recruitment and retention problem.

These are but some of the problems affecting the continuum of care or nursing home industry. After providing an overview of the nursing home setting, this chapter offers a close-up discussion of the human resources issues related to nursing homes including recruitment and selection, retention, compensation, benefits, training and education, performance evaluation, unionization, and legal and regulatory issues.

OVERVIEW OF THE SETTING

The continuum of care includes institutional and community-based services outside of the acute care setting. Long-term care institutions are defined as those facilities that have an average patient length of stay of more than 30 days. Along the continuum of care, a variety of inpatient and outpatient (ambulatory) services are available to the long-term care patient that can be utilized individually or in tandem with each other. Services available on an outpatient basis to assist the patient and his or her family include the following:

- Adult day care: a daytime program providing nursing care, therapies, and social services to adult clients for a certain number of hours per day or per week. Clients return to their homes in the off-hours. The Medicare program is investigating the possibility of paying for these services. Demonstration projects are currently under way. Some states' Medicaid programs provide reimbursement for these services.
- Home health agency: an organization that provides nursing, therapy, homemaker, and social services to patients in their own homes. Patients must be unable to leave their homes safely to visit physician offices or other healthcare facilities. The Medicare and Medicaid programs pay for these services.
- Respite care: a temporary service provided either in the home by home health workers or at an adult day care facility, or sometimes within an institution, so that the regular caregiver can have some time off from caring for the patient. The Medicare program pays for these services, with certain limitations on the number of days of coverage.

As the patient progresses along the continuum of care pathway, there may come a time when he or she can no longer live alone or be taken care of by family or friends in a home setting. At that point, the continuum of care follows an institutionalized path offering these services, usually in the following order:

- Retirement housing: a residential setting that provides architecturally friendly facilities for the elderly or disabled. Some social activities and personal care services may be provided. However, nursing care and rehabilitation services are generally not provided to these residents. The Medicare and Medicaid programs do not pay for these services.

- Assisted living (residential care): a residential setting that provides activities of daily living personal care services, 24-hour supervision, scheduled and unscheduled assistance, social activities, and some minor nursing care services. Some states refer to these types of services as "sheltered care." The Medicare and Medicaid programs do not pay for these services.
- Intermediate care facility: a residential setting that provides daily living personal care services, nursing services, and 24-hour supervision. The Medicare program does not pay for these services. Individual state Medicaid programs may reimburse for these services.
- Skilled nursing facility: a licensed regulated facility that provides regular skilled nursing, rehabilitation, and other specialized services to patients. The Medicare and Medicaid programs pay for these services.

When the patient has been diagnosed as terminally ill, the patient and his or her family may make the decision to employ hospice services to ease the dying process.

- Hospice: a cluster of special services for the dying that can be rendered in the home or in a facility. Hospice care provides palliative management of pain and medical, spiritual, legal, financial, and family support services. The Medicare and Medicaid programs pay for these services.

While some nursing homes specialize only in skilled nursing and rehabilitation care, many others offer a comprehensive array of services, including sheltered care, intermediate care, skilled nursing and rehabilitation care, and hospice services. Certain efficiencies can be achieved by sharing administrative and support services, such as laundry, dietary, business office, and plant operations. However, each service would have separate and distinct nursing units and assigned nursing and support personnel. This array of services is beneficial both to the facility and to the resident. For the facility, it provides a ready source of resident referrals as the resident transitions within the same facility for more complex care. The resident stays in the same familiar facility and continues to be able to maintain contact with fellow residents.

The past decade has seen changes in the traditional delivery of continuum of care services. The average occupancy rate for traditional nursing home services has declined to approximately 88%.[1] Nursing homes have gone from having an eager waiting list of potential residents to competing with alternative delivery services for the potential client. Due to limited commercial insurance coverage, restricted governmental reimbursement methodologies, climbing per diem costs, perceived poor-quality-of-care issues, and changing family values, the growth of alternative systems—such as adult day care, home health care, assisted living services, innovative private care agencies, and companion services—has negatively affected the utilization of nursing home facilities.

Contrary to common belief, the Medicare program plays a limited role in long-term care. Medicare Part A pays for long-term care services only after an initial three-day acute hospital stay, and only for skilled nursing and skilled rehabilitative services. The major portion of the cost of long-term care is paid by each state's Medicaid program. In 2000, the average client mix was as follows:[1]

- Medicare: 8.7%
- Medicaid: 67.7%
- Other payers, which are mostly self-pay: 23.7%

Approximately 53% of these patients are 65 years of age or older (the "elderly"), 44% are of working age, and 3% are children. Besides rendering care for the illnesses of aging, the continuum cares for handicapped patients, victims of traumatic injury, AIDS (acquired immunodeficiency syndrome) patients, and those suffering from mental illness or mental retardation.[2] Ninety percent of nursing home residents are elderly. Patients younger than 65 years of age are usually residents of mental hospitals, homes for the developmentally disabled, and/or home care or hospice patients.

The Center for Medicare and Medicaid Services (CMS) collects long-term care data through its Online Survey, Certification, and Reporting (OSCAR) system. Its database includes operating statistics, patient demographic data, and health deficiencies for each facility. State survey agencies collect and enter the data into this federal database. Unfortunately, data from different sources are not compatible. For example, OSCAR data cannot be reconciled with data produced by the National Center for Health Statistics (NCHS) through its National Nursing Home Survey. OSCAR data include only Medicare, Medicaid, and combined Medicare/Medicaid-certified facilities. The National Nursing Home Survey also includes noncertified private facilities.

From the 1999 National Nursing Home Survey, published by the National Center for Health Statistics (NCHS), the following nursing home data have been released:[3]

- There were 18,000 nursing homes.
- The average number of beds per nursing home was 105.
- The average facility occupancy was 87%.
- The discharge rate was 134 patients per 100 beds.
- The average length of stay for current residents was 892 days.
- Sixty-five percent of residents were admitted from a hospital, 22% from a private or semiprivate residence, and 5% from another nursing home.

From the March 2000 OSCAR survey, statistics reflected the following ownership characteristics:[4]

- Independently owned: 44.6%
- Multi-facility owned: 55.4%
- For profit: 65.2%
- Nonprofit: 28.3%
- Government owned and operated: 6.5%

The latest available data for home health care are out of date. Although NCHS statistics are available for 2002, changes in home health reimbursement have negatively affected both the number of agencies and the patient utilization rate. Many of the "mom-and-pop," privately owned agencies have been forced to close or sell out to larger for-profit chains, as "caps" have been placed on the number of visits the Medicare program will pay for and the amount of reimbursement available for each episode of care. NCHS data for 2000 reported the following statistics:[5]

- 1.4 million patients
- 7.2 million discharges
- 69 days average length of service
- Most common primary diagnosis: heart disease (13% of discharges)
- 20,000 agencies (approximate)

Staffing

According to estimates developed by the U.S. Bureau of Labor Statistics (BLS), more than 3.85 million workers were employed in the nation's long-term care delivery system in 2003. Among the nearly 2.2 million direct-care workers, 545,690 were professionals (registered nurses and licensed practical nurses), and 1.65 million were paraprofessionals, defined to include nurse aides (also known as nursing assistants), home health aides, and personal care workers. The remaining 1.65 million workers were physicians, therapists, support, and administrative staff.[6]

Approximately one-third of the long-term workforce is employed by home-based services. Home healthcare workers for non-hospital-based agencies are mostly home care aides (49%). The remaining staff is composed of registered nurses (19%), licensed practical nurses (6%), physical and occupational therapy staff (3%), and other workers (23%).[7]

Nursing homes are staffed with a mix of professional nurses and trained aides. Federal studies have suggested minimum staffing ratios to achieve best care. Indeed, some states mandate minimum staffing ratios. The issue of minimum staffing issues has been hotly debated, however. In its "Report to Congress: Appropriateness of Minimum Nurse Staffing Ratios in Nursing Homes Phase II Final Report,"[8] CMS concluded it had "serious reservations about the reliability of staffing data at the nursing home level and with the feasibility of staff ratios to improve quality, given the variety of quality measures used and the perpetual shifting of such measures." The report stressed that "related issues of management, tenure, and training of staff may determine quality, [and] the reality of current nursing shortages, and operational details, such as the difference between new nurses and experienced nurses, staff mix, retention and turnover rates, and staff organization" could also influence quality assessment.[8]

Effective January 1, 2003, Omnibus Budget Reconciliation Act (OBRA) regulations required nursing homes to publicly post the number of nursing staff they have on duty to care for patients on each daily shift. Licensed and unlicensed staff, including registered nurses, licensed practical nurses, and nurse aides, must be accounted for. The sign must be at least 8.5 by 14 inches and printed in a font size large enough to be easily seen. This sign should be posted in a public area (preferably in the lobby). The OBRA requirement may open the facility to possible fines or punishment if actual (as posted) staffing does not meet the minimum criteria. Additionally, if actual staffing does not meet the staffing levels stated on the sign, the facility may be fined or punished not only for failure to meet minimum criteria, but also for falsification of records.

The care of nursing home residents falls mainly to certified nurse aides, also known as certified nursing assistants (CNAs). Under the 1987

OBRA, which was enacted in 1990, these caregivers must receive at least 75 hours of training and must be certified by a state agency as having received such training within four months of employment. They must also satisfy continuing education requirements. The initial training may be offered through community colleges, in commercial for-profit educational institutions, or within larger health organizations.

Licensed practical nurses (LPNs) may also be known as licensed vocational nurses (LVNs). These individuals usually have a 9- to 12-month education period, followed by state licensure. Additionally, they must satisfy continuing education requirements. The initial training is usually offered through community colleges or commercial for-profit educational institutions.

Registered nurses may be diploma nurses (three years of training) or have a four-year bachelor of nursing degree. These individuals must be licensed in the state in which they practice and must satisfy continuing education requirements. The initial training may be offered through community colleges and universities or through a facility's nursing school. However, it has become increasingly rare for healthcare facilities to operate their own nursing schools. Many of these schools have closed, and more facilities now enter into cooperative educational agreements with local traditional educational institutions.

Table 9-1 shows the allocation of direct care staff and the average direct care staff hours per resident-day in a nursing home. Suggested minimum federal staffing standards recommend 2.00 CNA direct hours per resident-day, a combined 0.75 direct hour per resident-day for RNs/LPNs, and 0.20 direct hour per resident-day for RNs. However, the preferred minimum levels of staffing are 2.00 CNA direct hours per resident-day, 1.00

Table 9-1 Allocation of Care

Type of Care Staff	Percentage of Care Provided/Day (%)	Hours of Care Provided/Day (%)
Certified nurse aide (CNA)	68.8	2.30
Licensed practical nurse (LPN)	21.5	0.72
Registered nurse (RN)	9.7	0.32
Total	100.0	3.34

Source: American Health Care Association. United States Nursing Facilities (OSCAR Data). 2004. Available at: www.ahca.org. Accessed November 23, 2004.

combined RN/LPN direct hour, and 0.45 RN direct hour per resident-day. Unfortunately, most facilities do not meet these standards, with 54% of facilities falling below suggested minimum federal staffing standards for CNAs, 23% for combined RNs/LPNs, and 31% for RNs only.[9]

A 2002 study of three states, released by the U.S. Department of Health and Human Services, indicates that a resident needs an average of 4.1 hours of direct care per resident-day: 2.8 hours of nurse aide time and 1.3 hours from registered nurses or LPNs. Its recommendations would require nursing homes to have one nurse aide for every five or six residents from 7:00 A.M. to 11:00 P.M. Current staff ratios have one nurse aide for every 8 to 14 residents.[10]

Staffing ratios for home care agencies are based on patient acuity levels and geographic service area. The average patient load is six to seven patient visits per calendar-day. Nurses (RN or LPN) typically spend 45 minutes to 1 hour with each patient, and up to 2 hours for the first visit. Nurses who are "high-tech" have a lower caseload, typically three to five visits per day. High-tech nurses handle total parenteral nutrition (TPN), IV therapy, or ventilator care patients. These nurses are supported by therapists (if needed and when a physician order is given), social workers, and/or home health aides. However, most home health visits are handled by home health aides.

Various home health agency productivity studies have been conducted over the years. These studies show an average of 5.0 patients per day, with RNs' productivity being slightly lower than those of LPNs and home health aides.[11]

A point often not factored into home health productivity statistics is the issue of security. In high-crime areas, home health professionals may require a security guard to accompany them as they make their home visits. The cost of this security is usually not reimbursable by third-party or private payers. However, because these healthcare professionals are in uniform and may be carrying drugs and syringes, they can be targets for the criminal element. Public government agencies may have the ability to use community police officers for this purpose. For private for-profit agencies, the most common form of security is the privately paid security officer.

RECRUITMENT AND SELECTION

The U.S. Bureau of Labor Statistics has reported that community care facilities for the elderly and residential care facilities will experience a 55%

growth in employment between the years 2002 and 2012. In fact, seven of the ten fastest-growing occupations between 2002 and 2012 are expected to be medically related. Growth rates for specific occupations during this period are 59% for medical assistants, 49% for social and human service assistants, 49% for home health aides, 47% for medical records and health information technicians, 46% for physical therapist aides, and 45% for physical therapist assistants. The ten occupations with the largest job growth for the same period include registered nurses (27%) and nursing aides, orderlies, and attendants (25%).[12]

The hiring and lay-off of healthcare personnel have ebbed and flowed as reimbursement rates have fluctuated. The economies of many states have limited increases in Medicaid reimbursement rates. Given that more than 60% of a long-term facility's costs are salary related (wages and benefits), these facilities have responded to such financial limitations by utilizing a combination of staff lay-offs and salary freezes. At the same time, government-mandated staffing minimums and overtime limitations have created a demand for new workers in the healthcare industry. This demand has been addressed by recruiting new employees or by utilizing temporary staff agencies. Healthcare providers are caught between having limited financial resources and being required to provide additional minimum staffing levels and specialized workers.

Methods of Recruitment

When a vacancy occurs, many organizations first carry out a search within the organization to identify possible candidates before turning to various outside sources. Individuals may be considered for promotion into the position, for lateral transfer, or, in some rare cases, for demotion.

In long-term care facilities and in healthcare organizations where there is an ongoing relationship with patients/residents, internal recruitment may provide positive benefits to the resident because the "known" caregiver continues with the facility, albeit in another position. This retention provides a stable continuing environment for the resident, rather than a frequent turnover of personnel and the appearance of many "new faces."

It is a common industry practice below the level of management to post vacancies by advertising them widely throughout the organization. Job posting provides an internal candidate pool for the advertised position. It entails placing an announcement of the vacancy on a bulletin board or in an "in-house" newsletter. In some cases, however, these methods may not generate a positive response.

Well-qualified individuals may fail to apply for consideration because they may fear reprisal from their current supervisors. With continued shortages of qualified personnel and high turnover within nurse aide positions, many supervisors are extremely resistant to supporting promotion from within, especially if it means that they would lose one of "their" employees. A supervisor may consider an employee's inquiry regarding another position as an indirect statement that he or she isn't happy with his or her current position or with operations of the department. If the applicant does not obtain the new position, he or she would have to remain in the current position, where the supervisor now knows that the employee is "looking" for other opportunities.

A low-cost and often effective recruitment approach is to encourage employees to publicize job vacancies and promote job applications among family, friends, and colleagues. This "word of mouth" approach is frequently found in the long-term care nursing home industry. A cash bonus is often paid to employees who recruit new staff, if the new hire remains with the organization for a specified period of time. Drawbacks to employee referrals may be the development of cliques within the organization, alienation of employees whose referrals do not work out and who therefore receive no bonuses, and the perpetuation of systematic discrimination as "like tends to refer like."[13]

Numerous external sources of recruiting exist:

- Walk-in and write-in applications
- Classified advertising
- Employment agencies and search firms
- Direct mail
- Career days and conventions
- Open houses
- School liaisons
- U.S. employment service/military outplacement, and government training programs[14]

As most nursing facility nurses are graduates of diploma nursing schools or community colleges, many home health and nursing facility organizations work closely with these educational institutions to develop student in-service clinical programs and internships. By providing clinical rotations, part-time employment, and scholarships while the student is in school, these institutions develop a ready source of potential full-time employment candidates once they graduate from their nursing programs.

Newspapers have traditionally been the most common method of healthcare external recruiting. They reach a large number of potential applicants at a relatively low cost per hire. Newspaper ads are used to recruit all types of employees, from unskilled to top managerial positions. These ads range from matter-of-fact information to large ads with illustrations or slogans and logos designed to attract notice. As more newspapers are now online, newspaper Web sites also carry classified employment advertising. In addition, such Web sites as www.monster.com and other job-finding services on the Internet have become popular recruiting methods.

Many larger healthcare organizations and long-term care nursing facilities have also created their own Web sites, which they use to post job openings and information about their facilities. Some sites even allow for online application for employment. Multi-facility organizations may provide a comprehensive list of job openings on their main Web site and direct the Web site visitor to individual facilities for further employment opportunities and information.

Hodes Research conducted a national survey on the success of nurse recruiting. In order of success, employee referrals, word-of-mouth, student clinical rotations, and Internet sources were found to be the best methods of nurse recruiting.[15]

Trade publications enable organizations to aim at a more specific group of potential applicants. Unfortunately, long lead times are required for these publications, and thus the ads can become outdated. Some healthcare organizations reserve this recruitment method for administrative positions or for specialized employees, such as physical therapists or dietitians.

Although organizations may utilize both external and internal sources of recruitment, they may not always obtain the desired number of applicants. This is especially true in competitive markets for highly skilled individuals. However, the organization may enhance its recruitment efforts by offering inducements such as relocation assistance by establishing auxiliary programs such as career development, child care, or spousal job placement assistance. The national survey undertaken by Hodes Research[15] showed that tuition assistance, paid time off, and student scholarships were strong enticements in recruiting nurses. Nurse sign-on bonuses were another draw. The Hodes survey indicated that 59% of facilities offered referral bonuses and 45% offered sign-on bonuses.[15] Besides increasing the pool of qualified job applicants, these added benefits might increase the probability that once hired, the applicant-employee will stay.

Most nursing and healthcare professionals commit to one segment of the healthcare industry. It is rare for a nurse to jump back and forth between acute care hospital employment, for example, and alternative healthcare services such as long-term care or home health services. Nursing facility nurses usually choose this segment of the industry because it offers the opportunity to develop long-term nurse–patient relationships and to have a more regular performance of duties rather than the "emergency/acute" nature of hospital nursing. As physician services are limited to periodic monthly visits or assessments, nurses have greater autonomy in the care of their patients. Any acute change in the patient's medical condition usually entails a transfer to the local hospital.

Methods of Staffing

With the downsizing, rightsizing, or reengineering of healthcare delivery systems in today's market, alternatives to recruiting new employees have emerged. Such alternatives may include subcontracting work originally done by employees, hiring consultants or temporary help, or paying overtime compensation to existing employees to cover the duties of the vacated positions. Some organizations replace full-time employees with a combination of part-time employees and overtime assignments. This strategy allows the organization to avoid paying full-time employee benefits, such as vacation/holiday pay, health insurance, and pension benefits, and, in some cases, enables it to offer a lower rate of pay for the position. It also allows the flexibility to expand and contract hours as needed.

Most healthcare organizations use outside nursing pool agencies to cover vacant positions or handle increased resident census. These agencies' labor rates are expensive—sometimes twice the going pay rate. Additionally, a substantial amount of time may be required to orient a pool nurse to the physical facility and the organization's policies and procedures. Many times, however, the pool nurse may be a long-term agency employee who has worked in the same facility on many assignments. Other facilities may organize their own "in-house" nursing pool of individuals who prefer part-time or as-needed employment.

In all circumstances, care must be taken as to how these pool workers are classified. Some organizations have classified these temporary workers as "contractors," rather than as employees. Employment relationships presume the organization controls the means by which the individual fulfills contractual obligations with respect to the result being accomplished. The existence of an employment relationship is relevant to the tax and professional liabilities of both the individual and the organization. Among the areas affected are federal and state income tax withholding, Social Security/Medicare taxes, worker's compensation, unemployment compensation, and immigration matters.

Although an independent contractor relationship presumes the organization controls the result to be accomplished, it does not confer responsibility for the methods by which the individual exercises professional judgment in fulfilling contractual obligations. The required absence of "control" is determined in relation to the nature of the work and the legal circumstances of both parties. Additionally, the Internal Revenue Service (IRS) determines the independent contractor status based on the individual's liability or the responsibility for business risk. The IRS publishes form SS-8, "Information for Use in Determining Whether a Worker Is an Employee for Federal Employment Taxes and Income Tax Withholding," to assist in determining employment status.[16]

This issue has become a hot topic for healthcare workers. Home health agencies had attempted to classify home health nurses and aides as independent contractors, as these personnel did not work within a physical facility, but rather visited individual patients' homes. However, the courts and the IRS have ruled that home health workers are employees, as they are assigned, controlled, and supervised by home health agency management.

Nurses who work on an irregular basis or on an as-needed basis are considered to be employees; they are considered to be a part of the facility's nursing pool. Again, these persons are assigned, controlled, and supervised by facility management. Nurses obtained from commercial nurse staff agencies are considered to be employees of the staff agency, not the nursing facility. They are scheduled and paid by the agency, and their payroll checks have federal and state withholding tax deductions made by the nursing agency.

Most nursing home facilities contract for other professional functions and use physical, occupational, and speech therapists and dieticians on a contractual basis. A facility frequently does not need full-time personnel to perform these functions. These individuals are considered to be independent contractors if they meet the following criteria:

- They have variable compensation arrangements based on time spent or procedures performed.
- They can directly hire and supervise their own assistants.

- They work for two or more organizations.
- They can schedule their assignments on a mutually agreeable basis rather than be told to report to work at a certain time.
- They can show any factors that tend to indicate that the person bears the business risk of his or her own practice. If the business fails, he or she is personally responsible for the debts of the business.

Conversely, these individuals would be considered to have employee status if they meet these criteria:

- They are paid a fixed salary, are prevented from substituting qualified licensed replacements for themselves, or are prevented from engaging in outside employment.
- They are required to have facility-determined work hours, and their time is controlled by a facility supervisor.
- They are required to follow facility policies, including wearing a facility name tag or a facility supplied uniform.
- They receive the same rights and privileges as the facility provides to its own employees, such as vacation, sick leave, holiday pay, pay raises, or being included in the facility insurance benefits plan.

Many healthcare organizations have established foreign recruitment programs. The Hodes survey[17] indicated that approximately 9% of facilities recruited registered nurses internationally. Recruiters go to such countries as the Philippines, Ireland, or South Africa to recruit nurses. [As an aside, an ethical question about the use of this practice is the concern that rich countries (e.g., the United States) are raiding poorer ones for nursing talent.] These recruiting trips do not render immediate results. Some nurses must wait 8 to 12 months for working papers from the U.S. Immigration and Naturalization Service and will require assistance in making the transition to the U.S. healthcare system. Since the September 11, 2001, terrorist attacks, stringent immigration policies and procedures have been enacted that have delayed the approval and entry of foreign nationals into the United States. New immigration laws limit the number of immigration visas allocated to each country. In the past, the Philippines and Ireland have exceeded their visa quotas for the year, and no additional visas have been allocated to them. This has caused problems in obtaining healthcare personnel from these countries. The 2005 U.S. Congress approved the transfer of unused visas from other countries (France and Germany) to be used to supplement the demand for Philippines' visas.

For registered nurses to obtain U.S. immigration visas, they must pass a three-part multiple-choice examination, the Certification for Graduates of Foreign Nursing Schools (CGFNS), that tests both English proficiency and nursing knowledge. Most U.S. State Boards of Nursing require this examination as a condition of licensure for internationally trained RNs. For nurses for whom English is a second language, the Test of English as a Foreign Language (TOEFL) may also be required. The U.S. nurse licensing examination, the Nursing Council Licensure Examination (NCLEX), may be taken only in the United States after the nurse has successfully passed the CGFNS.[17]

The hiring of newly immigrated nurses has presented some problems for the long-term care industry. Because many of these immigrants are from Asia and speak English as a second language, communication problems have resulted with the elderly resident population who are not Asian and may not have had much interaction with other nationalities or cultures. Language and cultural differences often cause the resident and his or her family to be fearful regarding "quality of care" and their perceived or real inability to receive and understand resident progress updates and communications.

To meet the challenge of the nursing shortage, some facilities are teaming up with nursing schools and community colleges to "grow their own" employees. Facilities provide scholarships to students in certified nursing assistant (or certified nurse aide) and nursing programs, in return for students' promises to work for the facility once they graduate from the program and pass the required licensing examination.

Shortages in the healthcare workforce exist beyond the well-known fact of nursing shortages. From pharmacists to radiology technicians to service workers in dietary and housekeeping departments, vacant positions have become harder to fill and, once hired, employees have become more difficult to retain.[18]

RETENTION

In Medimorphus.com's "Recruitment Trends within Healthcare Professions"[19] survey, which was published December 2000, respondents cited the following reasons for looking for a new job:

- Low pay (67%)

- Better work environment (45%)
- Better benefits (42%)
- Advancement opportunities (38%)
- Change of career (28%)
- Different location (25%)

Even with the economic downturn that began in 2002, staffing vacant positions in hospitals, nursing homes, and home health agencies continues to be a major problem. Many employees have found that there is "another world" out there. In other words, there are alternative means of employment in ancillary healthcare-related companies that do not require mandatory overtime, stress-filled workdays, or professional liability concerns.

> Additionally, the major changes taking place in the healthcare industry have made nurses reluctant to remain in nursing and have caused prospective nursing students to make other career choices. Nursing, traditionally a woman's profession, has been slow to incorporate men, while medicine has been successful in recruiting women to fill a large percentage of medical school classes.[20]

Another public rating agency, Fitch Ratings Ltd., has concerns regarding the nursing home industry outlook:

> Although Fitch's industry outlook for the acute care (hospital) sector and CCRCs (continuing care retirement communities) has improved, the industry outlook for freestanding nonprofit nursing homes remains negative due to significant challenges in the industry that will continue to pressure already weak financial performance. The challenges include inadequate Medicaid reimbursement; rising insurance, labor, and benefits expense; and increased capital needs. Fitch expects labor expenses to increase at a higher than inflationary rate due to the nationwide nursing shortage and the difficulty in recruiting and retaining staff. Turnover rates are extremely high in this field, especially for certified nursing assistants and licensed practical nurses.[21]

Low-paid support workers in dietary and housekeeping positions have found that they can earn just as much in the fast-food industry, with better benefits and opportunities for advancement. Clerical, billing, and collections personnel have found better-paying jobs in the insurance industry, again with better benefits.

Nursing Shortage

The American Association of Colleges of Nursing has identified several concerns regarding the future of nursing care in the United States:

- The number of first-time U.S.-educated nursing school graduates who sat for the NCLEX-RN examination decreased by 20% from 1995 to 2003.[22]
- The shortage of nursing school faculty is restricting nursing program enrollments. More than 16,000 qualified applicants were turned away in 2003 due to insufficient faculty, clinical sites, classroom space, clinical preceptors, and budget constraints.[23]
- The average age of the RN is climbing. According to a July 2001 report released by the U.S. Government Accounting Office, *Nursing Workforce: Emerging Nurse Shortages Due to Multiple Factors,* 40% of all RNs will be older than age 50 by the year 2010.[24]
- The changing demographics signal a need for more nurses to care for an aging population.[24]
- The high nurse turnover and vacancy rates are affecting access to health care.
- The impact of nurse staffing on patient care includes a direct correlation between number of staff, healthcare quality, and clinical outcomes.[25]

Vacancy rates of staff nurses at nursing homes, which average approximately 19%, are higher than in hospitals. With limited financial resources and flexibility, nursing homes are at a significant disadvantage when competing for nurses, who are in high demand by other healthcare providers that can offer better salaries in a more favorable environment.[26]

A crucial study, "Results of the 2002 AHCA Survey of Nursing Staff Vacancy and Turnover in Nursing Homes," prepared by the American Health Care Association, was released February 12, 2003.[27] According to this study, vacancy and turnover rates vary from state to state and from urban to rural facilities. The largest number of vacancies and highest turnover rates are found in urban facilities. This can be attributed to both the volume of residents/patients and health professionals' ability to easily find alternative employment with other healthcare facilities or with alternative delivery systems.

National vacancy and turnover rates in nursing homes for 2002 are shown in Table 9-2. Although the vacancy rate for certified nurse aides was 8.5%, the turnover factor has caused great recruiting problems in nursing homes throughout the United States. These positions provide most of the direct hands-on nursing care in these facilities. Facilities in the South and Southwest regions of the United States reported the greatest problems in vacancies and turnover. This trend may be attributable to the population growth in these states, as well as the shifting population, as the aging population retires to the states with more temperate climates. In Arizona, the number of retired "snow birds" who temporarily relocate to the state for the winter months has caused swings in the demand for healthcare services during the December through April period.

A combination of industry and government efforts has focused on the nurse shortage problem. The federal Nurse Reinvestment Act of 2002 provided for the expansion of loan repayment programs to include healthcare facilities, whereby nursing students can work to meet their loan obligations. It also funded recruitment programs and provided scholarships, career ladder programs, and nurse mentoring programs. Individual states and local governments have developed programs to address the specific nurse shortage problems in their geographic areas.

Media campaigns are being used by the healthcare industry to encourage young people to "join the nursing profession." For example, Johnson & Johnson underwrote a national "Campaign for Nursing's Future" to promote careers in nursing.

Table 9-2 National Vacancy and Turnover Rate in Nursing Homes

Position	Vacancy Rate (%)	Turnover Rate (%)
Director of nursing	4.8	49.7
Administrative RN	8.1	35.5
Staff registered nurse	15.0	48.9
Licensed practical nurse	13.2	48.9
Certified nurse aide	8.5	71.1

Source: American Health Care Association. The 2002 AHCA Nursing Position Vacancy and Turnover Survey. 2002. Available at: www.ahca.org. Accessed December 4, 2004.

COMPENSATION

"In 2003, the median hourly wages for paraprofessional direct-care workers was $9.20, compared with median wages of $13.53 for all U.S. workers. According to the Health Resources and Services Administration, 20% to 30% of paraprofessional direct-care workers are employed on a part-time basis, and one-fifth of all paraprofessional direct-care workers earn incomes below the poverty level."[28] These workers make up 75% of the direct-care workforce and 43% of the entire workforce in long-term care settings. According to the U.S. Bureau of Labor Statistics, 90% of these workers are women with an average age of 39. One-quarter to nearly one-third are unmarried and living with children.[29] Table 9-3 shows salary data for these direct-care workers.

Hospitals are strong competitors for nursing personnel. They usually pay higher hourly wages and offer better and more comprehensive benefits. Earnings data collected for 2003 reported the median hourly earnings of nursing aides, orderlies, and attendants to be $10.27 per hour. Pay rates ranged from a low of $6.98 per hour to a high of $11.39 per hour in 2002.[29]

Median hourly earnings of home health aides were $9.08 in 2003. Pay rates ranged from a low of $6.56 per hour to a high of $10.37 per hour in 2002.[29]

Similar statistics can be found for registered nurses and licensed practical nurses. However, with the shortage of professional registered and

Table 9-3 Median Hourly and Mean Annual Wages of Direct-Care Workers

Occupation	Median Hourly Wages	Mean Annual Wages
Registered nurses	$23.82	$51,230
Licensed practical and vocational nurses	$15.57	$33,210
Nursing aides, orderlies, and attendants	$8.77	$21,050
Home health aides	$9.22	$19,180
Personal and home care aides	$7.91	$17,020

Source: U.S. Department of Labor, Bureau of Labor Statistics, Occupational Employment Statistics (OES) Survey. May 2003.

licensed practical nurses, the gap between acute facility and long-term care facility nursing wages has been shrinking.[29]

New overtime legislation enacted in 2004 further defined which workers are exempt from overtime pay. "Fact Sheet 17N: Nurses and the Part 541 Exemptions under the Fair Labor Standards Act (FLSA)"[30] addressed the issue of exempting healthcare personnel from overtime standards. To qualify for exemption, employees must meet certain tests regarding their job duties and be paid on a salary basis at not less than $455 per week ($21,100 per annum).

"Licensed practical nurses and other similar healthcare employees generally do not qualify as exempt learned professionals regardless of work experience and training, because possession of a specialized advanced academic degree is not a standard prerequisite for entry into such occupations."[30] Registered nurses may be deemed to be "learned professionals," as their work requires advanced knowledge in a field of science or learning, and is acquired by a prolonged course of specialized intellectual instruction.

However, this new legislation does not require registered nurses not to be paid overtime. Indeed, a healthcare facility that attempts to eliminate overtime pay for registered nurses may find it faces mass resignations as these individuals move to other facilities that continue to offer overtime pay. Additionally, overtime provisions in current union contracts can continue to be enforced.

All time actually worked counts toward overtime, even if the work is performed before or after the regular shift. Examples of such work include the following activities:

- Preparation for work, such as setting up equipment
- Changing clothes or wash-ups, if required or necessary
- Caring for equipment such as computers or tools
- Time spent on required training

Fast-food chains can offer competitive entry-level wages and, in many cases, better benefits to food service workers and housekeepers. A White Castle restaurant in suburban Chicago, for example, is currently offering $7.50 per hour to start, with a salary increase after 90 days of employment (2004).

Compensation surveys may be found in professional journals or be undertaken by professional associations. Precise surveys may be conducted by facility human resources management personnel or by the use of consultants who will collect and analyze data for the facility. Several Web sites also offer access to current salary information, including www. careerjournal.com, www.payscale.com, www.salary.com, and www. salaryexpert. com.

To determine the appropriate rate of pay, other factors besides average industry pay rate per job class must be considered: the prevailing wage rates in both the healthcare industry and in other industries that compete for the same employee; the power of the union in negotiating pay rates; the level of required productivity and stress, as compared to other facilities; government constraints; and labor market conditions. In general, hospitals have better pay rates and benefits than long-term care facilities and organizations. Some inner-city facilities already suffering financial difficulties have found they must pay premium hourly rates to entice workers to come into their geographic areas.

The Bureau of Labor Statistics reports that demand for health service managers is expected to grow faster than the average for all occupations through the year 2008.[12] Due to the aging of the U.S. population and the shift of some healthcare services out of hospitals, the demand is likely to be greater for managers who work in long-term care settings, physician practices, and other alternative delivery systems. The term "health services manager" is generic: "It may refer to persons who work in community outreach, marketing, finance, human resources, or general management. They may manage clinical areas, such as nursing, therapy, or surgery, or work in non-health departments, such as information management or dietary."[12]

Salaries in this field vary widely. Nursing home administrators may earn from $55,000 to $100,000 per annum, which is substantially less than what one can earn in a similar position within a hospital. Ultimately, all salary rates are determined by the individual's education, experience, certification status, and the size of the facility. Executive compensation in for-profit nursing home chains may be substantially higher when the position is at the corporate level, as is compensation in a privately owned facility in which the chief executive officer is also the owner or an investor. Additionally, managers in for-profit facilities may have profit-sharing bonuses, stock options, and deferred compensation arrangements that increase their overall compensation packages.

BENEFITS

Employee benefits are additional compensation above and beyond the hourly wage rate or annual salary. Some benefits may be tax-free; others are taxable to the employee. In terms of benefits offered, all employees are not created equal. There may be different employee benefits packages for full-time employees versus part-time employees, and different employee benefits packages for hourly workers versus professional employees. In addition, different benefits packages may be provided to hourly workers based on union–employer wage and benefits agreements.

Unfortunately, besides lower base compensation, long-term care facility workers tend to have less generous benefits packages. This is again attributable to the financial constraints that these facilities now face due to restricted Medicare and Medicaid reimbursement policies. While acute care facilities (hospitals) can still rely on commercial insurance and managed care contracts to subsidize the low government reimbursement rates, nursing homes, in particular, have few nongovernmental reimbursement residents. Currently, there is a move to encourage the purchase of private long-term care insurance policies that may prove financially beneficial to nursing homes, as these policies could supply increased average daily reimbursement above those rates paid by government payers. However, these policies are expensive, and many of them have preexisting conditions clauses and maximum payment amounts.

Employee benefits may provide several advantages to the employer and the employee. Time-off benefits may reduce fatigue and job burnout. They may discourage labor unrest by making total compensation packages comparable to those of other organizations and industries. Benefits plans may also aid in recruitment and retention of employees.

In general, benefits can be grouped into several categories: legally required, insurance related, retirement related, payment for time not worked, and other benefits. The costs of these benefits are a major expense for healthcare institutions. Many hospitals' benefits programs cost 18–20% of direct wage and salary expense. Long-term care facilities' benefits programs may cost 15–18% of direct wage and salary expense, as their benefits packages are usually less extensive than those offered by hospitals.

To compare compensation packages between facilities, one must consider more than the direct salary expense. While an employment candidate may be offered a salary of $40,000 at both facilities, one facility may have a better total compensation package (a combination of salary and benefits expenses) than the other facility. Even if one facility offers a lower salary, it may have a better total compensation package overall. Government healthcare facilities, in particular, may offer lower salaries but provide greater employee benefits, including more vacation, more holiday pay, better pension benefits, and greater sick leave benefits.

These days, medical benefits, life insurance, and retirement plans are expected employee benefits. For healthcare facilities looking to recruit and retain employees, however, these benefits may not be enough. To maintain a competitive edge, facilities are beginning to offer benefits tailored to each employee. To single, childless employees, medical benefits may not seem as important as vacation time, flexible scheduling, or tuition reimbursement. Married employees or those who have children may place greater importance on benefits that offer security to their families, such as long-term disability benefits and health insurance. Dual-working couples may wish to coordinate benefits packages to avoid duplicate medical coverage; if one parent carries family medical insurance coverage, the other working parent might not need medical coverage as an employee benefit. As workers approach retirement age, early retirement options and supplemental retirement benefits may become important benefits.

Some healthcare facilities have instituted nurse staff scheduling programs that allow direct-care workers to work ten-hour workdays over a four-day period. An employee–employer work agreement allows the employer not to pay overtime for the additional two hours per day. Such a schedule allows the employee to have three days per week off. Some employees may use the additional days off to "moonlight" at other healthcare facilities or to attend daytime college courses.

Because most healthcare facilities are 24/7 employers, flexible scheduling allows a facility to maintain minimum or mandated staffing coverage. Many facilities have found that employee productivity and morale go up when employees can work the hours best suited to them, and allow employees to bid for their desired shifts. Some employees may actually prefer to work the third shift or weekend shift for a variety of reasons, including childcare issues, continuing education course schedules, or simply being a natural "night owl."

Job sharing may also be a desirable benefit. As the healthcare industry is predominantly female, working mothers (or others) may be allowed to "share" a full-time job and receive pro rata benefits of the full-time employee. For example, the chief executive officers at Advocate Christ Hospital Medical Center in Oak Lawn, Illinois, shared this key administrative job.

Nursing home and home health employees may consider the "slower pace" of alternative care to be a quality-of-life benefit. Rather than face the intense pressures of medical and surgical procedures in taking care of an acute hospital patient, these employees may have the opportunity to develop long-term relationships with their patients and patients' families. However, with the growing shortages of personnel, required overtime, and increased resident workload to care for these long-term patients, most nursing home and home health employees currently may not agree with this statement.

Mandated Benefits

Legally mandated employee benefits include Social Security, Medicare insurance, unemployment, and worker's compensation. Some long-time governmental and nonprofit organization employees are covered under "private" retirement plans. Therefore, employers and employees do not pay into the federal system; instead, payments are made into a private retirement fund. This does not automatically eliminate these employees from receiving Social Security benefits upon retirement. If these employees have worked under the Social Security system with other employers (for a total of 40 calendar-quarters), they may also collect Social Security payments from the federal government. Each person must review his or her own private retirement plan. There may be a "coordination of benefits" requirement that reduces private retirement pension payments when the person also collects Social Security. Medicare insurance tax payments would still be deducted from new employees' paychecks.

Healthcare employers may purchase commercial worker's compensation insurance policies or participate in group self-insurance plans offered by healthcare organizations, such as the Metropolitan Healthcare Council of Chicago. The cost of each worker's compensation claim, plus an administrative fee, is charged to the facility as the Council processes and pays claims. Each state has its own unique worker's compensation laws that apply to all companies and organizations within the state. Payments to employees cover the loss of income and reimburse or cover medical expenses.

Healthcare employers may participate in the administrative unemployment management program provided by organizations such as the Metropolitan Healthcare Council of Chicago, or they may use the State Unemployment Department process to pay unemployment claims. Former employees are eligible to receive unemployment payments only if they meet two criteria: they lost their jobs through no fault of their own and they are seeking other full-time jobs.

Unemployment compensation is usually available for only a certain number of weeks (currently a maximum of 26 weeks). During certain recessionary periods, this period may be increased in increments of 13 weeks. With the nursing and personnel shortages within the healthcare industry, states' unemployment departments usually have few healthcare industry-related claims; if they do, the claims period is usually relatively short in duration.

Retirement-Related Benefits

Contrary to popular opinion, an employer is not required to offer a retirement pension plan. In addition, part-time employees may not be eligible for retirement pension coverage if they work less than an average of a certain number of hours per pay period or per year. Unless the long-term care worker is employed by a multi-facility chain or a governmental facility, in most cases the employer does not offer an employer-paid retirement plan. If a retirement plan is offered, it is usually funded by employee contributions into a 401(k) plan or its equivalent.

Insurance Benefits

Besides medical coverage, other insurance benefits may include dental, vision, or mental health coverage; long-term disability payments; life insurance; and legal insurance. Medical services may be offered by the healthcare institution through an employee health services program. However, many healthcare employees prefer to have their own medical care provided by a third party to protect their privacy.

Payment for Time Not Worked

No federal or state regulations require employers to offer vacation, sick, or holiday pay. However, laws do regulate employer payments for days off for jury duty or military reserve duty. Additionally, state requirements may govern rest periods (breaks) and lunch periods.

The employer may impose restrictions regarding the use of vacation time, including time limitations ("use it or lose it") before the end of the year, maximum accrual of unpaid vacation time, or certain minimum use of vacation time, such as in full-workday periods. Although many healthcare institutions have stated vacation policies, flexibility for both the facility and its employees has generally been incorporated into these plans to accommodate needed personnel requirements for patient census loads and for special projects, such as JCAHO survey visits. In most states, accrued vacation benefits are a legal right. When the employee leaves the organization, he or she will receive payment for any unused vacation time. This is called a "vested" benefit.

Sick pay is compensation paid to the employee for time not worked due to employee illness. Some employers may also allow employees to be paid for time not worked due to family member illness. Restrictions may apply to the use of sick time, including maximum accrual of unpaid sick leave or certain minimum use of sick time, as in full-workday periods. In the healthcare industry, some organizations may also allow for the "vesting" of accrued sick leave. When an employee terminates employment, he or she may receive a portion of the accrued sick leave benefit as additional compensation (e.g., 50%) or, in some cases, 100% reimbursement of accrued sick leave benefits. Smaller organizations, such as nursing homes and physician practices, usually do not pay for any unused sick benefits.

Although vested sick pay is a great benefit for employees, it may have disadvantages for the employer. Among these disadvantages is the payment, at current wage rates, for prior earned benefits, and employees who attempt to accrue as many sick days as possible. If the employee comes to work when he or she is sick so as to maintain the benefit for future use or for additional termination compensation, then the employer has a sick employee who may infect others and may not be especially productive.

Some healthcare organizations have unique vested sick pay programs. After "banking" a certain number of sick days, the employee receives payment for additional accrued unused sick pay on a periodic basis, such as every six months or annually.

Other Benefits

An organization may offer its employees a multitude of additional benefits. Among these employer-paid benefits may be educational assistance, financial services (discounts or free care), credit unions, and stock purchase programs or stock options for for-profit organizations.

Healthcare employees frequently receive reduced-charge or free cafeteria meals, free or reduced-charge parking, use of recreational or exercise facilities, and childcare or adult-care services. Well-care programs are relatively new benefits. They include free care and sponsored employer programs to encourage employee wellness, including paying for fitness facility membership dues and fees, stop-smoking and obesity programs, and "eat right" dietary classes, which are frequently located in the facility's site.

TRAINING AND EDUCATION

Initial training is the orientation of the employee to the organization, work unit, and job. There are two levels of orientation: overall organization orientation, which is usually performed by the human resources management department, and individual department and job orientation, which is usually performed by the department manager or supervisor.

Direct patient care personnel attend one- to three-week orientation classes before being permanently assigned to a nursing unit. During this period, through a combination of in-class and on-floor sessions, newly hired personnel are instructed on charting procedures (writing in the patient's medical chart), patient transfer policies and techniques (e.g., transfer from bed to chair or commode), medical care techniques (e.g., starting and monitoring IV solutions), and institution-specific patient policies and procedures.

Corporate orientation includes an overview of the healthcare facility, discussion of key policies and procedures, compensation/performance review schedules, fringe benefits, safety and accident prevention programs, employee and union relations, and a tour of the facility. It may also include a discussion of the current healthcare delivery system and its impact on this particular facility.

An orientation kit should include a map of the facility, an organizational chart showing the reporting structure of the organization, a policy and procedure manual and an employee handbook, a pay and holiday calendar, a sample performance appraisal form, required payroll forms, a current newsletter, copies of the insurance plan and other benefits programs, and a list of telephone numbers.

During general department orientation, the manager or designated person should discuss department duties and functions, specific job duties and responsibilities of the new employee, and department-specific policies, procedures, rules, and regulations. In addition, he or she should give a tour of the department and provide an introduction to department employees. A copy of the employee's job description should be given to the new employee.

Employee handbooks can be great tools for managers and human resources personnel. The employee handbook is the most efficient and consistent way to convey to all employees the policies and rules of the organization. Easy-to-read handbooks spell out compensation and benefits policies, the handling of health and medical issues, standards of conduct, federal and state laws and resulting antidiscrimination and nonharassment policies, and disciplinary procedures.

In a landmark decision issued on January 30, 1987 *(Duldulao vs. St. Mary of Nazareth Hospital Center),* the Illinois Supreme Court ruled that an employee handbook could amount to a binding contract with employees. Therefore, handbooks should be carefully worded to adequately describe the facility's policies and procedures. Handbooks must be reviewed frequently and updated as needed to reflect current policies. Any changes or amendments must be transmitted to all employees. Employers may prominently display disclaimers that the handbook is not intended to be a contract and that it does not alter the "employment at will" status. Also, a statement should be included that policies can be changed without notice, subject to the provisions of union contracts, if applicable. Each employee should sign a form acknowledging receipt of the initial employee handbook, and this signed form should be retained in the employee's personnel file.

Training is a learning process that involves the acquisition of skills, concepts, rules, or attitudes to increase the performance of employees. Training must be directed toward the accomplishment of some organizational objectives, such as more efficient production methods, improved quality of services, or reduced operating costs. Training needs may be determined by the following techniques:

- Reviewing resident/patient and family complaints
- Reviewing state inspection surveys and JCAHO recommendations
- Reviewing incident reports that indicate problems in patient care or violations of policies and procedures

- Interviewing supervisors and managers
- Designing and conducting a questionnaire survey for both supervisors and employees
- Analyzing personnel files and conducting a personnel inventory of skills
- Reviewing management requests
- Observing on-the-job behavior
- Analyzing results of tests
- Reviewing results of consultants' reports
- Reviewing quality-control standards and results outside of established parameters (e.g., a higher rate of patient infections or bed sores)

In May 2004, *USA Today* published a special week-long series on the state of nursing homes and assisted living facilities. An analysis of state inspections showed that low pay and high turnover contributed to staffing and training problems. Of the 5,305 facilities' inspection reports reviewed by the newspaper, 28% had training violations. "More than one in four was cited at least once for training violations, such as failing to ensure that staffers had adequate instruction in first aid, emergency procedures, or patient rights."[31]

Most states have online databases that list monthly nursing home violations. Type "A" violations—the most serious licensure violations—are listed by facility and by type of violation. For example, the State of Illinois Department of Public Health releases a Nursing Home Violation Report for each month at www.idph.state.il.us/public/press. Details of the violations can be found in the link "Statement of Violation." According to the July 2005 news release, an example of a Type "A" violation states

> _____, a 106-bed intermediate care facility located at _____ in _____, has been fined $5,000 (<u>Statement of Violation</u>) for failure to prevent a resident from leaving the facility unnoticed. Staff were unaware of the resident's disappearance until notified by a local hospital that she was wandering around the emergency department. The facility has not yet requested a hearing, but is still within the allotted time to do so.

These Type "A" violations require that the facility submit a plan of correction to the state. They should also form the basis of corrective training programs, as well as revised policies and procedures, and be used in employee personnel evaluations.

Specific areas to be covered in employee training and education in nursing facilities and home health agencies should include abuse and neglect; advance directives; confidentiality and privacy; infection control; medication errors; pain management; patient and employee safety, including transferring procedures; and handling special needs and behaviors of specific patient age-groups and populations served. In particular, home health workers should be trained to observe signs of possible patient neglect or abuse, home safety problems or violations, and resident–family interactions and relationships while performing their visit duties.

Training may include such methods as on-the-job training, job rotation, apprenticeship training, and on-site and off-site classroom training. Common training techniques in the healthcare industry for direct-care workers include lecture, video presentation, and role-playing. Because these facilities operate around the clock, training must be undertaken on each of the three work shifts and include weekend and as-needed personnel. Evaluating the success of these techniques includes reviewing the reaction of the employees to the training exercises, using feedback techniques and/or behavior or results improvement. A review of the quantity and severity of Type "A" violations should be undertaken pre- and post-training to ascertain the success of the training process in reducing the number and severity of the cited problems.

All employees should be evaluated and assessed for advancement potential. Additionally, employees should be evaluated for employee obsolescence—that is, when an employee no longer possesses the knowledge or abilities to perform the functions successfully. As the healthcare industry is constantly changing thanks to the development of new medical technology and new government regulations, employees should receive additional training to develop the skills needed to meet these emerging challenges. New procedures in patient lifting and transfer, insertion of IV lines, and changes in acceptable vital signs (blood pressure and blood sugar) require additional training.

Mentoring involves a relationship with an experienced, usually older person who coaches, supports, guides, and helps a protégé, usually in the same line of work.[32] The mentor may be an immediate superior, a professor, or someone with extensive experience in the field. The American College of Healthcare Executives' (ACHE) professional policy statement states that "healthcare executives have a professional obligation to mentor both those entering the field as well as mid-careerists preparing to lead the healthcare system of tomorrow."[32] Besides working with facility employees, mentoring includes working with students who are pursuing healthcare management careers by lecturing classes and providing meaningful practicum or residency opportunities. Many for-profit long-term care facilities have established one-year residency programs for newly hired administrative employees. Working under a licensed administrator, the employee is rotated throughout the departments of the facility. Once the residency program is successfully completed, many of these employees become administrators of their "own" facilities.

Continuing education may be mandated to maintain certification or licensure, to maintain or enhance professional and technical skills, or to foster personal growth and development of employees. In most healthcare facilities, nurse education departments provide in-house continuing education in new techniques or review existing care and reinforce current nursing procedures.

Continuing education can be expensive. Given the limited financial resources available to nursing facilities and home health agencies, most continuing education for these nurses and paraprofessionals takes place in-house. Many long-term care professional associations and JCAHO have continuing education and training packages that facilities may use to develop their own in-house programs. Education in these facilities stresses such currently hot issues as confidentiality and privacy (HIPAA), infection control, medication errors, pain management, patient safety, and restraints and seclusion policies.

In allocating limited training/education resources, one may consider the level of the position; allow registration on a first-come, first-served basis; or limit off-site education to a maximum dollar reimbursement per annum. Off-site academic education may be subject to such limitations as after-the-fact reimbursement based on a minimum course grade, reimbursement for only job-related courses, attendance at an accredited program, or seeking an approved degree that supports the employee's current position. Requiring an employee to remain with the institution for a specified length of time after receiving tuition reimbursement has legal ramifications. Recent court rulings have allowed employees to leave an institution before completing required continuing employment. In these cases, the former employee was allowed to make a pro rata refund of tuition reimbursement to the facility (usually based on a three-year period following reimbursement). For example, if an employee terminated employment one year after receiving tuition reimbursement, the employee would owe two-thirds of the tuition reimbursement to the former employer.

Unlike hospitals, which have no licensing requirements for executive management, a unique requirement for nursing home administrators is the requirement to successfully pass a federal and state licensing examination before assuming the position of the chief executive officer. (*Note:* Some states also require assisted living facility administrators to be licensed to assume the position of chief executive officer.) Additionally, continuing education requirements must be met to maintain licensure. Each state has its own minimum requirements to qualify to "sit" for these examinations. Some states may require only a high school diploma or equivalent and passing four required post-secondary level courses (Illinois). Other states may require the minimum of a bachelor's degree in a specialized field of study and practical experience.

The National Association of Boards of Examiners of Long-Term Care Administrators (NAB) is responsible for administering the national licensing examination. The exam is based on five domains of practice: resident care and quality of life, human resources, finance, physical environment and atmosphere, and leadership and management.[33]

PERFORMANCE EVALUATION

Among the appraisal factors to be considered in evaluating a healthcare employee are clinical skills, resident/patient/family relationships, dependability and reliability, accuracy and appearance of work, productivity, teamwork and cooperation, utilization of time, supervision required, job knowledge, and initiative.

Because the long-term resident–staff relationship is so prevalent in nursing homes, the opinions of residents and their families may be appropriate in caregiver appraisal. Specific resident/family comments or letters should be given some (minor) weight in the appraisal process.

Observation of the certified nurse aide's performance by supervisors should be given major weight in the appraisal process. Such duties as general nursing care, resident personal care and appearance, interactions with residents and their families, and compliance with patient and facility safety standards should be criteria for evaluation.

Performance evaluation of home health aides is a more difficult task, as supervisors are usually not present during home health visits. Patient and family comments and satisfaction surveys should be given additional weight in evaluating these employees' performance.

Appraisal and reward systems are designed to measure the effectiveness of an employee's job performance, assess the employee's value in relation to the facility's total performance, and determine the appropriate reward as payment. It is this reward for performance that reinforces the behavior and provides the motivation for future performance or, conversely, that causes the employee to seek other employment opportunities.

Some managers tend to use performance appraisals as a management tool, rather than as a source of information. They may inflate ratings to boost the spirits of an employee who has been distracted by a personal problem, to avoid confrontation with a difficult employee, to get a difficult employee promoted out of their department, to hide department problems from senior officials who are reviewing the appraisals, or to encourage a marginal employee who has just begun to show some improvement. In the long-term care industry, positive evaluations may be given in an effort to retain the employee, as replacing him or her while facing severe personnel shortages could lead to below-minimum staffing levels and/or the occurrence of expensive overtime pay. Conversely, managers may reduce ratings to subdue a troublesome employee, to use fear as a motivation to improve performance, to encourage a problem employee to resign, or to create a record to justify an impending discharge.

Among future-oriented appraisal methods are self-appraisals, psychological appraisals, criteria appraisals (such as the JCAHO methods), and "management by objective" approaches.

Performance appraisals may also mete out punishment for policy or job performance violations. Disciplinary action should be like the penalty from touching a hot stove: with warning, immediate, consistent, and impersonal.

Discipline is management's action to enforce an organization's standards. It has two purposes:

- Preventive discipline is used to encourage employees to follow standards and rules, so that infractions are prevented.
- Corrective discipline follows a rule infraction and seeks to discourage further violations, so that future acts are in compliance with standards. Typical corrective action may be a penalty (e.g., warning or suspension without pay).

Most employers follow a policy of progressive discipline, in which stronger penalties are given for repeated offenses. The purpose of such a policy is to give an employee an opportunity to take corrective action before more serious penalties are applied. However, whenever discipline is given, it must be documented, documented, documented.

Some systems allow minor offenses to be removed from the record after one to three years, allowing employees to return to step 1. Specified critical offenses are usually exempted from progressive discipline, and employees are discharged immediately.

An example of a discipline policy by Manor Health Care includes three classifications of offenses: critical, major, and minor. Examples of critical offenses include the following:

- Loss or suspension of personal licensure
- Patient abuse or neglect
- Unauthorized copying of facility records, including patient/resident medical charts or violation of patient confidentiality standards
- Theft
- Threatening, intimidating, or coercing patients or others
- A felony conviction
- Physical assault on fellow employees anywhere on the facility's premises
- Omission or falsification of information on the employee's employment application or facility's records

Major offenses are violations of a lesser degree than critical offenses. They necessitate immediate disciplinary action in the form of at least a written warning and/or a suspension. A second violation within a one-year period would result in immediate termination of employment. Examples of major offenses may include the following:

- Refusal to work, without good reason, when needed in an emergency, disaster, or patient emergency, either on an unscheduled day or on overtime
- An act of national origin/ancestry or sexual harassment
- Smoking in restricted areas
- Soliciting monetary contributions or distributing non-work-related materials in patient/resident care areas
- Soliciting or accepting tips from residents or their families
- Use of inappropriate language

Minor offenses are normally small breaches of policy that can be simply corrected without serious disciplinary measures. Supervisors may verbally reprimand employees for minor violations, with an emphasis on correcting the behavior. Examples of minor offenses could include excessive break time, excessive excused absenteeism or tardiness, or failure to wear required uniforms or identification badges in the appropriate manner. A record of oral reprimands should be recorded on the employee's disciplinary record and placed in the employee's personnel file. Progressive discipline is warranted for repeated violations.[14]

Unfortunately, because many nursing facilities face major nursing shortages, an honest performance evaluation using developed criteria may end up being curtailed or modified, so as to "not rock the boat." With state and federal minimum staffing requirements, it may be better to have a marginally competent employee rather than to have no employee at all. A vacant position would then require mandatory overtime from existing personnel, the additional cost of purchasing hours from an external nurse staffing agency, or a possible violation of minimum staffing levels.

Additionally, a marginal employee with seniority may not have the "best" clinical or employee skills but may be much "loved" by residents and their families. The termination of such an employee could cause much consternation among residents and families and disrupt normal resident activities.

UNIONIZATION

A labor union is an organization of workers formed to further the social and economic interests of its members. Since the passage of the Wagner Act of 1935, workers have had the right to organize and to bargain collectively. Collective bargaining provides the vehicle by which management and workers' representatives attempt to reach mutual agreement on solving, and avoiding, problems relating to wages, hours, and other conditions of employment.

Approximately 20 million workers (13.5% of the workforce) in the United States belong to unions.[29] Although union membership has dropped sharply from past membership rates, there has been a growing trend in service industries to effectively lobby and organize workers. In healthcare, particular issues that have caused attempts at unionization and increases in union membership include job security, staffing levels, working conditions, quality of care, and wages.[34] According to Hospitals and Health Network (HHN), current RN union membership is 17%, and membership is projected to increase to 33% by the year 2006.[34]

"Perhaps the most visible and aggressive healthcare organizer is the Service Employees International Union, which claims to represent more healthcare workers than any other union. The group says its rolls include almost 100,000 nurses, both RNs and LPNs. That's second only to the state affiliates of the American Nurses Association, which have 200,000 members in collective bargaining units."[34] Currently, both unions are co-operating in organizing tactics throughout the United States. The Service Employees International Union has more than 600,000 healthcare members, including 15,000 physicians.

The healthcare sector is facing ever-more-challenging problems as federal government and managed care health insurance plans reduce payments to medical care providers. Workers may feel pressure from management to control costs, increase productivity, and work outside their traditional job descriptions. Because most nurses carry their own professional liability insurance, they are concerned about quality-of-care issues that may translate into potential liability issues from handling ever-increasing patient loads and working mandatory double shifts due to nursing shortages.

In 1995, there were four strikes by registered nurses. In 2000, there were ten such strikes. During the first six months of 2001, there were seven RN strikes.[35] One result from these strikes and labor unrest by nurses has been the introduction of mandated nurse–patient staffing ratios by certain states.

California is currently reviewing its legislation relating to mandatory nurse–patient staff ratios. The implementation of this law (on January 1, 2004) has caused numerous problems in staffing nurse units and financial problems for healthcare facilities. More than a dozen states have either enacted or proposed similar legislation. Some legislation requires the state to mandate minimum staff levels. Other states' proposed legislation allows nurses to decide needed minimum staffing levels. The American Nurses Association supports the concept of nurses deciding needed staffing levels. It wants other factors—for example, the number of support staff, patient acuity of illness, and physical layout and design—to be considered when determining staff levels. Additionally, some states (e.g., New Jersey) have enacted overtime limitations that have led to staffing shortages and financial deficits.

Factors affecting staff size and composition include licensing requirements, Medicare/Medicaid requirements, philosophy of care, labor union contracts, skills-level mix, task assignments, physical layout, labor-saving equipment, disposable supplies, availability of family members, teaching programs, and the use of volunteers.

Some unique labor laws are applicable only to healthcare organizations:

- *8/80 Rule (Back-to-Back Work Agreement).* Healthcare workers are paid overtime under this provision if they work more than 8 hours in one day or 80 hours in a two-week period. Therefore, an employee may work 10 days straight, take the next 4 days off, and receive no overtime pay. This rule may be modified if a labor union contract is in effect.
- *Companionship Service Exemption.* This U.S. Department of Labor ruling exempts workers in home care from overtime pay if the worker provides fellowship, care, and protection for persons who, because of their age or disability, are unable to care for themselves. Maids and other domestic-in-service employees are covered under overtime provisions of the Fair Labor Standards Act. This ruling has been affirmed in the 2004 overtime revisions.

The 1974 Health Care Amendments to the National Labor Relations Act (Taft-Hartley Act) were enacted to prevent or minimize work stoppages or strikes. The amendments require additional notification and negotiation periods:

- *Ninety-Day Notice Requirement.* In collective bargaining contracts involving healthcare institutions, any party desiring to terminate or modify the agreement must give a 90-day notice to the other party and a 60-day notice to the Federal Mediation and Conciliation Service (FMCS) before the contract expiration date. The requirement for other industries is a 60-day notice to the other party and a 30-day notice to the FMCS.
- *Mandatory Mediation.* Parties to a dispute in the healthcare industry can be required to participate in mediation if the FMCS director believes that a threatened or actual strike will "substantially interrupt the delivery of healthcare in the locality." The director may appoint a board of inquiry to investigate the dispute, stipulate the facts discovered, and issue nonbinding recommendations.

- *Ten-Day Strike Notice Requirement.* A labor union may conduct a strike or picket a healthcare facility only after it has given the employer a 10-day written notice specifying the exact date and time that such activity will commence. If notice is not given, the employees engaging in such actions may be terminated. This requirement is intended to give healthcare institutions time to arrange for continuity of patient care. A union is released from this obligation if a healthcare institution has abused the 10-day notice by hiring worker replacements for employees it believes may strike, or by taking extraordinary steps to stock up on frequently used supplies. There are no specific examples of what constitutes "preparatory steps" that would justify a union being released from this 10-day strike notice.
- *Conditions Retaining Neutral Status.* This ruling applies to secondary strikes. If another neutral institution accepts transfer patients from the facility being struck or supplies services and/or personnel to a struck institution, the neutral institution may not be picketed, and the union may not request that the neutral institution's employees show solidarity and strike their own facility.
- *Nonsolicitation Rules.* The National Labor Relations Board (NLRB) adopted regulations stating that employees may not be solicited during working hours. Union representatives may not leave labor/union organizing materials in patient areas, including patient/resident rooms and sitting rooms on patient floors. Solicitation can occur during nonwork hours or outside of patient care areas.[14 (pp. 240–241)]
- *Number of Bargaining Units.* On April 21, 1989, the NLRB enacted regulations outlining specific bargaining units for hospitals: physicians, registered nurses, other professionals, technicians, clerical, skilled maintenance, other nonprofessionals, and security. This ruling was upheld on appeal by the U.S. Supreme Court on April 23, 1991. Nursing homes and other long-term care facilities can limit their bargaining units to four distinct units: nursing, other professionals, clerical, and maintenance/nonprofessionals. (*Note:* This legislation defines hospitals as facilities with less than a 30-day average length of stay.)
- *U.S. Supreme Court Ruling (NLRB vs. Kentucky River Community Care Inc., May 29, 2001).* In a 5–4 decision, the court ruled that registered nurses who use independent judgment in directing employees are supervisors, thereby exempting these positions from inclusion in

the bargaining unit. Employees are deemed to be supervisors if they practice one of 12 functions: authority to hire, transfer, suspend, lay off, recall, promote, discharge, assign, reward, discipline, or direct other employees, or to adjust their grievances. This ruling, in effect, could consider all RNs to be supervisors, given that they may direct nurses' aides and licensed practical nurses in their duties. Another case currently under review may clarify this issue.

LEGAL AND REGULATORY ISSUES

The National Institute of Occupational Safety and Health (NIOSH) "Guidelines for Hospital Occupational Health and Safety Program Evaluation" requires hospitals (and long-term care facilities) to provide the following services: pre-placement physical examinations, periodic health assessment examinations, health and safety education, immunizations, care for illness and injury at work, health counseling, environmental control and surveillance, and a health and safety records system. NIOSH studies have reported the most common causes of healthcare injuries, in order of frequency, to be strains and sprains, back injuries, puncture wounds (from needle sticks), and abrasions and contusions.

The Centers for Disease Control and Prevention published AIDS guidelines in July 1991.[36] The guidelines include the following provisions:

• All healthcare workers should adhere to universal precautions.
• Healthcare workers who perform exposure-prone procedures should know their human immunodeficiency virus (HIV) and hepatitis B virus (HBV) status.
• Mandatory testing of healthcare workers is not recommended.
• The public health benefits of notifying patients who have had exposure-prone procedures performed by healthcare workers infected with HIV or HBV should be considered on a case-by-case basis.
• Healthcare workers who are infected with HIV/HBV should not perform exposure-prone procedures unless they have sought counsel from an expert review panel. The panel would advise the workers under what circumstances, if any, they may continue to perform these procedures. Such circumstances would include notifying a patient of

the worker's status before the patient undergoes the procedure, and exposure-prone procedures should be identified by medical/surgical/ dental organizations and institutions at which the procedures are performed.

Effective October 1991, the Illinois Department of Public Health (IDPH) requires that it learn the name and type of practice of a healthcare provider who has AIDS. If the type of practice involves invasive procedures, and the healthcare provider does or has performed invasive procedures, then the IDPH will perform a risk assessment to determine whether these procedures constitute exposure-prone invasive procedures and whether the practice involves any other potential risk of HIV transmission to patients. If either inquiry yields a positive result, then either the healthcare provider must notify his or her patients or the IDPH will make the notification. This Illinois AIDS notification law has been heavily litigated, based on confidentiality and discrimination statutes. Healthcare providers have been encouraged to document their consistent use of universal infection precautions and to be prepared to show what types of procedures they perform.

Effective January 1, 1992, the Illinois Drug Free Workplace Act (P.A. 86-1459) required employers with 25 or more employees that receive state grants of $5,000 or more per year to make a good-faith effort to maintain a drug-free workplace. (Medicaid payments constitute state contracts.) Federal legislation also requires all states to implement employer/employee drug programs that must be at least as stringent as the federal legislation. States are allowed to enact more stringent requirements.

Under the Illinois law, a statement must be published notifying employees that it is illegal to manufacture, distribute, dispense, possess, or use a controlled substance in the employer's workplace. The legislation also specifies the actions that will be taken against employees for violations of the act and tells employees they must notify the employer of any criminal drug conviction arising from a violation committed in the workplace, no later than five days after the conviction. Each employee must receive a copy of the statement, and the statement must be posted in a prominent spot in the facility.

Employers must establish a drug-free awareness program that informs employees about the dangers of drug abuse in the workplace; the employer's policy of maintaining a drug-free workplace; any available drug counseling, rehabilitation, and employee assistance programs; and penalties that may be imposed for drug violations.

If an employer receives notification of an employee's conviction for workplace drug incidents, it must notify the state Medicaid program within 10 days and impose a sanction on the convicted employee, up to and including termination, or requiring satisfactory participation in a drug abuse, assistance, or rehabilitation program. Employers must have a trained referral team available to assist employees.

If an employer violates the act, its state contract may be suspended or terminated. Employers violating the act may also be barred from entering into contracts with the State of Illinois for at least one year, but no more than five years.

Regulations Specific to Long-Term Care

As U.S. employers, long-term care facilities are required to meet both national and state labor laws. These industry-wide laws can be reviewed in any labor relations textbook. In addition, healthcare-specific laws and regulations apply to long-term care institutions. Following are brief discussions of some of these unique regulations. (Note that this list is not meant to be all-inclusive.)

The federal Older Americans Act requires the appointment of a long-term care ombudsman who will protect and promote the rights and quality of life for persons who reside in long-term care facilities. This key individual may be an employee of the facility or a regionally designated individual who is responsible for several facilities. This person serves as a resident advocate who protects resident/family rights, resolves complaints, provides information, and advocates for quality individual care plans.

Limited English proficiency (LEP) regulations require a provider that accepts patients covered by Medicare Part A, Medicaid, or S-CHIP to provide, at no cost, an interpreter during the encounter. They must also supply appropriate translated forms and post signs in appropriate languages that state LEP patients have a right to an interpreter and to translated forms. This requirement also applies to hearing-impaired patients/residents who need sign language interpretation. This legislation may influence recruitment criteria (requiring an applicant to be bilingual) or mean that a facility must conduct foreign-language classes for its existing employees.

Some states have enacted "English as the official language" legislation. Federal law overrules this state legislation in cases of medical/nursing care. Healthcare facilities and workers must continue to offer translation services and forms written in the most common languages of the service area community.

As mentioned earlier in this chapter, nursing home staffing notification became effective January 1, 2003. As a result of this regulation, nursing homes must publicly post the number of nursing staff on duty to care for patients on each daily shift. Licensed and unlicensed nursing staff include registered nurses, licensed practical nurses, and nurse aides. The sign must be at least 8.5 by 14 inches and printed in a font size large enough to be easily seen. The sign must be posted in a public area (preferably the lobby). This requirement may expose the facility to possible fines or punishment if actual (as posted) staffing does not meet minimum criteria. Additionally, if actual staffing does not meet the staffing levels stated on the sign, the facility may be fined or punished not only for failure to meet minimum criteria, but also for falsification of records.

On the state level, the Illinois Health Care Worker Background Check Act of 1996 applies to all individuals employed or retained by a healthcare employer as home healthcare aides, nursing aides, personal care representatives, private-duty nurse aides, student nurses, day-training personnel, or any similar health-related occupation. Those employees already licensed by the Department of Professional Regulation of the Department of Public Health (e.g., registered nurses) are not included in the act, but are covered under similar legislation. Effective January 1, 2006, Illinois House Bill 2531 requires healthcare facilities to initiate background checks for employees who have any contact with residents. Therefore, any employee who comes in contact with residents, including admission and business office personnel, maintenance workers, and laundry or dietary workers who deliver meals or linen to the units, is required to undergo a background check. This new law is part of the National Healthcare Background Check Pilot Project administered by the Center for Medicare and Medicaid Studies (CMS).

Federal legislation requires similar legislation in all states. A healthcare facility may not knowingly hire, employ, or retain any individual in a position with duties involving direct patient/resident care who has been convicted of committing or attempting to commit one or more prohibited offenses. Such prohibited offenses include first- or second-degree murder, involuntary manslaughter and reckless homicide, kidnapping, unlawful restraint, child abduction, assault (including domestic battery), criminal sexual assault, financial exploitation of an elderly or disabled person, retail theft, robbery, burglary, arson, or controlled substances abuse.

A facility must initiate a non-fingerprint-based criminal history record check pursuant to the Uniform Conviction Information Act (UCIA) whenever a conditional offer of employment is made to a healthcare applicant. Under the 2005 National Healthcare Background Check Pilot Project, administered by CMS, seven states (including Illinois) are required to conduct a fingerprint-based criminal history record check for all direct-care licensed and nonlicensed staff.

As a result of new specific legislation, the Vulnerable Adults Protection Act of 2005, the State of Illinois will now require that residents also undergo background checks that would identify registered sex offenders, criminal parolees, and those on probation or court-ordered supervision. This act requires the long-term care facility to identify, assess risk, develop a care plan, and establish treatment and discharge policies for violent offenders. Residents and their families must be informed of such individuals when they are admitted to the facility. This law amends the Illinois Nursing Home Care Act and the state's Code of Corrections.

The Worker Adjustment and Retraining Notification Act (WARN) became effective February 4, 1989. Employers with more than 100 employees must give an advance 60-day notice if more than 50% of the workforce will lose their jobs for 30 days or more. Notification is required if employees will suffer a six-month layoff or a 50% reduction in work time during six consecutive months. Employers that fail to give such notice can be forced to compensate workers for wages and benefits over the 60-day period in which the notice should have been given. Employers are also subject to civil penalties of $500 per day.

In this era of healthcare financial uncertainty, more than 100 hospitals, nursing homes, and home health agencies are closing their doors each year. Besides complying with the WARN Act, healthcare facilities are required by their states to provide prior closing notice to the State Public Department of Health. In Illinois, the facility must also obtain approval to discontinue services from the Illinois Health Facilities Planning Board. This Board requires the facility to submit a patient transfer and relocation plan, and to disclose where patient records, x-rays, and billing records will be stored, and how any hazardous waste (nuclear, medicine/gases) will be disposed of.

The Occupational Safety and Health Act (OSHA) details specific rules and regulations for healthcare organizations. It establishes safety and health standards for all organizations. Even if no specific standards have been issued, employers must provide employees with a safe place to work, free from recognized hazards that cause, or are likely to cause, serious physical harm or death.

Worker's compensation laws are intended to compensate for injuries and illnesses already received. OSHA laws provide no compensation, but rather are intended to prevent or remove hazardous conditions before they lead to injuries or illnesses. Worker's compensation laws use the threat of increased insurance premiums as an incentive for employers to improve job safety and health. By contrast, OSHA uses a system of standards, inspections, citations, and financial penalties to encourage compliance.

The concept of "equal pay for equal work" became law with the passage of the Equal Pay Act of 1963. This statute states that if jobs require equal skill, effort, and responsibility, and if working conditions are equal, then employers must pay men and women performing these jobs at the same rate. A healthcare industry example is the job classification of "aide" versus "orderly." Historically, women were classified as nurse aides and men were classified as orderlies. Orderlies were paid a higher salary than aides, even though both jobs required lifting and transferring patients. If both jobs require equal skill, effort, and responsibility, under equal working conditions, then persons of different sexes performing these jobs must be paid at the same rate unless the employer can establish that the differences in rates are based on a seniority system, merit program, measures of quality or quantity, or differentials in pay based on a factor other than sex.

In the aftermath of the September 11, 2001, terrorist attacks, employers must be aware of their legal obligations to military reservists. Many healthcare personnel who are members of active reserve units or who have an unfilled military obligation have been called to duty to serve in the Middle East. "Federal legislation passed in 1994 gives those who serve in the reserves the right to request re-employment once they return from military service up to a period of five years from their release date. In many cases, they must be given preferential hiring status. If their specific job is not available, they must receive preferential hiring status for a comparable position. If absent for less than 91 days, employees should be reemployed in the same position they held before they were called up."[37]

Employers must provide certain pension, health, and other benefits to those who are on military leave and to reemployed veterans. Workers covered by defined-benefit pension plans must be credited for the time they were on military service. For any vesting purposes, it is as if they never left.

"Federal law does not require an employer to pay an employee's salary while he/she is on military leave. In some cases, if a worker is on leave for less than a week, employers may be required to continue paying his/her salary. Employees must give advance notice of their military call-up unless circumstances make it impossible."[37]

CONCLUSION

The future of U.S. health care is dependent on the healthcare workforce. As part of the national, state, local, and facility planning processes, all of these entities must review the composition of the current healthcare workforce, academic and technical training of the future workforce, competition for healthcare workers within and from outside the industry, and technology demands and changes that will influence the delivery of health care in the United States.

Human resources management problems in the nursing home and home healthcare industries will not be solved in the short run. Some factors that will negatively affect the future of the continuum of care process are as follows:

- An aging U.S. population, which will require more long-term health care
- The rapid growth of the elderly population as the baby boomer population ages
- A longer life expectancy, which means health care will be needed for a greater number of years
- A shrinking birth rate, which will reduce the number of future healthcare employees
- Immigration restrictions, which will reduce the number of current and potential healthcare employees
- An aging nurse workforce, which will reduce the number of nurses in the profession as they retire
- Fewer individuals entering the nursing profession

During his second term, President George W. Bush and the U.S. Congress will attempt to address the issue of the aging of the U.S. population and its effects on the Social Security system. Along with this endeavor, the federal government, state and local entities, and the healthcare industry itself need to make greater efforts to address the long-term healthcare issues of this population, including the question, "Who will take care of this segment of the population?" This population is our grandparents, parents, and ourselves. The clock is ticking.

REFERENCES

1. American Health Care Association. United States Nursing Facilities, 2001 and 2002. Available at: www.ahca.org. Accessed November 23, 2004.
2. Pratt JR. *Long-Term Care: Managing Across the Continuum*. Second Edition. Sudbury, MA: Jones and Bartlett Publishers; 2004.
3. National Center for Health Statistics. NCHS—Publications and Information Products—The National Nursing Home Survey—1999. 1999. Available at: www.cdc.gov/mchs/data/. Accessed December 15, 2004.
4. American Health Care Association. United States Nursing Facilities (OSCAR Data). 2004. Available at: www.ahca.org. Accessed November 23, 2004.
5. National Center for Health Statistics. National Home and Hospice Care Survey—2000. 2000. Available at: www.cdc.gov/nchs/data/. Accessed December 24, 2004.
6. U.S. Department of Labor, Bureau of Labor Statistics. Occupational Employment and Wages, November 2003. 2004. Available at: www.bls.gov. Accessed December 17, 2004.
7. National Association of Home Care. Home Care and Hospice Staff Productivity. 2001. Available at: www.nahc.org. Accessed December 30, 2004.
8. Center for Medicare and Medicaid Services. Report to Congress: Appropriateness of Minimum Nurse Staffing Ratios in Nursing Homes. Phase II Final Report. 2001. Available at: www.cms.hhs.gov/medicaid/reports/default.asp?. Accessed December 17, 2004.
9. Nursing Home Statistics—AHCA. Available at: www.efmoody.com/longterm/nursingstatisics.html. Accessed July 28, 2004.
10. U.S. General Accounting Office. *Nursing Homes: Quality of Care More Related to Staffing Than Spending* (GAO-02-431R). Washington, DC: 2002.
11. National Association of Home Care. Facts & Stats. 1997. Available at: www.nahc/Research/research.html. Accessed December 30, 2004.
12. U.S. Department of Labor, Bureau of Labor Statistics. The 10 Fastest Growing Occupations, 2002–2012. Available at: www.bls.gov. Accessed December 17, 2004.
13. Lombardi DN. *Handbook of Personnel Selection and Performance Evaluation in Healthcare*. San Francisco: Jossey-Bass; 1998.

14. Cirn JT, Gellatly DL. *Long-Term Care Human Resources Management: The Personnel Touch.* Arlington, VA: Association of University Programs in Health Administration; 1989.
15. Bernard Hodes Group. Health Care Metrics Survey—National Sample. 2003. Available at: www.hodes.com. Accessed December 28, 2004.
16. Internal Revenue Service. Form SS-8: Determination of Worker Status for Purposes of Federal Employment Taxes and Income Tax Withholding. Available at: www.irs.gov. Accessed December 28, 2004.
17. Hart KA, Christmas K. International Nurse Recruitment: Issues and Answers. Bernard Hodes Group. 2002. Available at: www.hodes.com. Accessed December 28, 2004.
18. American Association of Colleges of Nursing. 2002 Healthcare Workforce Survey. 2002. Available at: www.aacn.nche.edu/Media/Survey/NursingShortage. Accessed December 4, 2004.
19. Recruitment Trends within Health Care Professions. 2000. Available at: www.medimorphus.com. Accessed January 7, 2002.
20. Standard and Poors Public Finance. Shortage of Nurses in the U.S. Could Have Long-Term Adverse Effects. 2001. Available at: www.standardpoors.com. Accessed August 30, 2004.
21. Fitch Ratings Ltd. 2004 Industry Outlook for Nonprofit Continuing Care Retirement Communities and Nursing Homes. 2004. Available at: www.fitchratings.com. Accessed November 23, 2004.
22. National Council of State Boards of Nursing (NCSBN). Quarterly Examination Statistics. Available at: www.ncsbn.org/pdfs/NCLEX_fact_sheet.pdf. Accessed December 28, 2004.
23. American Association of Colleges of Nursing. Nursing Shortage Fact Sheet. 2004. Available at: www.aacn.nche.edu/Media/Factsheets/NursingShortage. Accessed December 4, 2004.
24. U.S. General Accounting Office. *Nursing Workforce: Emerging Nurse Shortages Due to Multiple Factors* (GAO-01-944). Washington, DC: July 2001.
25. Buerhaus PI, Staiger DO, Auerback DI. Implications of an aging registered nurse force. *Journal of the American Medical Association.* 2000; 283:2948–2954.
26. Fitch Ratings Ltd. Nursing Shortage Update. 2003. Available at: www.fitchratings.com. Accessed November 23, 2004.
27. American Health Care Association. The 2002 AHCA Nursing Position Vacancy and Turnover Survey. 2002. Available at: www.ahca.org. Accessed December 4, 2004.
28. U.S. Department of Labor, Bureau of Labor Statistics. Occupational Employment Statistics (OES) Survey. 2004. Available at: www.bls.gov. Accessed December 17, 2004.
29. U.S. Department of Labor, Bureau of Labor Statistics. November 2003 National Occupational Employment and Wage Estimates. Available at: www.bls.gov. Accessed December 17, 2004.

30. U.S. Department of Labor, Employment Standards Administration, Wage and Hour Division. FairPay Fact Sheets by Occupation Under the Fair Labor Standards Act (FLSA): Fact Sheet 17N: Nurses and the Part 541 Exemptions Under the Fair Labor Standards Act (FLSA). 2004. Available at: www.dol.gov/esa/regs/compliance/whd/fairpay/fairpayprintpage.asp?REF=fsl7n _nu. Accessed September 10, 2004.

31. McCoy K, Appleby J. Problems with staffing, training can cost lives. *USA Today.* May 26, 2004:1, 3B.

32. American College of Healthcare Executives. Responsibility for Mentoring. 1999. Available at: www.ache.org. Accessed August 30, 2004.

33. National Association of Boards of Examiners of Long Term Care Administrators. Nursing Home Administrator Licensing Examination. 2004. Available at: www.nabweb.org/home/default/aspx. Accessed December 10, 2004.

34. Hospital and Health Networks. Workforce. 1998. Available at: www.hospitalconnect.com. Accessed December 17, 2004.

35. American Nurses Association. Strike Statistics. United American Nurses, AFL-CIO. 2004. Available at: www.ana.org/uan. Accessed December 17, 2004.

36. National Institute of Occupational Safety and Health. Updated U.S. Public Health Service Guidelines for the Management of Occupational Exposures to HBV, HCV, and HIV and Recommendations for Postexposure Prophylaxis. 2001. Available at: www.cdc.gov/niosh/topics/bbp/. Accessed December 17, 2004.

37. Murphy T. Reservists Have Job Rights. September 25, 2001. Available at: www.cnn.com/2001/business. Accessed December 17, 2004.

CHAPTER 10

Human Resources Management in Community Health Centers

Gretchen Gemeinhardt

VIGNETTE

Northeast Community Health Clinic (NCHC) is a brand-new, federally qualified health center (FQHC) that will provide primary care to individuals in northeast Houston. This area has been designated as a medically underserved area (MUA), as well as a health professional shortage area (HPSA), with access to primary and other healthcare services currently being somewhere between minimal and nonexistent. NCHC's mission is "to provide primary and preventive healthcare services to improve the health of underserved and vulnerable populations." The newly formed board of directors consists of more than 51% consumers from the service area and others with business and historical ties to the area. Among other professions, they represent small businesses, social services, healthcare services, and education. Most board members live or work in the target area.

The board members have been responsible for providing leadership and developing policies and procedures pursuant to the Bureau of Primary Health Care guidelines for FQHCs. They are looking forward to the opening of the clinic. A full-time physician is currently being recruited by the NCHC board, and several others are under consideration. The board members understand their role as primarily providing fiduciary and programmatic oversight and realize that it is time to think about hiring a clinic director. In thinking about what kind of person they need to hire for the director position, they have given some thought to the human resources challenges that any community health center director might face.

This chapter provides NCHC's board of directors and other readers with background and approaches for addressing human resource challenges in community health centers. After providing an overview of the health center setting, we discuss such human resources issues as staffing, employment, retention, compensation and benefits, performance evaluation, safety training and education, and legal and regulatory issues.

OVERVIEW OF THE SETTING

Originally known as neighborhood health centers and now known as federally qualified health centers (FQHCs), community health centers are local, nonprofit, or public healthcare providers serving low-income and medically underserved communities. For nearly 40 years, FQHCs have provided high-quality, affordable primary and preventive care services. Today, there are 1,000 FHQCs, with 5,000 sites located in all 50 states, Puerto Rico, the District of Columbia, the U.S. Virgin Islands, and Guam. About half of health center patients reside in rural areas; the others live in economically depressed urban areas. These centers are located in areas where care is needed but scarce, and services are provided regardless of individuals' ability to pay or insurance status. In addition to medical care, many community health centers provide on-site dental, mental health, and substance abuse services and pharmacy.

To receive funding, community health centers must meet certain statutory requirements:

- They must be located in a federally designated medically under-served area (MUA) or serve a federally designated medically under-served population (MUP).
- They must have nonprofit, public, or tax-exempt status.
- They must offer services to all ages and all populations, regardless of patients' ability to pay, and offer a sliding fee scale for clients.
- They must provide comprehensive primary healthcare services, referrals, and other services needed to facilitate access to care, such as case management, translation, and transportation.
- They must remain open at least 32 hours per week, with provisions for emergency coverage.
- They must have a governing board, the majority of whom are patients of the health center.[1]

The requirement that a majority of the board members be health center patients makes these clinics unique (Table 10-1).[2] This requirement is

---

Table 10-1 Health Center Boards: Federal Requirements

- The board must have at least 9 members, but no more than 25 members.
- At least 51% of the board's members must be users of the health center.
- Half of the remaining members of the board (49% or less) cannot earn more than 10% of their income from the healthcare industry.
- The remaining members of the board (49% or less) must represent the area served by the center and have expertise in community affairs; federal, state, and local government; accounting; health administration; health professions; business; finance; banking; legal affairs; trade unions; insurance; and personnel management, as well as social services, such as religion, education, and welfare.
- Board members must reasonably represent the individuals served by the health center in terms of demographic factors:
  - Ethnicity
  - Race
  - Sex
  - Migrant/seasonal farmworker
- Employees of the center and their spouses, children, parents, or brothers or sisters (blood or marriage) cannot be members of the board.

Source: U.S. Department of Health and Human Services, Health Resources and Services Administration, Bureau of Primary Health Care. *Governing Board Handbook.* Bethesda, MD: 2000:40.

designed to ensure that the centers remain responsive to community needs. It can prove challenging to develop and maintain this board composition in high-need, underserved communities. The requirement generally prevents health centers from being part of a larger enterprise, such as a hospital, local government, or religious order. Health centers that exclusively serve migrants or homeless patients do not have to meet the majority consumer board requirement.

Health centers are staffed by a combination of clinical and administrative personnel (Table 10-2).[3] Typically, they are managed by a chief executive officer or program director, chief financial officer, chief information officer, and clinical director. The functions associated with these positions may be combined or performed by more than one individual. Depending on the size of the patient population, the clinical staff consists of a mixture of primary care physicians, nurse practitioners, physician assistants, nurses, and substance abuse and mental health specialists. Another

Table 10-2 Health Center Staff and Related Patient Visits

	Full-Time Equivalents	Patient Visits
Primary care physicians	6,487.6	25,325,866
NPs/PAs/CNMs	3,693.1	10,414,386
Nurses	8,075.5	3,091,731
Dentists	1,586.5	4,365,671
Dental hygienists	547.8	760,986
Mental health and substance abuse specialists*	2,548.0	2,732,571
Pharmacy	1,633.7	N.A.
Total Enabling Services†	8,575.0	3,842,581
Other Staff‡	50,541.0	N.A.
Total	**83,688.2**	**52,323,834**

*Includes psychiatrists, psychologists, and licensed or credentialed behavioral health providers.
†Includes health educators, case managers, translators, transportation, and eligibility workers, among others. Not all staff has related patient visits. Does not include workers for other social services, such as WIC, Head Start, housing assistance, food banks, and employment counselors.
‡Includes specialists and other medical, dental, and professional personnel, as well as administrative, patient services, and other staff.
Source: National Association of Community Health Centers, Inc. *Health Center Fact Sheet United States, 2004.*

unique aspect of the community health center is that physicians are employees of the organization.

Community health centers face unprecedented challenges as public funding sources decrease while the demand for care from a growing indigent population increases. To support this shift organizationally, clinic administrators must figure out how to recruit and retain well-qualified staff in all areas of clinic operations. Steps to meet this challenge include the following:

- Ensuring that salary levels are competitive through periodic review
- Developing training opportunities and incentives for employee skill enhancement
- Developing systems for recognizing and rewarding productivity of all employees
- Implementing training programs for all employees, including in-service and specialty workshops

In the labor-intensive delivery of healthcare services, the effective management of human resources assumes considerable importance. Management of human resources encompasses many functions, the extent of which depends on the size and scale of the health center and whether it is a stand-alone operation or part of a larger system of healthcare delivery. However, a number of human resources functions are common to all community health centers:

- Recruiting, selecting, and training employees
- Maintaining records to meet legal requirements of employment
- Developing procedures and policies related to work performance and evaluation
- Establishing equitable compensation and fringe benefits
- Monitoring and administering employee health and safety standards
- Formalizing grievance procedures to resolve conflicts

STAFFING

Clinical staffing patterns vary among community health centers. All staffing arrangements are designed to lead to the desired outcomes of availability, accessibility, quality, comprehensiveness, and coordination of services for health center patients. Generally, FQHCs maintain a staffing level that allows for between 4,200 and 6,000 visits per year for each full-time equivalent (FTE) healthcare provider. The federal guidelines recommend a physician-to-patient ratio of 1:1,500 and a midlevel practitioner-to-patient ratio of 1:750.[4] Physician staff should be board certified or residency trained. Other clinicians, such as nurses, nurse practitioners, and physician assistants, also need to be licensed and certified as appropriate under state law.

The individual job is the starting point in managing the employee. Each employee's job must be completely described, specified, and analyzed, and its role in the organization must be clarified.

Job Description

The job description is a statement providing an overview of the job and its relationship to the organization. The essential functions of all positions should be clearly laid out in health centers' job descriptions. For example, the description of a medical records clerk position would include a title, summary statement of the job, list of specific duties, and delineation of the limits of authority and responsibility. The format of the description should be standardized for all positions. Many job descriptions also include a "catch-all" phrase that allows modification of the descriptions as necessary. Although health centers are not legally obligated to develop comprehensive job descriptions, job descriptions are a good risk management tool because, when properly developed, they define the health center's expectations and may prevent any subsequent disagreements about job responsibilities. Health centers should regularly review their job descriptions to ensure that they accurately reflect the center's positions and that they comply with the ever-changing judicial or EEOC interpretations of the requirements under the Americans with Disabilities Act (ADA).[5]

Job Specification

The job specification carries the job description one step further by outlining the required qualifications for the job. Generally, job specifications include the following elements:

- Education and technical qualifications
- Experience levels required
- Responsibility limits, including authority to make decisions and organizational accountability

- Physical effort, including dexterity, special skills, and degree of effort required
- Mental effort, including level of initiative required
- Number of employees directly managed
- Chain of command, including an outline of relationships with other functions or departments

Job Analysis

Job analysis takes the description and specification yet another step by providing a factoring or ranking system that assigns values to each of the specification categories. The total value over all categories provides a weight that is useful in comparing jobs on the basis of responsibility and performance. Job analysis can also provide a system of measurement to assist in establishing performance standards for productivity. Such analysis can be conducted by existing staff or outside consultants.

THE EMPLOYMENT PROCESS

The employment process involves recruitment, employment applications, interviewing, reference checks, hiring, credentialing, advancement and promotion, and separation. Each of these aspects of employment is addressed next.

Recruitment and Selection

The recruitment process consists of interrelated steps aimed at attracting qualified primary care professionals to practice and support staff to work at a community health center. While the principles of recruitment are the same for both professionals and nonprofessionals, there are some particular challenges that health centers face in recruiting professional staff, because they are often located in areas that healthcare professionals might not find attractive. Additionally, community health centers are perceived as having poor working conditions and inadequate salaries, and working with the populations served by community health centers is not respected by many in the medical profession.

Recruiting can be costly. The Rural Physician Recruitment Survey Report estimates that the majority of private recruitment efforts cost approximately $10,000 per physician practitioner recruited.[6] Therefore, community health centers need to have a recruiting budget that will support the cost of staff time involved in recruitment efforts, advertising costs, and site visits. It may also be necessary for health centers to retain the services of a professional recruitment company, so the recruiting budget needs to cover that firm's fees.

A number of sources may be utilized to recruit professional and nonprofessional staff. Employee recruitment can take the form of advertising in the local newspaper, on Internet job boards, or in professional journals. Professional associations should be contacted, as they are an excellent source for primary care professional recruitment and cover a variety of disciplines, including physicians, physician assistants, nurse practitioners, certified nurse-midwives, dentists, dental hygienists, psychiatrists, clinical psychologists, licensed clinical social workers, licensed professional counselors, marriage and family therapists, and psychiatric nurse specialists. Search firms can also be retained. In addition, local colleges and universities can be useful sources of recruits. The types of staff positions that health centers are trying to fill influence how searches are conducted in terms of the recruiting methods used and the extensiveness of the search undertaken. Using multiple sources for recruitment is probably best, but organizations need to consider the costs associated with each of these sources. A longer-term recruitment strategy that has worked for many community health centers has been to send a clinic employee for physician assistant or nurse practitioner training.[6] Also, the National Health Services Corp Scholarship Program (Table 10-3) offers federal support-for-service in training to become a physician, dentist, nurse practitioner, or physician assistant.[7] Table 10-4 details how physicians themselves search for jobs.[8]

The communities that have had the most success in attracting healthcare professionals to their facilities have concentrated their recruitment efforts on the following types of candidates:

- Practicing primary care practitioners who currently reside in or come from the area or a similar environment
- Students originally from the area or a similar environment
- Seasoned or retired professionals
- Practitioners who do not want to assume the financial responsibility of a private practice
- Nurse practitioners and physicians assistants in training who are seeking clinical rotations

Table 10-3 National Health Services Corps Program

The National Health Services Corps (NHSC) has a number of programs that support the goal of recruiting and retaining healthcare professionals to serve in a health professional shortage area (HPSA).

- *NHSC Scholarship Program.* Students pursuing primary care careers as allopathic/osteopathic physicians, nurse practitioners, physician assistants, certified nurse-midwives, and dentists receive tuition, fees, and monthly stipends for up to four years. They must serve one year for every year of financial support received, with a two-year service minimum.

- *NHSC Loan Repayment Program.* The loan repayment program targets already-trained health professionals. It is open to allopathic/osteopathic physicians, nurse practitioners, physician assistants, certified nurse-midwives, dentists, dental hygienists, and mental health professionals, including psychiatrists, health service psychologists, clinical social workers, licensed professional counselors, marriage and family therapists, psychiatrists, and psychiatric nurse specialists. In exchange for a two-year minimum commitment to serve in a federally designated HPSA, the NHSC will assist in the repayment of educational loans.

Source: Taylor J. *The Fundamentals of Community Health Centers.* National Health Policy Forum; 2004.

- NHSC Scholars and/or those interested in the NHSC Loan Repayment Program[6]

Employment Applications

Employment application forms completed by job applicants serve as an initial employee record. The application form is an objective screening tool in that it permits the health center administrator to determine whether the applicant possesses the skills and background needed to perform the job. Application forms should include questions on personal

Table 10-4 How Physicians Search For Jobs

Sources of Job Leads	Frequency of Use
Personal and professional referrals	50%
Physician recruiters	43%
Online job sites	42%
Ads in print journals	40%
Mailings to physicians	34%

Source: Williams G. NAS Insights: Physician Recruitment Report. 2005. Available at: http://www.nasrecruitment.com/MicroSites/Healthcare/Articles. Accessed October 22, 2005.

data, experience, education, previous employment, and references. It is important to remember that laws determine the type of questions that employers may and may not ask on application forms. Questions relating to race, color, religion, national origin, age, disabilities, or marital status are usually illegal.

Interviewing

The opportunity to meet a job applicant face to face is a critically important aspect of the hiring process. To be an effective tool, interviewers need to be knowledgeable about the position and its requirements, so that they can gather information that will allow them to form a complete picture of the applicant and his or her appropriateness for the position. Having a carefully tailored standard set of interview questions for each vacant position will help the hiring manager to compare the strengths and weaknesses of each job applicant. A standard set of questions will also give the interviewer little opportunity to stray off course, thereby ensuring that the interview serves the health center's objectives and complies with employment discrimination laws. While some questions should not be asked during an interview, it is perfectly permissible to ask these questions after an offer of employment is made.

Reference Checks

Reference checking is an important part of the employment process. Telephone reference checks are far more reliable than written letters of reference, but it is important to ask similar questions for all telephone reference checks. Questions should be asked about the applicant's strengths and weaknesses and his or her reason for leaving the employment of the reference. It is useful to ask if the reference would rehire the applicant. The applicant should provide written permission for reference checking. Federal credit laws place restrictions on the scope of questions that can be raised, and the manager should review these limitations with an attorney to assure conformance with the law.

Hiring

Hiring constitutes employer commitment, and the commitment should spell out clearly the new employee's compensation and benefits and the employer's methods and timing of performance evaluation. Typically, a verbal offer will be quickly followed by a written offer of employment.

One of the biggest mistakes made by many centers is failure to clearly define their offers. The offer, which may be discussed and a number of items negotiated, needs to specify the terms of employment, length of employment, financial agreements, fringe benefits, and relocation support.

Most organizations have a probationary period during which the employee can be terminated for noncompatibility or inadequate performance. It is usually easier to terminate an employee during the probationary period than after the conclusion of probation.

Adequate orientation of the new employee is a critical aspect of hiring. Studies of turnover rates indicate that a large number of separations occur shortly after employment, due to the false representation of the position or poor orientation into an organization. A well-planned orientation is designed to help an individual feel welcome, less apprehensive, and more knowledgeable about the new environment and his or her position. In smaller organizations, orientation is often based on a buddy system, in which the new employee is assigned to a senior employee for orientation and training. Supervisors should oversee orientation to assure that good work habits are established. In larger organizations, the human resources department may provide formal sessions at which policies and procedures are reviewed in detail. Such sessions also cover the history, mission, and organization of the clinic; benefits; vacation and sick time; and other appropriate information.

The length of time it takes to orient a new healthcare provider will depend both on the position within the organization and on the individual. In the case of an existing facility, an effective orientation period may range from two to three months. In the case of a solo practitioner, it will probably take three to six months before the new person's practice actually affects the health of the community.

Credentialing of Clinical Staff

Health centers need to have defined standards for assessing the training, experience, and competence of their clinical staff so as to assure the clinicians' ability to qualify for hospital privileges and payer credentialing. This process needs to include a review of the individual's original credentials when a practitioner joins the staff, as well as recertification and/or reappointment. In the initial credentialing process, centers want to verify that the practitioner has a current license to practice and clinical privileges in good standing at any hospital where the clinician has admission privileges.

In addition, practitioners need to show current, adequate malpractice insurance and professional liability claims history. Generally, the credentialing process includes querying the National Practitioner Data Bank and verifying education and licenses. Credentialing and privileges processes need to meet the standards of national accrediting agencies, such as the Joint Commission on Accreditation of Healthcare Organizations (JCAHO) and Accreditation Association for Ambulatory Health Care (AAAHC).

RETENTION

Promotion and Job Changes

Adequate record keeping and a clear understanding of employee work performance are important for advancement and promotion decisions, particularly when comparisons are made between existing employees and applicants from outside the organization. Employees who exhibit initiative and demonstrate growth potential should be monitored and provided with opportunities for advancement.

Empowering Health Center Staff

The inability to empower staff plagues more organizations than community health centers, but the administrator of one community health center in a large metropolitan area believes the ability to empower staff is among its greatest challenges.[9] A large health center with more than 40,000 patient encounters per year, this facility experiences bureaucratic quagmires that directly result from the healthcare system's traditional top-down hierarchical system.

Barriers to staff empowerment often result from organizational beliefs regarding authority and status. If the organizational culture views authority and power—as opposed to expertise and ability—as the motivation to accomplish the goals and objectives of the organization, empowerment of employees is not possible.

Not only must the organization's culture support and encourage empowerment, but employees must have the desire to assume more responsibility and implement critical thinking skills. Thinking "outside the box" and making independent decisions are not skills commonly expected from nursing and ancillary staff. To support staff taking initiative and being creative, management must commit to an empowerment philosophy. This commitment requires enthusiasm, time, imagination, and resources.

Empowering staff has become a major goal for this community health center.[9] Paul Shank, administrator at Strawberry Health Center, believes that his staff has much to contribute and has set up his organization so as to empower his staff. He has divided the center into pods, with each pod having its own team leader. Team leaders have complete responsibility for managing the day-to-day operations of their pods. This scheme has freed the physicians, who did not necessarily have the business and interpersonal skills needed to operate successful centers, from operational responsibilities. The team leader structure has allowed the physicians to focus on their area of expertise, which is treating patients. In addition, the center uses its monthly in-service training days to discuss opportunities for process and operations improvement. Morale, cooperation, and communication have increased as a direct result of the in-service training days.

Procedures for changing from one job to another within the organization should be developed carefully. Lateral transfers can sometimes solve problems of incompatibility between employees in a particular area. At other times, an employee may request a lateral transfer because the change in work is perceived as a promotion. For example, a change from the records department to the front office might be perceived in this way. Such transfers can work to everyone's advantage. However, if transfers encourage the best employees of a department to leave for other positions within the clinic, then the message sent to remaining employees can be misinterpreted. Job enrichment is important, but reasons for transfers should be clearly understood. Care should also be taken not to transfer an employee who is a proven poor performer. Chances are high that the poor performance will be repeated in the new department.

Separation

Administrators and supervisors must have the courage to take action when separation is required. Whenever an employee is placed on probation, it is essential that a decision be made at the end of the probationary period whether to terminate the employee, extend the probation, or remove the employee from probation. The separation process for an employee who is past the probationary stage must be handled more carefully than that for an employee who is in the probationary period. Personnel records should clearly document meetings held with an employee who is not performing up to expectations. Such documentation should refer specifically to the employee's deficiencies, and the employee should acknowledge in writing that the problems were discussed. Documentation of a problem with no proof of what was discussed with the employee has little or no value.

Firing an employee is not only an unpleasant task, but can potentially be a legal minefield. If it is not done correctly, a wrongful termination lawsuit could result. The health center's personnel policies will be the backbone of its defense in such cases. Two approaches are possible: at-will statements and just-cause proof. If the health center is an at-will employer, an employee can be dismissed at any time for any reason. There should be no problem terminating an employee, whether it is his or her first or fifth offense. Conversely, if the health center operates in a state that does not recognize at-will statements, the health center must prove just cause for firing the employee. In this scenario, it will have to rely on documentation to prove that the staff member was fired for a valid reason.

It is good business practice to have all departing staff members leave with a sense of pride. Meeting with the departing person says that the organization has noticed his or her departure. Departing employees have high visibility, because the rest of the staff are watching how they are treated. An organization wishing to impress on its staff members that it cares about them should implement a policy such as the exit interview.

Reasons that employees voluntarily leave an organization can be determined with exit interviews. Employees may be reluctant to state their real reasons for leaving (perhaps out of fear of jeopardizing future references), so probing questions may be needed. While the median tenure of primary care physicians in community health centers is three years,[10] inadequate salary is not a primary reason for leaving. Instead, physicians and dentists cite dissatisfaction with job security and professional autonomy and lack of cooperation among major healthcare providers[11, 12] and poor relationships with administrators as reasons for leaving.[13]

Impact of Losing a Physician

All health center staff play a role in physician retention, and losing a physician can have an enormous impact on the center, both financially as well as personally for staff, board members, and patients.[14]

Loss of Patients and Revenues
Although studies that estimate the specific economic losses to health centers have not been reported, corporations estimate that losing an executive costs

two to four times the individual's salary. The cost of replacing a physician, including the search, screening, and interview processes, is estimated to be $60,000. A signing bonus, moving expenses, and promotion costs are additional expenses that are part of turnover.

In addition, there is a phase-out period during which the departing physician is terminating his or her care of patients. Some of these patients may choose to seek care elsewhere, and the center may see a reduction in users. During the recruitment period, the health center may have to retain a locum tenens physician at an estimated cost of $600 to $900 per day plus expenses. Other costs may include a loss of revenues as a result of reduced productivity of a new physician. In total, the financial loss associated with losing a physician may be estimated at between $150,000 and $300,000, depending on the physician's length of the search and the amount of lost revenues to the center.

Loss to the Community

Less quantifiable losses are also associated with a physician's departure. For example, the community may tend to view the health center as having "transient physicians"—an image that is not especially positive. Also, given that most Americans view themselves as having a relationship with their personal physicians as opposed to an entity such as a clinic or health center, the loss of a physician can disrupt stable physician–patient relationships.

Loss to Health Center Staff

The loss of a physician can also negatively affect the morale of the health center staff. Because quality care to the center's patients is provided by a team of caregivers, the exit of a critical member of that team can be a grievous loss. In addition, staff members may be anxious about the possibility of not finding a replacement physician and the subsequent effects on the health center's financial status and their own job security. Staff may also be anxious about how the replacement physician will relate to the current provider team. Will a new provider make changes in the way the team has traditionally functioned?

Loss to the Board of Directors

Health center boards may likewise feel abandoned when a physician leaves. Given that the board may not be aware of the reasons for a physician leaving the center, an exit interview by the board or with select board members may help the board gain a better understanding of physician retention issues at the center.

Source: Wilhide S. *Physician Retention in Community Health Centers.* National Association of Community Health Centers; 2004.

Turnover rates should be monitored as an early warning sign of organizational or supervisory problems. It must be kept in mind, however, that turnover rates also reflect the economy. A recession, for example, tends to reduce the rate of turnover.

COMPENSATION AND BENEFITS

The level of compensation and the duties associated with the position are closely related. Likewise, the qualifications of the employee are important considerations for determining compensation. Ideally, compensation levels and qualifications will have a close relationship. Placing an overly qualified applicant in a position that is viewed by the employee as unreasonably low in stature contributes to unnecessary turnover. Clarification of duties and responsibilities assigned to a particular position in the organization is therefore important.

Compensation

Factors affecting compensation include the rate of compensation in the marketplace, the relationship between supervisors and employees in the center, and assessments of employee capabilities. In terms of the marketplace, the level of compensation should be similar to that offered by other organizations for similar jobs. Typically, community health centers pay below-market rates. Data from the National Association of Community Health Centers suggest that primary care physicians who work in rural community health centers earn perhaps 9% to 12% less than similar doctors do nationally.[15] Staff cannot be expected to be compensated significantly less than their colleagues, especially given that health centers are taking care of some of the most difficult patients in our society. Salary surveys should be undertaken frequently to delineate equitable compensation ranges. In addition, the salary ranges for a particular position should relate to the health center's internal job structures. Ideally, jobs carrying the same level of responsibility should receive equivalent compensation. Even under the most rational compensation system, however, exceptions may be necessary to attract or retain employees who are particularly skilled or to recruit replacements for hard-to-fill positions.

Compensation relationships between supervisors and employee staff must also be considered when making compensation decisions. At times, supervisors working on a straight monthly salary may be at a salary disadvantage, if hourly workers in the same department receive higher pay because they work overtime hours at premium rates. Such factors should be considered in revising salary ranges.

More-capable employees may be paid better in recognition of the higher quality of their work. In such cases, evaluation systems used to set pay ranges must be understood by employees. Otherwise, differences in pay may be interpreted as favoritism or special privilege, which may lead to dissension among employees. Although systems oriented toward merit or incentive pay for special performance are highly desirable, they are difficult to implement and maintain in a community health center. For example, in evaluating a nurse aide who is responsible to a specific physician, the evaluation may be heavily weighted by the physician's personal opinion of the employee. The evaluation may include such statements as "best nurse aide I ever had" or "worth more than anyone else in the clinic."

An inability to evaluate employees accurately and objectively in comparison with other employees can lead to compensation based on favoritism. Because of the difficulty in establishing merit systems that are fair, larger organizations are increasingly using step-and-range pay systems. Step-and-range pay systems compensate employees on the basis of tenure. A range of pay is established for each position, and then pay increases are given regularly until a maximum rate of pay is reached. These ranges are also adjusted to compensate for inflation and other market factors. Within the range, pay differences among employees reflect differences in tenure, not performance. When such a system is used, employees must be monitored closely in the first 90 days of employment so that weaker employees can be weeded out before they move into tenured positions.

The administration of any compensation system requires attention to a number of procedural factors. One critical issue is confidentiality. From the organizational viewpoint, keeping salaries confidential is important to avoid internal friction. However, adoption of a step-and-range pay system, as well as the process of recruitment, requires salary ranges to be made public. Although a given individual's salary may be confidential, considerable information about salary may nevertheless be exchanged by employees. For these reasons, it is important that the salary system avoid any practice that might be construed as leading to favoritism or special privilege.

In maintaining equity, reevaluating existing positions, and establishing pay for new positions, a credible salary administration program needs to be established by a compensation committee. This committee should include managers and supervisors at all levels. It must be a consistent group of individuals who have the organizational scope and commitment to maintain the system fairly.

Benefits

Managers and employees sometimes focus too much on direct compensation and fail to recognize the importance of fringe benefits. Benefits may vary according to employee position, tenure in the job, and other factors. They may include retirement, life and accident insurance, disability insurance, medical and dental health insurance, vacation time, worker's compensation, tuition reimbursement, sick leave, professional organization memberships, and other benefits.

Structuring of benefits must take into account the age of the employees as well as the external marketplace. The types of benefits that are most attractive to employees, for example, may depend in part on the age of employees. Younger employees may be more interested in dental coverage and wages, for instance, than they are in retirement benefits. Older employees, by contrast, may be more interested in retirement benefits than in life insurance. To gauge how the marketplace is evolving, benefit and compensation surveys should be carefully performed and analyzed.

One benefit offered at community health centers that helps them retain healthcare professionals is coverage of those employees under the protective liability coverage through the Federal Tort Claims Act (FTCA). In essence, malpractice liability shifts from the individual health center to the federal government, with the costs being paid out of the federal health center program's annual appropriation. Health centers deemed eligible by the Health Resource and Services Administration (HRSA) qualify for FTCA coverage. The eligibility process covers credentialing of health center providers, the health center's risk management systems, and the center's past claims history. Once a center is deemed eligible, any officer, board member, or employee of the health center is covered by FTCA.[8]

PERFORMANCE EVALUATION

Problem Identification and Employee Counseling

Problems can be identified by a variety of mechanisms that are broadly classified as either operational or environmental. An example of a mechanism for operational identification of a problem is an employee complaint to a supervisor or other member of the staff about a specific problem. An example of an environmental mechanism is review of employee turnover rates and exit interviews. Other mechanisms for identifying problems include monitoring absenteeism rates, which assumes that unhappy employees tend to take more time off from work, and reviewing regular operating reports, in which supervisors are asked to list problems.

Personal contact with employees can also reveal problems with job satisfaction. The enthusiasm of employees can be measured in many ways if managers are keenly attuned to this aspect of job performance. In some organizations, employers conduct employee attitude surveys. To be most effective, these surveys should be administered by an outside party. Such surveys can produce excellent information about employee perceptions of the effectiveness of supervisory structures and the level of job satisfaction. A commitment to change based on the findings of the survey is essential to the success of this process.

These and other indicators provide managers with a sense of the state of employee morale. Of course, a lack of specific problems encountered on a day-to-day basis should not be taken by itself as an indicator of high morale. Perhaps managers are so distant from the operation that they are oblivious to employees' true feelings. Thus the lack of recorded problems, such as failure of the supervisor to monitor employee absenteeism, may actually be an indicator of a serious problem.

Counseling

Job-related counseling helps build a productive, smoothly working team. Essentially, two counseling approaches exist: directive counseling and nondirective counseling. Directive counseling is a fact-finding process relating to a specific problem. The supervisor weighs the facts, advises the employee, and attempts to motivate the employee to adhere to the advice given. Nondirective counseling focuses on the person being counseled rather than on the problem to be resolved. This approach takes a broader view. Typically, the organization selects the counseling approach that best matches the problem being addressed. More generally, a good manager tends to favor approaches that build rapport and contribute to the employee's understanding of the larger picture. The manager must sort the facts of the problem from the projected attitudes of the employee. It is important to distinguish between factual information and information that is biased by the employee's viewpoint.

There are several requirements for effective counseling. The most important considerations are to set the stage carefully, create rapport, and permit the employee to engage in a meaningful dialogue with his or her manager. It is also important to determine in advance, whenever possible, when and how closure should take place. This effort requires that the manager carefully think through strategies that might successfully meet the employee's needs.

Performance Appraisal

The continuous process of providing information to a person about his or her performance is critical to ensure desirable behavior. Organizations will typically have mechanisms for both informal and formal performance appraisal. Informally, employees will need to hear with some regularity about how their work is perceived by others—particularly co-workers, managers, and patients.

A formal semiannual or annual system of performance review also needs to be in place. Any evaluation process involves three basic components: understanding by both the employer and the employee of the employee's assignments that are subject to evaluation; processes and procedures for conducting the evaluation; and feedback to the employee about the outcome of the evaluation. Obviously, the effectiveness of the evaluation process depends on having adequate job descriptions and reaching agreement among all parties regarding the objectives to be evaluated. The absence of feedback on performance can seriously jeopardize the evaluation process. Ideally, the evaluation should be documented in writing and signed by the supervisor and employee, because the employee may attend to only selective information in an evaluation conference.

Discipline

Disciplining an employee is a complicated process that includes recognition of the problem and careful assessment as to whether a policy or practice has been violated. When disciplinary action is in order, disciplinary policies must be followed carefully to maintain morale and equity of personnel relationships. The first step in disciplinary action is often a warning. Careful documentation of any verbal or written warning is essential. The extent and degree of further intervention by management in disciplinary matters depend on the magnitude of the problem. Management also must assure that a deviation from norms is, in fact, taking place.

Sometimes many employees may be violating the same rule, but only one employee is being disciplined. Once disciplinary action has been initiated, the organization must set a timetable for resolution of the problem. For example, if the employee is put on probation, the organization must specify a definite length of time for the probationary period.

A particularly challenging situation is disciplining employees for abusing drugs or alcohol in light of a health center's obligations under the ADA. A health center can discipline employees for illegal use of drugs that affects job performance, for conduct that violates workplace health and safety requirements, and for violations of the Drug-Free Workplace Act. The regulations implementing the ADA specifically state that the terms "disability" and "qualified individual with a disability" do not include individuals currently engaging in the illegal use of drugs when an employer acts on the basis of such use. Most health centers are required to comply with the Drug-Free Workplace Act as a condition of receiving federal funds. As such, the heath center can prohibit the illegal use of drugs and the use of alcohol at the workplace by all employees, and it may require that employees not be under the influence of alcohol or engage in illegal use of drugs at the workplace.[5]

SAFETY

Community health centers are usually located near their patients or target markets. Often these locations are in lower socioeconomic areas, which may have higher crime rates. One community health center in a large metropolitan area experienced multiple challenges regarding patients' as well as staff members' safety.[16] This facility experienced a number of violent and nonviolent crimes within a year. Violent crimes ranged from abduction and murder across the street from the center to bullets shot through an employee's office window. In addition to the violent crimes, theft of money, purses, wallets, and radios had occurred within the center's building.

The health center's limited ability to provide a safe environment for its patients and staff created numerous problems. Patients perceived that the center was not a safe environment and stopped seeking much-needed healthcare services. Staff recruitment and retention—already a challenge for the health center—were made even more difficult by the perception that working at the center was dangerous.

Several solutions were proposed and implemented by the community health center's administrator, but had only limited success in increasing the overall safety at the center. Resources were simply not available to hire security officers. Requesting more funding was a laborious process and required time before resources became available. During the wait, the community clinic administrator wanted to provide as safe an environment as possible with the clinic's limited resources. The following solutions were implemented:[16]

- Held an annual safety and awareness training
- Trained supervisors on how to handle hostile patients
- Posted "no soliciting" signs around the building
- Installed self-closing and locking door pushbars at entrance and exit points
- Increased interior lighting and placed outdoor lighting on sensors
- Established agreements with the constable's department to provide immediate constable response when alerted
- Created staffing assignments so that three to four employees were present at all times

The administrator also proposed implementing some additional solutions:[16]

- Providing self-defense classes conducted by local law enforcement officers for all staff members
- Installing door signals with on and off switches to limit access during less-staffed hours

In an attempt to convince city and county officials of increased crime in the area where the health center was located, as compared to other areas, the community clinic director prepared a crime report.[16] Ideally, these data would show that crime was a major problem at the health center and the need for security officers would be supported.

TRAINING AND EDUCATION

The process of adequately orienting a new employee so that he or she becomes a valuable, informed member of the staff is just the beginning of employee training. Recruiting experienced health professionals makes this initial training easier, but the new employee must still be indoctrinated with an adequate sense of the organization's culture. Once the well-oriented employee is fully productive, the health center must provide continuing education opportunities so the employee can remain current in the conduct of his or her professional and practice activities. Research has shown that members of a highly educated workforce are likely to remain interested in developing their skills and knowledge over their entire careers.

One area of training needed in community health centers is in the provision of culturally effective care. Health centers serve culturally and linguistically diverse communities, and their policies and procedures, as well as staff members, need to respect and respond to the cultural diversity of the communities and clients served. To do so effectively, healthcare providers and nonprofessional staff alike must have a firm understanding of how and why different belief systems, cultural biases, ethnic origins, family structures, and other culturally determined factors influence the manner in which people experience illness, adhere to medical advice, and respond to treatment.[17] Being culturally competent is a way to interact effectively with diverse patient populations, reduce healthcare disparities, and improve the quality of care for all patients. Experts draw clear links between cultural competence, quality improvement, and the elimination of racial or ethnic disparities in care.[18] Hiring staff with language skills and backgrounds that reflect the communities served is not always possible. Currently, few professional training programs provide any formal education about culture and its relationship to health, so many healthcare providers enter the workforce with little or no training in psychosocial issues. Community health centers need to offer training programs to equip their staff with the tools and skills needed to be competent to provide appropriate, culturally effective care. Such programs should include educational modules that emphasize cross-cultural training, effective communication, and an awareness of the impact of social and cultural factors on health beliefs and behaviors.

Family Healthcare Center

The Family Healthcare Center (FHC) is a community health center and residency program providing primary care to underserved populations in Cass County, North Dakota, and Clay County, Minnesota, where 45,000 people live below 200% of poverty.[17] Thirty-five percent of clinic patients are members of a racial/ethnic minority group. Clinical services and programs, including dental care, are targeted to special populations, including homeless, refugee, migrant, and Native American clients. FHC is the primary care provider for refugees resettled in the community each year from Europe, Asia, and Africa by the Office of Refugee Resettlement and local agencies.

In collaboration with the University of North Dakota School of Medicine, WIC, Migrant Health Services, Head Start, public health, Lutheran Social Services Refugee Programs, and area mental health agencies, the FHC successfully recruits minority providers and clinic staff and maintains cultural diversity with attention to the unique needs of its patient population. The FHC/University of North Dakota Medical School family practice residency collaboration enables family practice residents to train in a culturally diverse environment. The residency actively and successfully recruits minority residents, including Native Americans.

FHC was the first health/human services agency in this largely Anglo, Scandinavian American region to use paid interpreters for all appointments with patients who speak languages other than English. Clinic staff participated in a task force to establish a community interpreter center, which serves as a formal training program for all interpreters. The clinic is the largest user of interpreter services in the community. Interpretation is built into the job descriptions of bilingual staff, and training and competence are assessed through the community interpreter program.

Source: U.S. Department of Health and Human Services, Health Resources and Services Administration, Center for Managed Care. *Cultural Competence Works.* 2001.

Educational opportunities are nearly limitless. Professional organizations, colleges, and continuing education seminars are all options for on-the-job training and job enrichment. Community health centers have a number of options, depending on the focus of the training program, the number of staff members involved, and available resources. The most popular options are probably sending individual staff members to off-site workshops and seminars, contracting with experts to train staff members on-site, and offering in-house training using the knowledge and skills of the center's own staff. Adherence to several general principles can help narrow the alternatives when deciding on an educational approach for staff members:

- Provide integrated training toward specific objectives, based on employee weaknesses and strengths and the organization's training objectives.
- Include money in the training budget to cover the significant costs of employee time for attending training programs.
- Establish policies for selecting employees to attend training and trainings that employees can attend.
- Require that employees who attend meetings share what they learn with others on the staff.

LEGAL AND REGULATORY ISSUES

Regulations affecting employment practices are extensive and beyond the scope of this chapter but are discussed elsewhere in this book. The following federal laws generally impact community health centers:

- Americans with Disabilities Act (ADA)
- Age Discrimination in Employment Act (ADEA)
- Title VII of the Civil Rights Act of 1964 (Title VII)
- Employee Retirement Income Security Act (ERISA)
- Group health plan coverage under the Consolidated Omnibus Budget Reconciliation Act (COBRA)
- Family and Medical Leave Act (FMLA)
- Fair Labor Standards Act (FLSA)
- Equal Pay Act
- National Labor Relations Act (NLRA)
- Labor-Management and Reporting Act (LMRDA)
- Immigration and Nationality Act (INA)
- Occupational Safety and Health Act (OSHA)
- Uniformed Services Employment and Reemployment Rights Act (USERRA)[19]

CONCLUSION

In a service industry such as health care, the workforce component assumes great importance. Hiring and maintaining a qualified, knowledgeable, hard-working, competent, and reliable staff is one of the most important aspects of any community health center's operations. Strong efforts are required now and over the next several years to recruit and retain sufficient health professionals, administrative, and other needed staff to sustain the workforce at current health centers while simultaneously meeting the demands for health center expansion.

REFERENCES

1. Bureau of Primary Health: Requirements of Fiscal Year 2003 Funding Opportunity for Health Center New Access Point Grant Applications. 2003. Available at: http://www.bphc.hrsa.gov/grants/newaccess.htm. Accessed July 22, 2005.
2. U.S. Department of Health and Human Services, Health Resources and Services Administration, Bureau of Primary Health Care. *Governing Board Handbook*. Bethesda, MD: 2000.
3. National Association of Community Health Centers, Inc. *Health Center Fact Sheet United States, 2004*. Washington, DC.
4. Bureau of Primary Health. Requirements of Fiscal Year 2004 Funding Opportunity for Health Center New Access Point Grant Applications. Available at: ftp://ftp.hrsa.gov/hrsa/04guidancebphc/hrsa04034.pdf. Accessed October 23, 2005.
5. National Association of Community Health Centers. *The Americans with Disabilities Act*. 2002.
6. National Health Services Corp. Site Development Manual. Available at: http://nhsc.bhpr.hrsa.gov/resources/SRM-toc.asp. Accessed October 12, 2005.
7. Taylor J. *The Fundamentals of Community Health Centers*. National Health Policy Forum; 2004. Washington, D.C.
8. Williams G. NAS Insights: Physician Recruitment Report. 2005. Available at: http://www.nasrecruitment.com/MicroSites/Healthcare/Articles. Accessed October 22, 2005.
9. Personal communication with author. August 8, 2004.
10. Singer JD, Davidson SM, Graham S, Davidson HS. Physician retention in community and migrant health centers: who stays and for how long? *Medical Care*. 1998; 36(8):1198–1213.
11. Conte SJ, Imershein AW, Magill MK. Rural community and physician perspectives on resource factors affecting physician retention. *The Journal of Rural Health*. 1992; 8(3):185–196.
12. Bolin KA, Shulman JD. Nationwide survey of work environment perceptions and dentists' salaries in community health centers. *Journal of the American Dental Association*. 2005; 136(2):214–220.
13. Cochran C, Peltier J. Retaining medical directors in community health centers: the importance of administrative relationships. *The Journal of Ambulatory Care Management*. 2003; 26(3):250–259.

14. Wilhide S. *Physician Retention in Community Health Centers.* National Association of Community Health Centers; 2004. Washington, D.C.
15. National Association of Community Health Centers. *Health Center Compensation and Benefits Report 2005–2006.* Washington, DC.
16. Personal communication with author. July 29, 2004.
17. U.S. Department of Health and Human Services, Health Resources and Services Administration, Center for Managed Care. *Cultural Competence Works.* Rockville, MD: 2001.
18. Betancourt JR, Green AR, Carrillo JE, Ananeh-Firempong O. Defining cultural competence: a practical framework for addressing racial/ethnic disparities in health and health care. *Public Health Reports.* 2003; 118(4):293–302.
19. National Association of Community Health Centers. *Classifying Workers as Employees or as Independent Contractors: Why It Matters and How To Do It Correctly.* Washington, DC: March 2004.

CHAPTER 11

Human Resources in Physician Practice Management

Daniel F. Fahey

VIGNETTE

It's 3:30 P.M. on Tuesday. Your administrative assistant informs you, the medical group administrator, that a patient is on the phone with a complaint regarding Dr. Swanson, her primary care physician. The patient tells you that she has tried to resolve her issues with Dr. Swanson, but without success. Her chief complaints are that Dr. Swanson is abrupt, does not answer her questions, and seems to disregard her request for a specialist referral. The patient is a member of one of the group's largest contracted managed care plans, and she intends to contact the HMO regarding Dr. Swanson. You assure the patient that you will investigate the matter and get back to her.

You have heard of other complaints regarding Dr. Swanson, but this is the first patient you have spoken with personally. After listening to the patient, you contact Dr. Price, Chief of Family Practice and Dr. Swanson's "boss." Dr. Price reminds you that Dr. Swanson is board certified in family practice, with more than 10 years experience. You ask Dr. Price if he has received any complaints about Dr. Swanson. He responds that he has heard some vague complaints in the past, but insists that Dr. Swanson is an outstanding clinician and the group is lucky to have his services.

After getting nowhere with Dr. Price, you investigate when Dr. Swanson's performance was last reviewed according to human resources (HR) policy. The HR director reports that there are only two or three brief scribbled notes in Dr. Swanson's personnel file, the last of which dates from more than four years ago. No documentation indicates that anyone has spoken with Dr. Swanson regarding his patient relations. Furthermore, the HR director informs you, this is not unusual. Few physicians in the group have undergone a formal performance evaluation. It appears that the situation with Dr. Swanson is symbolic of a larger issue—the tip of the iceberg, so to speak. As administrator, what do you do to address this situation?

INTRODUCTION

The Medical Group Management Association (MGMA), formed in 1926, defines a medical group as a formal affiliation of three or more physicians who share income, expenses, facilities, equipment, and staff.[1] Currently, more than one-third of all physicians in the United States practice in over 19,000 medical groups with over 226,000 physicians.[2] Medical groups are usually identified as either single specialty (such as anesthesia, radiology, or orthopedics) or multi-specialty (where physicians with varied expertise join together for common benefit). Group ownership may be nonprofit, part of a large integrated delivery system, or affiliated with a health plan, such as Kaiser Permanente. In the United States, the majority of physician group practices are for-profit and are owned by the physicians participating in the group.

While medical groups such as the Mayo Clinic and Scripps Clinic have existed for decades, the evolution from private, fee-for-service insurance plans to employer-paid managed care plans created a "strong force driving physicians to join group practices."[3] Large medical groups not only enjoyed certain economies of scale, thereby reducing their overhead costs, but, more importantly, were able to negotiate effectively with aggressive managed care health plans.

This chapter focuses on the practical knowledge, skills, and tasks necessary to effectively manage the human resources function of a small to medium-sized physician practice, with specific emphasis on single-specialty and multi-specialty medical group practices in the range of 50 to 200 employees. While the challenges of managing a solo physician office practice with several employees are significant, a fully organized human resources department does not become a necessity until the operation reaches a critical mass of perhaps several dozen employees. Medium-sized group practices may employ more than 100 clinical and support staff. When a group expands to this size, the need for a more formal approach to salary and benefits structure, job classifications, policy and procedure manual, job training, performance evaluations, and a grievance procedure becomes apparent. No longer are informal communication methods adequate to meet the needs of the practice. Often, one or more full-time human resources professionals are employed to handle the myriad tasks associated with managing a multi-million-dollar payroll, an increasingly diverse workforce, and the demands of a highly competitive and complex business.

For the purposes of this chapter, the terms "physician practice," "physician group practice," "medical group," and "physician organization" are used interchangeably.

The human resources function of a physician group practice can be approached from a number of perspectives. This chapter follows a format selected by the American College of Medical Practice Executives (ACMPE), the professional credentialing organization of the MGMA. In 2001, the ACMPE created *The ACMPE Guide to the Body of Knowledge for Medical Practice Management*.[4] The *Guide* sets forth the essential skills and knowledge necessary to be an effective physician practice executive. It encompasses skills, tasks, and knowledge in a variety of areas, including finance, planning and marketing, information systems, governance, business and clinical operations, and human resources. While mastery of each of these areas does not guarantee success in managing physician practices, failure to understand and apply the basic knowledge, skills, and tasks contained in the *Guide* will most likely ensure an abbreviated management career.[5] Therefore, the chapter topics will parallel those found in the ACMPE *Guide* under "Human Resources Management."

OVERVIEW OF THE SETTING

According to the U.S. Department of Labor,[6] more than 1.9 million professional and support staff are employed in physician practices and clinics in the United States. The annual expenditure for physician services in the United States in 2002 was approximately $340 billion, according to a report published by the American College of Healthcare Executives.[7] As the population in the United States continues to age, it is anticipated that the growth in physician practices will likewise continue, making this sector of the healthcare industry a consistent source of employment for the foreseeable future.

Unfortunately for many physician practices, the cost of operations, including employee salaries and benefits, has increased faster than reimbursement over the past decade.[8] While total medical revenue increased 52% from 1992 to 2002, total operating costs increased almost 67% in the same period. During this time period, physician compensation rose by only 33%.[8] According to the MGMA Cost Survey, the primary reasons for this disparity are increased numbers of support employees per full-time physician and increased salaries and benefits for those employees.[8] MGMA suggests that multiple reasons explain this trend: a shift of services from hospitals to physician offices, the increased complexity of medical procedures performed in physician offices, and an increased demand for more administrative documentation and compliance measures.[8] As increasingly more medical services are performed on an outpatient basis due to this practice's lower charges and greater customer convenience, physician practice costs will likely continue to grow despite improvements and clarifications to the federal self-referral laws (the so-called Stark laws).[9] Stark laws prohibit physicians from referring Medicare patients to medical services in which the physician has a financial interest or from receiving a financial inducement to admit patients to a hospital or other healthcare setting. Exceptions are made under "safe harbors" provisions for physicians in group practice, formal hospital affiliation, or managed care plans. Because the Stark laws are very technical, seeking legal advice in this area is recommended.

Physician practice administrators and human resources directors are also encouraged to consult several helpful publications available through the MGMA:

- *Rightsizing: Appropriate Staffing for Your Medical Practice,* by Deborah Walker and David Gans, 2003.
- *The Essentials: 2003 MGMA Survey Results* (set of four), including physician compensation, cost survey, performance standards, and management compensation survey.
- *Group Practice Personnel Policies Manual* (set of two), by Courtney Price and Alys Novak, 2001.

Major Employment Categories

The following is a more detailed breakdown of major employment categories in physician practice organizations. Ask almost any physician practice administrator what he or she needs in terms of human resources, and you will get substantially the same answer: more qualified nurses, better-trained office staff, and caring physicians.

Nurses. There are approximately 2.5 million registered nurses in the United States.[10] Despite this seemingly large number, a national shortage of nurses has been well documented.[11, 12] It is estimated that the demand for registered nurses exceeded supply by 6% in 2000. This shortfall is expected to double by 2010 and to increase to almost a 30% shortfall by 2020.[11] Fortunately, this shortfall should have minimal impact on physician practices, as most offices can provide appropriate nursing care within existing state laws by employing certified nursing assistants (CNAs) or licensed vocational nurses (LVNs). These individuals are more readily available than their registered nurse counterparts, because the amount of training required is substantially less and compensation is correspondingly lower. For the most part, physician practices do not require the same level of training or sophistication as hospitals do. There are exceptions, of course: Oncology practices, dialysis centers, or certain surgical specialties may require registered nurses whose enhanced training and skills warrant their greater expense. Generally speaking, most primary care physician practices and clinic settings do not need a full contingent of registered nurses, which is a significant cost saving to the practice.

Physician Extenders. One unique feature of physician practices is the use of physician extenders or mid-level providers in the form of physician assistants (PAs), nurse practitioners (NPs), and others.[13] Experts have identified 10 types of nonphysician clinicians.[14] The physician practice needs to be cognizant of recruiting opportunities associated with these highly compensated and often certified or licensed professionals. Like physicians, these physician extenders are considered employees, but they are often treated as a distinct category. They are typically exempt from overtime rules and may be eligible for performance bonuses, along with their physician counterparts.

Over the past 10 years, the number of graduating PAs and NPs has increased by almost 50%.[13] In 2005, there were more than 106,000 nurse practitioners and more than 60,000 physician assistants in the United States.[13] These mid-level practitioners and physician extenders are highly sought after by physician practices for several reasons. First and foremost, they are able to perform a significant number of duties traditionally performed by primary care physicians at less than half the salary cost of an M.D.[15] The rapid rise of managed care since the early 1990s encouraged physician practices to employ NPs and PAs who are fully capable of handling routine primary care problems, leaving the physician more time to devote to patients with more complex problems.[13, 16] Nurse practitioners and physician assistants also tend to spend more time with patients, have a greater focus on preventive care, and are more interested in patient education than their physician colleagues.[17]

Other Clinical Staff.   Depending on the size, specialty, and sophistication, the physician practice may employ a number of licensed or registered clinical support staff, such as pharmacists, radiology and laboratory technicians, and physical and respiratory therapists. Physician practices must compete with hospitals and other healthcare organizations for these highly trained professionals, who are in short supply. Some physician practices choose to "outsource" or contract with professional agencies that provide clinical staff on an "as needed" basis. If the need for clinical staff is consistent and an adequate supply of qualified staff is available within the community, it makes economic sense to hire such individuals. In contrast, if the volume of work is sporadic or qualified staff is in short supply, contracting may be more cost-effective and expedient. Each situation should be assessed on its own merits.

Office Support Staff.   A frequent lament of physician practice administrators is the lack of qualified office staff to work in areas such as reception, billing, appointment scheduling, and medical records. In an era of relatively low unemployment rates and numerous alternative opportunities, work in a physician office practice, with its typical low pay, high stress, and limited promotional opportunities, needs to be enhanced to attract and retain qualified individuals. Another factor complicating the availability and hiring of office staff is the age variation and cultural diversity in the United States. Some physician practice administrators contend that the work ethic among younger employees is different than that found among older employees.[18] Likewise, the influx of foreign-born immigrants to the United States, with accompanying language challenges and cultural differences, places additional burdens on the human resources environment. The result is potential misunderstanding and conflicts, and "in some cases, outright animosity."[19] (p. 7) Nonetheless, attracting and retaining a cadre of patient-friendly and technically competent office support staff is crucial to the successful operation of any physician practice.

Kennedy[19] identified the following age-related staffing concerns for physician practices:

- *A management deficit.* Younger workers don't want to be managers, with the attendant pressures and longer work hours.
- *Lack of loyalty to the employer.* Experienced staff have multiple job opportunities and are quick to leave a job that offers little incentive to stay.
- *A shortage of medical personnel at all levels.* This shortage includes nurses, physician therapists, pharmacists, and billers and coders.

The HR department can make a substantial contribution in this area by arranging for multicultural and diversity courses to be offered to employees. Often, university faculty have designed courses that may be customized for physician practices.

Caring Physicians.   Another deficit in human resources is caring physicians. Physician dissatisfaction with the business of medicine in the modern era, which is often focused on health maintenance organizations (HMOs), is well known and thoroughly documented in the literature.[20–23] As managed care, Medicare, Medicaid, and private insurances have reduced reimbursement for professional services, while at the same time patient demand for services and the threat of malpractice suits have multiplied, it is no wonder that physicians have become frustrated and angry over their loss of autonomy and income. According to a recent MGMA survey,[24] physicians are working longer hours for less compensation than in previous years. To make up for this loss of income, physicians have resorted to seeing more patients during office hours, meaning that they spend less time with each patient. The result is reduced patient satisfaction, increased physician hostility, and increased staff turnover—a lethal combination. Physicians are leaving medical groups, looking for more satisfying practice situations, and medical groups are seeking to hire physicians who have not yet "burned out."

Physician Influence in Human Resources

Managing human resources in physician practices is especially difficult due to the unique presence and influence of physicians within the practice. As Mertz states when referring to physicians, "When not governing, they are, essentially, employees."[25] (p. 23) Unlike hospitals or other healthcare organizations in which the physician is often an infrequent visitor, attending to his or her patients before and after a busy office practice, physicians in medical group practices spend the majority of their time in the office, surrounded by staff who are technically or nominally in their employ.

This proximity to the workplace can be either good or bad, depending on the organizational culture, attitudes of the physicians, stress tolerance of the practice administrator, and other factors. It is not uncommon for a physician/owner of a medium to large practice to attempt to treat the practice as his or her own fiefdom. Such an attitude creates havoc with the HR department, which is responsible for supporting myriad rules and regulations. The most common problem is the physician who wants to "fire" or transfer his or her nurse for some real or imagined infraction, without benefit of any prior counseling or warning. The HR staff must be firm but diplomatic in dealing with the physician/owner, preventing both a blowup by the physician and a lawsuit filed by the employee for an unlawful termination. A periodic review of HR policies and procedures at appropriate physician committees and board meetings is one method of reducing the potential for embarrassment—or worse.

Physicians add a level of complexity to the human resources function that does not exist in most other healthcare enterprises. For example, physicians tend to reward or sanction employees based on their personal perception of the situation and/or relationship with the employee; they are not necessarily concerned with consistency or due process. Physicians are more concerned—as they should be—with the direct effects they and their employees have on patient care than with the subtleties of employment law, job classification, or salary structure. Physician/employee issues tend to take on a more personal tone rather than an organizational perspective. This scenario makes managing the human resources function of a 10- to 50-physician group practice extremely challenging. As the group expands into the 100-plus physician range, the issues tend to change and become more like those of a hospital or more traditional healthcare organization. In very large medical groups, the organization becomes more bureaucratic and the individual physician is less likely to behave like an entrepreneur or owner.

Legal Structure

While this chapter will not go into the legal structure of physician practices in depth, it is necessary to acknowledge that medical groups may be organized in a variety of legal ways: single proprietorships, partnerships, shareholderships, limited liability corporations, subchapter "S" corporations, and medical care foundations, among others.[9, 26] Some or all of the physicians participating in the medical group may be "owners" of the practice; others may be "employees"; and still others may be serving under a personal services or independent contractor agreement. Each of these arrangements presents different challenges to the human resources function and further differentiates physician practices from other healthcare organizations. Regardless of the type of ownership, the human resources policies and procedures for the medical group should include provisions for dealing with employment issues generated by physicians. Therefore, this chapter will make special note of issues unique to the employment of physicians by medical groups.

STRATEGIC PLANNING

A well-organized human resources department can be of significant benefit to physician practices in the area of strategic planning. Because the majority of a medical group's assets are found with its employees, a careful analysis of workforce issues may help the group identify its current and future needs, such as physician and management succession planning, employee skills inventory, potential training needs, and competition for highly trained individuals. The HR department can be helpful in identifying difficult-to-recruit and -retain staff, compensation and benefits trends, and general performance evaluation deficiencies to enhance the workforce and help the group achieve its strategic initiatives.

COMPENSATION AND BENEFITS

The oft-repeated phrase from the movie *Jerry Maguire,* "Show me the money," also applies to physician practice management. Employees in every job classification, including physicians, are understandably interested in earning the maximum possible compensation. The employer, whether physician- or corporate-owned, is often interested in paying the minimum possible compensation while attracting and retaining competent personnel. The trick is to balance these two competing priorities while staying within legal bounds and competitive market pressures. Thus compensation and benefits design is one of the most critical and complex tasks handled by the human resources function.

Right or wrong, most of us equate our value to an organization to how much we are paid, especially in relation to others within and outside the organization. Unless we are independently wealthy, so that travel or golf in Hawaii is perhaps an option, most people have to work for a living during the bulk of their productive lives. What we are paid for our efforts is a reflection of our "worth" in the market and the value placed on our efforts by the organization. Maintaining the appropriate balance between personal and organizational values is critical for both attracting and retaining qualified employees.

In the healthcare industry, physician practices typically compensate their employees at a level somewhat below their counterparts in hospitals and other sectors of the industry.[27] The counterbalance to this inequity is that physician practices tend to have more predictable work hours, are often open 9 A.M. to 5 P.M. on weekdays, and place a less demanding physical workload on employees due to the ambulatory nature of the patients. Regardless of the merits of this debate, the reality is that physician practices must compete for employees within the same basic labor market as other healthcare organizations. Therefore, it behooves the practice to formalize a compensation and benefits plan that is consistent, is internally equitable, is affordable within the financial realities of the practice, rewards employees for meeting organizational goals, and is competitive within the local market.

Compensation Strategy

Strategically, the physician practice may wish to compensate its employees at a rate higher than the average in the community. This approach will most likely attract more qualified applicants and retain quality personnel, but may conflict with the desires of the physician owners to maximize their income. Generally speaking, any profit derived from the activities of the physician practice belongs to the physician owner(s), unless the practice is nonprofit or owned by a corporation. (Physician compensation will be addressed later in this chapter.) By contrast, achieving a reputation as the lowest-paying practice in the market will discourage highly qualified candidates and may contribute to excessive turnover, which is both expensive (due to recruitment and training costs) and disruptive to patients and other staff. Striking a happy medium is, therefore, often the goal of physician practices.

Several methods may be used to ensure that the practice is attractive and competitive from a compensation perspective. The easiest (but potentially risky) is to establish an informal relationship with the nearest competitors and share information. Discussions about compensation ranges, rather than specific rates, are less problematic and preserve individual confidentiality while achieving the intended purpose. Anonymous surveys—especially when they are conducted by third parties, such as regional, state, or national healthcare trade organizations like the MGMA—offer objective salary and benefits data to members. Another informal approach is to have current employees respond to job ads to obtain salary ranges, although this strategy could have unintended (and unhappy) consequences. Finally, if exit interviews reveal that your employees are leaving mainly for salary reasons, it is a tipoff that your compensation plan needs an overhaul.

Compensation Plan Approval Process

From the HR department's perspective, it is important to establish a written compensation and benefits policy and procedure. To avoid chaos, and perhaps a lawsuit, it is critical that the organization develops a formal approval process that delineates who has the authority to set salaries or salary ranges, who approves changes to benefits, which specific compensation model is to be utilized by the practice, and who approves individual pay increases. In a small physician practice, it may be acceptable to pay different staff members different rates of pay, based on their longevity, skills, and perceived value to the practice. In large groups, it is highly problematic to pay differentially for anything other than objective and verifiable reasons. It is acceptable, however, to offer a "pay for performance" bonus or to tie compensation to incentives or specific job skills. For example, if an employee meets certain preestablished performance goals or secures a certificate or credential to perform certain tasks beyond the normal scope of the position, additional compensation is justified and appropriate to retain a motivated employee. Schneck[28] suggests a variety of incentives, including bonuses, profit sharing, stock ownership, and gain sharing, depending on the legal structure of the specific physician practice.

Every practice should establish a consistent approach to modifying the compensation system, granting salary increases, or changing benefits. Either the governing authority, such as the board of directors or the executive committee of the board, or the chief executive officer, on behalf of the governing authority, should periodically review and approve any changes to the compensation and benefits plan. Groups are advised to seek qualified legal counsel in the form of a labor attorney to review both the initial plan and any subsequent material changes.

Compensation Models

As with many other healthcare organizations, a number of models may be used to determine employee compensation in a physician practice organization. Specific methodology and examples are provided elsewhere in this book. Generally, the job description of each position determines the pay grade, as job titles may be misleading.[29] Often, a large medical group will have dozens of job classifications and pay grades.

Some of the more common compensation models used by physician practice organizations include the following:

- *Benchmarking,* where positions are usually those that (1) are important to the organization and represent a cross section of the organization; (2) vary in job requirements, skills, and training; (3) do not change over time; and (4) are generally used in the industry to track wages and benefits[29]

- *Market-driven approach,* which pays whatever the market demands for a given position, especially in highly competitive areas
- *Broad-banding,* which uses fewer but broader (hence the name) pay grades; is simpler to use and thus less cumbersome than the more traditional multiple pay grade method; and is found in flatter, less hierarchical organizations
- The widely used *point system,* which is based on a series of compensable factors, such as education, job knowledge, job skills, experience, credentials, and working conditions, broken down into compensable factors that are weighted by points
- *Pay for performance,* which closely aligns the organization's mission, values, and goals with individual employee performance to produce a "win/win" outcome

Physician Compensation and Benefits

There is an old saying in medical group practices: "There are three physician compensation plans—last year's, this year's, and next year's." Simply stated, the variety and complexity of physician/owner compensation plans is too great for an in-depth discussion in this general chapter on human resources. Several texts and articles, including those by Benedict,[30] Fried and Johnson,[31] Gulko,[26] Keagy,[32] Poplin,[33] and Ross, Williams, and Pavlock,[34] offer more extensive explorations of this topic. However, a brief discussion here is warranted, due to the importance of this topic in physician practices.

When it comes to hiring physicians for a large medical group practice, compensation and benefits are often treated separately from those of other employees. However, the same caveats apply. Be sure to have a written and approved compensation and benefits plan that is both competitive and internally consistent. Physicians talk to each other, both inside and outside the medical practice. They are quite knowledgeable about salaries and benefits, and they are not shy about confronting management and the governing authority regarding a real or perceived inequity.

Regional and national physician group associations, such as the MGMA, maintain current comparative salary and benefits data, so that member groups may offer competitive compensation. Typically, an employed physician will be offered a professional services agreement that stipulates a monthly salary, fixed benefits (e.g., paid health care, disability and life insurance, three to four weeks vacation per year, perhaps a paid week or two for continued medical education), and perhaps other benefits such as a retirement plan. In many cases, the initial salary, while important, is less critical than the chance to become an owner of the medical group. With ownership comes the opportunity to share in the profits of the practice instead of working by the hour. However, an associated downside risk comes with ownership: If the physician practice experiences severe financial difficulties, the owners may have to personally fund any deficits.

Alternative Compensation Methods

Several methods of physician compensation other than straight salary exist. Some medical groups choose to compensate their physicians based on productivity, especially if the practice receives a majority of its income from fees for service. Some groups combine salary with a percentage of each physician's collections and/or relative value units.[35] These groups will argue that a straight salary arrangement does not motivate a physician either to see more than the average number of patients or to seek ways to increase ancillary revenue. Conversely, pay based solely on productivity may lead to "churning" (i.e., bringing back patients for unnecessary visits) or encourage redundant or perhaps unnecessary ancillary tests and procedures. At best, a productivity-based model places greater risk on the individual physician that may be problematic for the newly hired physician.[26] If the medical group has a high percentage of patients enrolled in HMOs, where compensation is based on capitation, or where a fixed monthly payment is made prospectively, the more care rendered that is not medically necessary and appropriate, the greater the negative impact on the group's profitability. For many physician practices, a reasonable combination of salary plus incentive bonuses based on productivity and patient satisfaction seems to be a satisfactory formula.

Regardless of the specifics of the plan adopted, it behooves the group to consider its financial position and method of reimbursement for the majority of patients before embarking on a new or revised physician compensation plan.

Redesigning a Physician Compensation Plan

Porn[36] (p. 293) suggests the following steps in redesigning a physician practice compensation plan:

1. Select the compensation redesign committee.
2. Determine the overall compensation philosophy and objectives.
3. Match the corporate strategy and alternative compensation formula components.
4. Develop a conceptual design for the proposed formula.
5. Model the proposed methodology.
6. Meet with key constituencies and highly affected specialties and individuals.
7. Determine the payout schedule and cash flow.
8. Design an appeals process.
9. Design a transition plan as necessary.
10. Roll out the compensation strategy.

This process may take as long as a year to implement fully. While some shortcuts may be possible, especially with a smaller, single-specialty physician practice, sufficient time should be allocated to this effort to avoid conflict and confusion. All key participants need to fully understand the impact of the new compensation plan, especially if it is substantially different from the previous plan. As Porn observes, "Equity of physician compensation is one of the most contentious issues that practices face."[36] (p. 309) The axiom, "Do it right or don't do it at all," should guide practice administrators who are unfortunate enough to be part of this process. Nothing will get a physician practice administrator fired more quickly than messing with physician compensation, so if there is a compelling reason to change physician compensation plans, following Porn's[36] strategy is good job retention advice for practice administrators.

Academic Practices

The problems of compensation are somewhat different if the physician practice is affiliated with an academic medical center or if it is traditionally hospital-based, such as an anesthesia, emergency, pathology, or radiology practice. In these situations, physicians are usually compensated by salary. They are often responsible for supervising other physicians in training or have certain administrative duties as program directors.

Academic center physicians are often affiliated with "faculty practice plans." This type of physician practice does not generally lend itself to bonus arrangements or ownership of the group. The "faculty practice plan" may receive a substantial proportion of its reimbursement from Medicare or Medicaid and perhaps research grants. For this reason, salaries are invariably lower than those in the private practice sector.[27] However, there are offsetting benefits to being associated with a medical school or teaching hospital, such as time for research and consulting and the prestige of working in a teaching or research center.

Physician Employment Agreements

While not legally mandatory, it is advisable for physician practices to create and implement a standard physician employment agreement. Because physicians are at the heart of the medical practice, are usually the most highly compensated employees, and may be owners of the practice as well as employees, it is advisable to engage legal counsel when preparing a physician employment agreement. According to Fitzgerald, Burkett, and Key,[37] this agreement should address a variety of issues: compensation, hours of work, benefits, malpractice insurance, hospital privileges, obligations of the physician, obligations of the employer, mutual obligations, terms and termination provisions, intellectual property, noncompliance clause, and regulatory issues. A well-formulated agreement will address substantially all of the relevant issues between the physician and the practice and, ideally, will establish expectations in advance of any problems. In many ways, the document can be thought of as a "prenuptial agreement" between the parties.

Independent Contractors

While employment is the most common method of securing a professional relationship with physicians, an alternative is to enter into a professional services agreement or independent practitioner contract. From the Internal Revenue Service's perspective, the key issue to consider is the degree of control exercised by the physician practice over the physician or other professionals.[38] Generally speaking, a "contracted" physician must comply with the practice's HR policies regarding treatment of staff. From the HR perspective, the relationship between the contracted physician or other professional and the employees of the physician practice must be handled somewhat delicately. For example, a nurse assigned to work with a contracted physician is professionally under the supervision of the contracted physician, yet an employee of the practice or group. It is generally a good idea for the practice to designate one employed physician—perhaps the group's medical director—to serve as a liaison with the contracted physician to ensure that all human resources policies and procedures are honored. As with other contracts, consultation with the organization's legal counsel is advised to avoid unpleasant situations.

RECRUITMENT

One of the most persistent problems in the healthcare industry is attracting and retaining qualified staff at all levels of the organization. Most difficult to recruit and retain are nurses and other highly trained professionals, who are in short supply and have numerous job opportunities. Every decade or so, a nursing shortage occurs and puts pressure on all segments of the healthcare industry to increase the number of nurses graduating from training programs, increase salaries and benefits for nurses, and create an environment that forces the industry to become more creative in its recruiting programs. The United States is currently in the midst of such a crisis. Nursing and other clinical professions are not the only positions in short supply, however. Billing and coding staff, data analysts, computer programmers, and others are also in great demand, and the healthcare industry has to compete with other industries for personnel to fill these positions. While they are often at a competitive salary disadvantage, physician practices must nevertheless recruit qualified staff to satisfy the demands placed on physicians from patients, insurance companies, and the government.

Recruitment Process

The recruitment process is one of the important components of the human resources program. After all, without an ongoing infusion of qualified and committed personnel, the physician practice will eventually grind to a halt. Fried[39] suggests that a human resources plan include the following elements:

- A specific recruitment strategy
- An understanding of the type of individual needed by the organization
- A systemized approach to recruitment and hiring

- A clear statement as to how human resources support organizational goals
- An understanding of past recruitment practices
- A skills inventory of internal employees

When all costs are taken into consideration, recruitment is very expensive and should not be approached haphazardly. Large healthcare organizations, including the larger medical groups, often have a well-thought-out recruitment strategy that accounts for the relative costs of advertising, referral bonuses, recruitment agency fees, travel and relocation expenses, and outsourcing. Additional costs in the recruitment process include examination fees, reference and security checks, drug screening, orientation, and training.

Internal Versus External Recruiting

Recruitment from within the organization may be more desirable and less costly than relying on external candidates. Some of its advantages follow:

- Job orientation and assimilation into the organization's culture may go more quickly.
- The organization already knows the work ethic of the candidate.
- Overall morale is enhanced when people are promoted from within.

However, there are some negative side effects:

- Morale may decrease among those not selected.
- Internal recruiting may discourage new ideas and promote "inbreeding."
- It may leave other holes to be filled by external recruiting.

The organization should seek to meet its staffing needs by balancing recruitment between internal and external candidates. As a practical matter, it is often impossible to select candidates exclusively from within the organization, especially in physician practices, because most existing employees do not have the skill sets or credentials to perform many of the tasks necessary. Nevertheless, it is important, for both legal and practical reasons, to post job openings before going to the external market. Perhaps there are talented and qualified internal candidates available who otherwise would not know of the job opening. This step also allows current employees to share information about the job opening with friends or acquaintances who may be interested in applying, thus saving some recruiting costs.

SELECTION

The next step in the process is the actual selection of a candidate for the available position. As a general rule, the physician practice should "maximize the possibility that the right candidate will select the organization after it makes a job offer."[39] (p. 126) Specific selection tools are often used to ensure that the candidate is qualified for the position. These tools should be both reliable, meaning that they are dependable, consistent, and valid, in that the tool measures the applicant's ability to perform the essential duties of the job. A valid tool might be to require that a laboratory technician applicant perform certain lab tests that demonstrate proficiency. Some organizations also require candidates to take psychological tests to determine attitudes, personality, or cognitive reasoning.

Reference Checks

Not surprisingly, some physician organizations are in such a hurry to place a candidate in the job that they ignore an important step in the selection process—namely, checking references from previous employers. Failure to adequately check references may result in hiring an unqualified or undesirable employee or—even worse—hiring a true liability, as any malpractice attorney will confirm.[40] Unfortunately for the physician practice seeking information from previous employers, often only dates of hire and termination, job title, and salary are given for the former employee. Given that an estimated 30% of individuals misrepresent or fabricate their résumés, obtaining a true work history is problematic.[41]

Reducing the Hiring Risk

There are several ways to substantially reduce the risk of giving and receiving references:[41]

- Ask the job candidate to sign a waiver or release to allow the prospective employer to contact previous employers for references.
- Never volunteer negative information or make unsolicited comments.
- Limit comments to those related to job performance.

- Fully document all attempts to secure references.
- Fully document all facts learned during a reference call.
- Give specific facts without labeling them as positive or negative.
- Inform terminated employees that the reason for the termination will be given to prospective employers if requested.
- If possible, say something positive about the former employee to reduce a potential claim of bias.
- Don't offer "off-the-cuff" remarks that are unsolicited or are not factual.

Rather than performing background checks themselves, some physician practices choose to use national companies for this purpose.[42] This tactic does not absolve the physician practice from making a hiring mistake, but it substantially reduces the risk of any misadventure.

Nurse Recruitment

While there is a continuing shortage of registered nurses nationally, medical group recruitment is somewhat easier than hospital nurse recruitment. For many nurses (the majority of whom are female), the regular and consistent working hours in physician practices are far superior to the varied shifts and overtime found in many hospitals. The working hours for many medical groups allow nurses to maintain reasonable working hours, allowing for family responsibilities. Seldom is overtime a requirement in medical groups, and the pace of work is more consistent and predictable. Compensation levels may be somewhat lower than those found in comparable jobs elsewhere, but lifestyle and working conditions often counterbalance the alternatives. Because most medical groups depend on nursing assistants for the bulk of their clinical activities, registered nurses are often employed in supervisory or technical positions that are less demanding physically.

Physician Recruitment

While hiring clerical or support staff is important for any physician practice, hiring physicians is a substantially more critical issue, because a physician is not only the primary care provider in the organization but also the primary generator of income for the practice. Thus the cost of physician turnover in a medical group practice is too great to endure anything more than reasonable change. One knowledgeable observer suggests that the true cost to a medical group of recruiting a physician often exceeds the cost of the physician's first-year salary.[43] An urban area that includes one or more medical residency programs may offer more opportunities for identifying and attracting new physicians to the group. Rural areas may have to rely on paid physician recruiters to identify potential candidates. If the medical group offers the prospective physician candidate the potential of a partnership or shareholder status, then the process for achieving that milestone should be well articulated during the initial interview. It is inappropriate, and perhaps unlawful, to do a "bait and switch" after the physician has performed satisfactorily for the required number of years with the expectation that a partnership or shareholdership will be offered.

Legal Issues in Recruitment and Selection

This chapter does not offer any detailed discussion regarding legal issues impacting recruitment and selection. Readers are encouraged to seek authoritative texts and articles or obtain legal advice on this topic. For the purposes of this chapter, however, it is relevant to comment on three federal laws that impact the hiring process: Title VII of the Civil Rights Act, the Equal Pay Act, and the American with Disabilities Act of 1990.

Title VII of the Civil Rights Act of 1964 prohibits discrimination based on gender, race, religion, or national origin. While overt discrimination is relatively easy to recognize and document, more subtle abuse is less readily apparent and more difficult to prove. It is unlawful according to the *Equal Pay Act of 1963* to establish different pay levels for males and females or for any other "class" of employees. The axiom, "Equal pay for equal work," should be the guideline for physician practices. Finally, the *Americans with Disabilities Act of 1990* stipulates that prospective employees with disabilities may request that the prospective employer make reasonable accommodations. The employer may legally decline to hire a disabled person if the disability would endanger the employee, other employees, or patients. The HR department should be versed in the nuances of this act, as it has far-reaching consequences for the physician practice.

Other Legal Issues

A number of other state and federal laws govern the conduct of physician practices. While all are relevant, several offer unique challenges to physician practices.

The *Family and Medical Leave Act* presents a specific challenge to physician practices, as a relatively large number of employees are female and tend to assume the primary responsibility for child rearing and, increasingly, care for aging parents.[44] Federal law requires that employers provide up to 12 weeks of unpaid leave for family or medical emergencies. During this time, the employee's job must be held for his or her return, and the employer must continue to pay most benefits, including medical insurance. Where state law regulating family and medical leave provides more protection to the employee, the state law prevails over federal law.

The *Age Discrimination in Employment Act of 1967* also places restrictions on physician practices, making it illegal to discriminate in employment of individuals 40 years of age and older. If the physician organization terminates or lays off older employees, it may be subject to legal action if it can be shown that the organization engaged in a pattern of age discrimination.

The *Fair Labor Standards Act* establishes the minimum wage and regulates which employees are exempt from receiving overtime for hours worked. Because physician practices often hire inexperienced, minimum-wage employees, and often require that employees work overtime due to the nature of the business, the Fair Labor Standards Act has significant implications for physician practices.

Exempt versus nonexempt employees relates to who is entitled to receive compensation for working overtime. Generally speaking, exempt employees, including management and most professionals, do not receive additional compensation for hours worked beyond the normal 8 hours per day or 40 hours per week. Nonexempt employees are usually entitled to compensation for working overtime or on holidays. Given that state laws may vary regarding to this issue, the HR department should be conversant with current law.

When in doubt as to the legality of employment practices within a physician group, consult the *Uniform Guidelines on Employee Selection Procedures* in the *Federal Register 1978*. These *Guidelines* help interpret the rules regarding compliance.[31]

TRAINING AND EDUCATION

Employee Orientation

A thorough employee orientation should set the tone for a long-lasting relationship between the employee and the organization. All too often, the practice is in such a hurry to put the new employee to work that key elements of the orientation are either ignored or delayed, creating a gap in the employee's knowledge of the practice and contributing to a limited assimilation into the new culture.

Ideally, orientation should occur before the employee begins his or her regular work. Such matters as fire and safety (OSHA) rules, workplace practices, explanation of benefits, discussion of the Employee Handbook (see Exhibit A), introduction to key services and individuals, and other important topics are usually covered during orientation. Waiting for days or weeks before orienting a new employee is not desirable for either the employee or the organization. As a practical matter, however, smaller physician practices may schedule orientation sessions only once a month or once a quarter. In this situation, the employee's supervisor or lead person in the department should provide the new employee with a basic orientation until such time as a full orientation can be arranged.

Physician Orientation

All too often, a new physician is hired, is assigned an office and staff, and starts seeing patients without sufficient orientation to the organization. Wendling-Aloi[45] suggests that the practice organization provide an opportunity for the new physician to engage in the following activities:

- Learn the history of the practice
- Learn its mission, vision, values, and strategic initiatives
- Understand the benefits package
- Meet the administrative staff as well as fellow physicians

It is important that new physicians be assimilated into the practice as soon as possible, not only to allow them to become economically productive, but also to avoid creating human resources issues with staff. A new physician, especially a newly graduated resident, may not be accustomed to functioning in a non-teaching setting, where patient satisfaction and efficiency of time and resources are critical for the success of the physician practice. According to Wendling-Aloi,[45] a thoughtful orientation program will achieve the following results:

- Reduce turnover and increase retention of all staff
- Improve productivity
- Improve patient safety
- Reduce penalties for infractions of governmental regulations

- Enhance communications
- Provide a mentor to the new physician
- Have profound, lasting results

From a practical perspective, appropriate patient charging, coding compliance, utilization and referral processes, laboratory and imaging services, transcription, medical records, and appointment scheduling are just a few of the many subsystems critical to the success of the physician practice. Any new physician should rapidly become familiar with them.

Organizational Culture Integration

Hanson[46] suggests that it is critical for the physician practice to develop methods to culturally integrate the new physician into the practice. Indicators that the practice exhibits cultural integration include the following:

- Willing to delegate authority and give up individual autonomy
- Able to work collaboratively to solve problems
- Committed and/or willing to follow group goals and directives
- Accepting of consolidation of practices and economies of scale
- Willing to share income, expense, and/or governance
- Focused on the long term and the short term
- Willing to deal with problems of other group physicians

As Wendling-Aloi observes, "strong leadership—both physician and administrative—must exist for a successful cultural orientation."[47] (p. 9) This leadership does not necessarily come easily, so significant effort must be expended to make the physician orientation process successful.

One of the important roles of the HR department is "improving the organization's effectiveness by providing employees with the learning needed to improve their current or future job performance."[48] Thus training is highly focused on knowledge, skills, and abilities. Knowledge is both remembering and understanding information; skills are the capacity to perform specific tasks; and abilities are the physical, mental, or social capabilities necessary to function at a certain level.

According to Leahy, "poorly trained front and back office staff cost practices plenty."[49] (p. 22) Not only are poorly trained staff less efficient in their use of time, but practices can experience failures to collect money through inaccurate documentation and billing, fail to receive authorization to treat under an HMO arrangement, and lose valuable customers due to rudeness or inattention. Employees at all levels in the organization can benefit from enhanced technical knowledge and skills and from greater attention to customer service needs. Physician practices should consider compensating employees who seek out employer-sanctioned education by various methods, including tuition coverage, release time, training reimbursement, and other methods. While employees benefit directly from additional training, so too does the physician practice.

Role of Trainer

Depending on the size of the physician practice, Leahy[49] suggests that it may be cost-effective to designate a full- or part-time trainer to achieve the following:

- Develop a training curriculum and materials to address specific needs of the practice
- Address staff questions as they occur
- Develop and document comprehensive training policies and procedures
- Train small groups in customer service
- Identify individual employee training needs
- Recheck employees on process and procedure to confirm that the initial training has been effective
- Establish benchmarks or targets for performance improvement

Where possible, it is desirable to appoint an internal candidate to the training position, assuming the employee is experienced in a variety of functions and has a positive attitude toward the organization. The training program should not only seek to enhance current knowledge and skills, but also anticipate the need for new knowledge and skills. For example, if a physician practice expects to acquire a new piece of diagnostic equipment or a new computer application, training should begin in a timely manner to take full advantage of the innovation. In some cases, new staff may need to be recruited and then trained to meet the demands of a new service or program. It therefore behooves the HR department to keep in touch with key operating departments to discover training needs in advance of implementation.

Training and Motivation

Linking job rotation, job sharing, and cross-training with enhanced employee motivation is one method of improving employee performance and enhancing organizational outcomes.[50] Casebolt and Barton[51] support this concept and take it one step further by suggesting that employees become more motivated when they are involved with redefining their jobs. Management should take the lead in providing coaching to employees to help staff identify how each job affects others and address ways to simplify or eliminate tasks so as to improve workplace processes. In physician practice settings, it is extremely economical to cross-train employees in front-office duties, such as receptionist, billing, scheduling, and other clerical tasks, rather than hiring temporary help to perform these duties. Fortunately, many medical assistants employed in physician practices have graduated from practical training programs that prepare them for the multiple assignments that are routine in most practices. Offering pay incentives to learn multiple tasks is one method of ensuring that employees are cross-trained in the event of illness, vacation, or other absences.

Job Rotation and Cross-Training

There may be value in considering cross-training or rotating employees who have been in their individual jobs for years. At a certain point, anyone may stop learning and become bored with relatively routine duties. If an employee has reached the top of his or her ability to be promoted, or no promotional opportunities are available, consideration should be given to rotating job assignments or reshaping jobs to match employee interests.[50] While this practice may appear costly initially, in the long run it encourages retention of superior employees, produces a more flexible and innovative workforce, and enhances job satisfaction, which in turn creates a more satisfying work environment for both staff and customers.

Positive Training Environment

The embrace of job rotation and cross-training would suggest that the physician practice should strive to become a positive training environment, in which top management and employees at all levels of the organization recognize the desirability of continuous learning to improve individual and group performance, to share knowledge and ideas, and to foster coaching and reinforcement of newly acquired knowledge and skills.[48] Training to enhance job performance and job satisfaction should permeate the organization; it should be consistent; and it should be rewarded. Unfortunately, training may be "put on the back burner" when resources become scarce, only to be resurrected when a new supervisor is appointed or turnover creates a shortage of experienced staff. Training, like quality improvement, should be constant and permeate the entire organization. It should not be viewed as a luxury, but rather as a necessity to enhance the organization's performance and employee retention.

RETENTION

The easiest and most cost-effective way of reducing the cost and uncertainty of recruitment is to retain valued employees. Many organizational behavior studies have concluded that money alone is not the ultimate or even a strong motivator for employees. Therefore, a physician practice must seek other means of retaining valued employees. According to Fabrizio,[52] this process starts with the initial interview. The practice should try to match the potential candidate with the culture of the organization to see if there is a potential "fit." The interviewer does so by explaining the mission, vision, and values of the practice, in an effort to determine whether the prospective candidate identifies with the organization's public statements. Another approach is to ask the candidate specific behavioral or situation-based questions to gauge his or her responses to hypothetical problems. It is also appropriate to ask candidates how they addressed actual problems or situations in their prior place of employment.

It is clearly more cost-effective to retain competent employees than to experience constant turnover. Employees respond much better to praise than to criticism, welcome constructive advice, value timely communication, and appreciate consistent decision making by supervisors. Most employees leave their jobs not for higher compensation, but because of dissatisfaction with the intangibles of the workplace, such as respect from their bosses, a congenial work environment, relative autonomy, and the opportunity for challenge.[53] Additional incentives for retention include enhanced benefits and educational programs.

Benefits Enhancement

Physician practices frequently reward employees for years of service by offering enhanced benefits, such as longer vacation periods, a higher contribution to the retirement plan, educational reimbursement, and other perquisites, to show appreciation for their loyalty and contribution to the organization. While it must remain ever mindful of laws prohibiting discrimination, a physician practice can provide meaningful benefits to encourage employees to remain with the organization.

Educational Incentives

Providing employees with incentives to continue their education is a double-edged sword. On the one hand, better-educated employees may potentially improve the services offered by physician practice. On the other hand, more education makes these employees more marketable to other employers. The most enlightened theory recognizes that good employees will often seek to enhance both their skills and their compensation, and helping the employee to facilitate educational advancement will generate loyalty toward the physician practice and encourage the employee to remain with an organization that recognizes and rewards initiative.

Employee Handbook

While each physician practice is encouraged to create its own Employee Handbook to deal with the unique requirements of a specific practice, Exhibit A outlines many of the issues identified as appropriate for most physician practices.[26] Discussion of the Employee Handbook should begin at orientation, if not before, and should focus on issues that are considered critical to the continued success of both the employee and the organization. Where legal, the HR department should require that the new employee sign an acknowledgment that he or she has received and read the Employee Handbook. Where the organization has a Compliance Policy, it should be mandatory that all employees read and sign the policy to safeguard the physician practice. For example, some organizations have a policy against sharing proprietary information with others, or accepting gifts of gratuities over a certain value. To the extent reasonable, the Employee Handbook should specify acceptable and unacceptable behavior in unambiguous terms. It is far better to advise employees in advance of any untoward situations than to live with the consequences of ignorance.

Personnel Files

Employment records are generally kept in employees' personnel files. Different states may have different requirements for employee record content and retention, so the material presented in Exhibit B is intended as a general guide.

Right to View Personnel Files

In most cases, employees have a right to view their personnel files upon request. The employer must make the personnel file available at the requesting employee's workplace within a "reasonable time period," generally within 10 working days. The employee should use his or her own time, such as a lunch break or after work, to view the file. A member of the human resources staff or other authorized representative should be in attendance during the entire process. Employees may also request a copy of the contents of their personnel file. An employee's right to view his or her personnel file does *not* apply to two items:

- Records relating to the investigation of a possible criminal offense
- Letters of reference

A few records should not be kept with the employee's personnel file, including any investigation of harassment claims, discrimination claims, and background or reference checks. As with most issues relating to the law, seeking sound advice from a labor attorney will save the practice heartache, time, and money in the long run.

PERFORMANCE EVALUATIONS

The performance evaluation is a "formal system of periodic review and evaluation of an individual's or team's performance."[54] [(p. 144)] There are multiple purposes for a performance evaluation: to evaluate adequacy of job performance, to determine compensation, to consider potential promotability, and to assist the employee with career development.

Unfortunately, too many managers procrastinate when it is time to conduct a performance evaluation for key employees. Perhaps this reluctance is avoidance of confrontation in situations where the employee is not performing satisfactorily, or perhaps the manager has not documented performance throughout the year and prefers not to meet with little to discuss with the employee. Whatever the reason, the need for the "boss" to do a performance evaluation on employees is often bounced back to the HR department to prod the supervisor to do his or her job. This awkward situation can be avoided by making performance evaluations mandatory and encouraging the board of directors to impose negative sanctions against managers who fail to perform this important task. Sending a list of overdue evaluations to the practice administrator or to the board of directors usually solves the problem, after first giving the appropriate manager a full opportunity to schedule and complete the evaluation.

Alternative Evaluation Methods

The most common form of performance evaluation is one in which the manager and employee meet one-on-one for a reasonable time period to assess the employee's strengths and weaknesses, suggest improvement, and outline a plan of corrective action (if necessary) over a specific time period. While this process can be punitive, it is more beneficial for all concerned if the performance evaluation session is constructive, objective, and focused on performance improvement. To achieve this mutually desirable outcome, it is incumbent on the manager to periodically document both positive and negative performance during the evaluation period (usually annually), so that the session is productive.

A second common method is the physician-employee evaluation. In medical group settings, nursing staff are often assigned to individual physicians. Nurses and nursing assistants are appropriately evaluated by the physicians with whom they work most closely. Physicians are often either reluctant or too preoccupied to conduct a formal performance evaluation on those who work with them side-by-side. A poorly performing nurse may therefore be allowed to remain with the organization for years, until a crisis situation prompts the physician to demand that the nurse be terminated or transferred, usually without prior documentation of any negative performance. It behooves human resources management to insist that physicians provide timely and comprehensive performance evaluations, so that all employees are dealt with in a fair and consistent manner, while at the same time maintaining a competent workforce.

Self-appraisal encourages the employee to self-assess his or her performance to determine whether the employee's perception of performance matches that of the manager. The performance evaluation can then focus on areas of difference, thus making the best use of the time available. This type of evaluation is highly beneficial to the organization in that it encourages employee development.[54]

A team-based appraisal is quite common in complex organizations, in which employees are assigned to teams to maximize performance. In situations where the employee's major contribution to the organization is serving as a member of a performance team, as opposed to working independently, it is both realistic and fair to evaluate the employee on the basis of his or her contribution to the team performance. One method of performance evaluation in these circumstances is to encourage the team members to evaluate or rate other team members. If team members know that their performance will be measured by others on the team, greater teamwork should result; the team may be more productive; and individual team members will be discouraged from trying to shirk their responsibilities.

Physician performance appraisals are often neglected in this process. In many cases, a formal evaluation of physician performance is either ignored or glossed over until problems develop. It is recommended that all physicians participate in a formal performance evaluation process, with specific emphasis on patient satisfaction, quality outcomes, and productivity. The traditional hospital peer-review process is appropriate for a technical evaluation of the physician's performance, but it does not touch on other important aspects of the physician's work as an employee of the practice and as a member of the clinical team.

A 360-degree appraisal is useful when the organization wishes to perform a comprehensive evaluation on an employee. Such an approach may be appropriate if the employee has limited interaction with managers or other employees, is based in a location distant from the majority of employees, or performs tasks for which there is a high degree of external customer involvement. In these situations, the human resources department may ask a variety of individuals to comment on the employee's performance, so that the evaluation looks at the full scope of the job and the individual's ability to perform. Hoffman[55] suggests that a 360-degree appraisal may be appropriate for several reasons, including supporting team initiatives, assessing developmental needs, identifying performance thresholds, and improving customer service.

Reverse appraisals, in which senior managers appraise their boss anonymously, are becoming increasingly common in large organizations. This kind of evaluation provides the chief executive officer and perhaps the board of directors with valuable input into the human relations performance with peers and subordinates. If the manager appears to be doing an effective job, but all of his or her subordinates hate working for the individual and will leave the organization given the opportunity, this information would be meaningful for those who are ultimately responsible for the success of the organization. The major drawback of this approach is the potential for a vindictive employee to provide a negative appraisal of his or her boss either to take the pressure off the employee or to cast the boss in an unfavorable light. If enough subordinates are afforded the opportunity to evaluate their superiors, a single negative evaluation should be discounted.

Performance Evaluation Elements

While there is no one best method of performance evaluation, and certainly no one best format, most evaluations generally include three elements: traits, behaviors, and results or outcomes.[54] Some performance evaluations use a graph to measure and rank traits or behaviors, especially where a number of individuals are performing essentially the same tasks (e.g., receptionists, billers, or nursing assistants). Some organizations will consciously seek to retain those employees who rank in the upper quartiles of performance by offering pay increases or bonuses, while providing training for those who fall below a certain performance level. In selected situations, the organization may encourage low performers to leave the organization.

There should be no surprises at the periodic or annual performance evaluation. A focus on the future during the performance evaluation is beneficial to both the employee and the organization. The employee needs to be reminded of his or her value to the organization and the performance needed to continue making a positive contribution. Likewise, the physician practice should expect the employee to continue to focus on achievable results and the manager to reinforce positive performance, which ideally will lead to promotion and advancement.

Task Performance Versus Behavior

Measurement of task performance, while often difficult, is relatively objective. The employee is either capable of performing the task within predetermined specifications or not. One aspect of performance that poses a challenge for measurement is behavior toward fellow employees and customers. Ability and willingness to please patients in a physician practice go beyond simply performing the elements of the job adequately. Patients may adore their physician but leave the practice due to rude or unaccommodating staff. The physician may not even be aware that employees in the practice are uncaring, combative, or just plain nasty to patients until the loss of patients becomes painfully obvious. Fried[54] suggests using a Behavior Observation Scale (BOS) to assess behavioral characteristics of employees, such as overcoming resistance to change, demonstrating a positive attitude, and engaging in effective communication with patients. An employee may be very efficient in performing the tasks associated with the job, but be ineffective in dealing with customers and patients. Most healthcare organizations, especially physician practices, cannot afford to retain employees who alienate current and potential patients.

Problems with Performance Evaluations

Some common problems occur when conducting performance evaluations. First and foremost, the evaluation process may be cursory at best, resulting in no change in performance or behavior. This is most often due to the manager's reluctance to confront negative issues with employee performance, a lack of documentation, or fear of employee retaliation. This failure to appropriately address performance does a disservice to both the employee and the organization. Minor deficiencies are not addressed and corrected while there is still time to salvage an otherwise valuable employee. The organization also loses in that a new employee must be hired and trained, resulting in significant unnecessary expense to the physician practice.

Performance evaluations are also vulnerable to personal bias on the part of the manager. This bias may take the form of either favoritism, whereby an incompetent employee is allowed to remain in the practice, or negative bias, which forces out a competent employee.

Performance evaluations may also be deficient if they do not address the core of the employee's performance. If the evaluation focuses on only the most visible aspects to the job and does not take a comprehensive approach, poor performance may be ignored, to the detriment of the practice.

Progressive Discipline and Grievance Procedure

It is critical to both the employee and the physician practice that unacceptable or inadequate performance be documented. In situations where the employee is covered under a collective bargaining unit (union), it is imperative that the organization adhere to the progressive discipline and grievance procedure, according to the agreement. Failure to properly document poor performance will most likely result in either a reversal of the employer's action or a lawsuit, or both. Because the majority of physician practices do not fall under collective bargaining agreements, both employer and employee may find it advantageous to establish a formal progressive discipline policy and procedure that spells out the process of informing the employee of unsatisfactory performance and time periods to grieve a negative evaluation. In many cases, the employee has 10 working days to formally challenge a negative performance evaluation or a warning notice. The HR department should include a specific statement in the Employee Handbook regarding the progressive discipline process, so that employees are fully aware of the process, their rights to challenge any personnel action, and the time period pertaining to each action.

CONCLUSION

All of the workforce issues confronting the healthcare industry now and in the future will be experienced by physician practice organizations. The aging of the U.S. population will put additional pressure on physician practices in dealing with chronic diseases. The number of foreign-born patients is also expected to increase, leading to new cultural and communication challenges for physician practices. The number of medically uninsured in the United States now exceeds 44 million and is rising. Pressures for healthcare cost reductions will continue, as will pressures to reduce physician reimbursement from government programs and private insurance plans. Shortages of nurses and other skilled workers will continue to create problems for the healthcare industry as a whole, but especially for physician practices, which may not be able to remain salary-competitive. We can also expect to experience higher malpractice costs, increased regulation and compliance requirements, and increased costly innovations in medicine and technology.[56] Despite these and other pressures on the healthcare industry, the fact remains that physicians and practice administrators have survived similar challenges for decades. They are expected to face these new challenges with the same degree of optimism, dedication, and innovation as their predecessors.

The pressures on health care will continue to mount well into the next decade, and physician practices will be prime targets for politicians, regulators, and employer groups intent on enhancing quality of care and patient satisfaction, while at the same time attacking the rising cost of health care. Issues involving medical ethics, healthcare rationing, and end-of-life decisions will accelerate, along with demands for universal healthcare coverage.

Physician practices are microcosms of the healthcare industry. While unique in some aspects, they reflect what is happening within the industry in terms of economics, politics, the professions, and employment trends. Physician practices are among the first places patients turn to in time of medical need. How the practice addresses those needs in a compassionate, comprehensive, and cost-effective manner will largely influence the patient's ultimate outcome. Ensuring that the physician practice is staffed with competent and caring employees is the primary bulwark in our defense against disease and one of the greatest challenges in our society. The human resources function is not just a mechanical process, but one that helps set the moral and ethical tone for the entire organization. Hiring inadequate staff, failing to compensate employees equitably, and ignoring poor performance are all unacceptable in dealing with the healthcare needs of our communities. We can and must be held to a higher standard.

REFERENCES

1. Medical Group Management Association (www.mgma.com). A guide to the body of knowledge of medical practice executives. Denver, CO: American College of Medical Practice Executives; 2004.
2. Schneck LH. Strength in numbers: medical group practices fill vital niche in U.S. health care system. *MGMA Connexion.* 2004; 4(1):34–43, 1.
3. Moser JW. Socioeconomic characteristics of physicians in alternative practice arrangements. *Journal of Medical Practice Management.* 1998; 13(5):223–224.
4. American College of Medical Practice Executives. *The ACMPE Guide to the Body of Knowledge for Medical Practice Management.* Englewood, CO: Medical Group Management Association; 2003.
5. Gans DN. Ockham's razor cuts confusion surrounding management. *MGMA Connexion.* 2004; 4(6):24–27.
6. Modern Healthcare. *Key Industry Facts.* 2003 Supplement.
7. American College of Healthcare Executives. *Key Industry Facts.* 2004.
8. Gans DN. Health care's dilemma. More staff, higher costs, little benefit. *MGMA Connexion.* 2004; 4(2):24–27.
9. Johnson BA. Stark II, phase II: what it means for physician compensation. *MGMA Connexion.* 2004; 4:43–48.

10. White KR, Clement DG. Healthcare professionals. In: Fried BJ, Johnson JA, Eds. *Human Resources in Healthcare.* Chicago, Ill: Health Administration Press; 2002.

11. Arsenault E. Impact of nurse workforce issues on the physician and practice manager. In: Keagy B, Thomas MS, Eds. *Essentials of Physician Practice Management.* San Francisco: Jossey-Bass; 2004.

12. U.S. Bureau of Health Professions. Projected supply, demand, and shortages of registered nurses: 2000–2020: 2002. Available at: www.bhpr.hrsa.gov/healthworkforce/rnproject/report.htm#chart1.

13. Keagy BA. The role of nonphysician clinicians in medical practice. In: Keagy BA, Thomas MS, Eds. *Essentials of Physician Practice Management.* San Francisco: Jossey-Bass; 2004.

14. Cooper RA, Laud P, Dietrich CL. Current and projected workforce of nonphysician clinicians. *Journal of the American Medical Association.* 1998; 280: 788–794.

15. Regan DM. Stretch capability: physician extenders can expand access cost-effectively. *MGMA Connexion.* 2002; 2(3):48–51.

16. Chung K, Bell R, Gellatly DL. How capitation and practice size affect health work force. *MGMA Connexion.* 2002; 2(4):62–66.

17. Davis RJ. When to consider a nurse practitioner. *Wall Street Journal.* April 23, 2002: D4.

18. Medical Group Management Association. Defining the profession: talk' 'bout your generation: *Medical Group Management Journal.* 2001; 48(4):24–26.

19. Kennedy MM. Boomer and busters: addressing the generation gap in healthcare management. *Healthcare Executive.* 1998; 13(6):6–10.

20. Stone DA. The doctor as businessman: the changing politics of a cultural icon. *Journal of Health Politics, Policy and Law.* 1997; 22(2)533–556.

21. Mechanic D. Changing medical organization and the erosion of trust. *The Milbank Quarterly.* 1996; 74(2):171–189.

22. Reinhardt UE. The rise and fall of the physician practice management industry. *Health Affairs.* 2000; 19(1):42–55.

23. Stevens RA. Public roles for the medical profession in the United States: Beyond theories of decline and fall. *The Milbank Quarterly.* 2001; 79(3):327–353, III.

24. *The Essentials: 2003 MGMA Survey Report.* Physician Compensation and Productivity Report. Englewood, CO: Medical Group Management Association; 2003.

25. Mertz G. Effective physician governance is not an oxymoron. *MGMA Connexion.* 2003; 3(1):50–53.

26. Gulko E. From the ground up: Guidelines for the development of a group practice. *MGMA Connexion.* 2003; 3(9):56–61.

27. Van Amerongen D. Physician compensation. In: Fried BJ, Johnson JA, Eds. *Human Resources in Healthcare.* Chicago, Ill: Health Administration Press; 2002.

28. Schneck LH. Incentive programs that drive your employees to excel. *MGMA Connexion.* 2001; 1(2):38–40.

29. Crisafulli J, Fried BJ. Compensation. In: Fried BJ, Johnson JA, Eds. *Human Resources in Healthcare: Managing for Success.* Chicago, Ill: Health Administration Press; 2002.

30. Benedict GS. *The Development and Management of Medical Groups.* Englewood, CO: Medical Group Management Association; 1996.

31. Fried BJ, Johnson JA, Eds. *Human Resources in Healthcare: Managing for Success.* Chicago, Ill: Health Administration Press; 2002.

32. Keagy BA. The role of nonphysician clinicians in medical practice. In: Keagy BA, Thomas MS, Eds. *Essentials of Physician Practice Management.* San Francisco: Jossey-Bass; 2004.

33. Poplin AC. Physician compensation—past, present and future: a literature review. American College of Medical Practice Executives Paper. Available at: http://www.mgma.com/acmpe/. Accessed August 2002.

34. Ross A, Williams SJ, Pavlock EJ, Eds. *Ambulatory Care Management.* Third Edition. Clifton Park, NY: Delmar Publishers; 1998.

35. Redling B. Focus on academic practice: compensation plan features flexibility, incentives. *MGMA e-Connexion.* March 2003; Issue 27.

36. Porn L. Physician compensation. In: Keagy BA, Thomas MS, Eds. *Essentials of Physician Practice Management.* San Francisco: Jossey-Bass; 2004.

37. Fitzgerald PE, Burkett SH, Key CM. An exercise in controversy. Case study: Revising a physician employment agreement. *MGMA Connexion.* 2003; 3(10):44–49, 1.

38. McGeorge AM. Taxation and physician practices. In: Keagy BA, Thomas MS, Eds. *Essentials of Physician Practice Management.* San Francisco: Jossey-Bass; 2004.

39. Fried BJ. Performance management. In: Fried BJ, Johnson JA, Eds. *Human Resources in Healthcare: Managing for Success.* Chicago, Ill: Health Administration Press; 2002a.

40. Redling B. How deep do you dig when checking out applicants? *MGM Update.* September 2000; 39(18).

41. White CS, Thibadoux GM. Defer to refer? Giving references and avoiding legal liability. *MGMA Connexion.* 2002; 2(2):60–63.

42. Fried BJ, Thomas MS, Goodrich LL. Human resource management. In: Keady BL, Thomas MS, Eds. *Essentials of Physician Practice Management.* San Francisco: Jossey-Bass; 2004.

43. Hekman KM. Hidden expenses: the true cost of adding a physician to your medical group practice. *MGMA Connexion.* 2004; 4(1):44–47, 1.

44. Price C, Strickler B. The Family and Medical Leave Act: making it work for practices and employees. *Personnel Postscript/HR Issues.* September 2002; 15(3).

45. Wendling-Aloi S. Plotting a path to success: developing a physician orientation program. *MGMA Connexion.* 2003; 3(3):42–46.

46. Hanson RD. What makes a successful medical group? *MGM Update.* 2001; 40(15):6.

47. Wendling-Aloi S. The link between physician retention and orientation. *MGMA Connexion.* 2003; 3(1):28–29.

48. Johnson JA. Training and development. In: Fried BJ, Johnson JA, Eds. *Human Resources in Healthcare: Managing for Success.* Chicago, Ill: Health Administration Press; 2002.

49. Leahy ME. Train 'em and reap: a structured training program for front and back office staff. *MGMA Connexion.* 2002; 2(2):34–37.

50. Redling B. Assembling a solid staff: job rotation, job shaping and cross-training help employee retention. *MGMA Connexion.* 2003; 3(3):38–40, 1.

51. Casebolt K, Thompson B. Reshuffle the deck: a simple plan for improving employee motivation. *MGMA Connexion.* 2003; 3(4):48–50, 1.

52. Fabrizio NA. Hire to fit: ask the right questions, reduce turnover. *MGMA e-Connexion.* February 2004: 4(2).

53. Fahey DF, Myrtle RC, Schlosser JR. Critical success factors in the development of healthcare management careers. *Journal of Healthcare Management.* 1998; 43(4):307–321.

54. Fried BJ. Performance Management. In: Fried BJ, Johnson JA, Eds. *Human Resources in Healthcare: Managing for Success.* Chicago, Ill: Health Administration Press; 2002.

55. Hoffman R. Ten reasons you should be using 360-degree feedback. *HR Magazine.* April 1995; 82–85.

56. Redling B. Workplace issues: New challenges facing medical groups. *MGMA Connexion.* 2003; 3(3):24–25.

Employee Handbook

5. Jury Duty
6. Military Leave
7. Health/Dental Insurance
8. Worker's Compensation/Accidents (Injuries on the Job)
9. Pension Plans/401(k)
10. Group Life Insurance

Section IV
1. Medicare/Medicaid Compliance
2. Personnel Appearance
3. Safety
4. Smoking
5. Solicitations and Distribution of Literature
6. Security Inspections
7. Use of Phone and Mail Systems
8. Use of Equipment
9. Emergency Closing
10. Visitors in the Workplace
11. Use of Computers and E-mail
12. Workplace Monitoring
13. Attendance and Punctuality
14. Public Relations

Section V
1. Alcoholism and Drug Use
2. Appearance
3. Attitude
4. Changes in Personnel Status
5. Complaints and Grievances
6. Sexual Harassment
7. Confidential Information

Section VI
1. Employment Conduct and Work Rules
2. Progressive Discipline
3. Termination of Employment
4. Layoffs
5. Unemployment Compensation Insurance

Personnel Files

The personnel file usually contains original documents pertaining to the employee's qualifications for hiring, promotion, a record of pay increases, employment anniversary date, benefit changes, disciplinary action, and termination:

- Application for employment
- Résumé
- Hiring documents (e.g., W-4)
- Job description
- Payroll change forms
- Performance evaluations
- Promotion recommendations
- Record of grievances affecting employment status
- Notices of warnings and disciplinary actions (signed by employee)
- Education and training records
- Notices of commendation
- Notices of layoffs
- Family/medical leave requests
- Worker's compensation records
- Return to work releases
- Medical restrictions
- Request for leave of absence (signed by employee)
- Exit termination notice

Personnel files are to be retained on the premises of the employee's workplace and should contain original documents. While record retention may vary from state to state, it is generally a good practice to keep records for at least five years following the date of termination.

CHAPTER 12

Human Resources Practices and Management in Public Health Clinics

Anne M. Hewitt

VIGNETTE

Sara pulled the curtain open and yanked the unruly shades up on the main front window of the Wood County Public Health Clinic. A newborn baby's whimper came from behind her, and she glanced to see Tishonda registering the first of at least eight clients in an impatient line coming through the door. Thursday was Child Care Day and was always busy for all of her co-workers. Sara hoped the Visiting Nurse Association had finally been able to fill its open position and that the clinic would be fully staffed today.

As she turned back to look into the sunshine, someone caught her attention across the boulevard. On the dirty side-walk, with his back to the corner of the alley, sat Rasheed, wrapped in newspapers. As manager of all the health clinics, Sara knew that Rasheed attended the tuberculosis (TB) clinic on Friday, and here he was a day early for his appointment. She wondered if the new full-service TB clinic and the proposed partnership with Memorial Hospital would be approved at the next county board meeting. Establishing linkages with the hospital for healthcare clinic services would free up her staff to attend to neglected outreach efforts, such as worksite screening and senior health fairs. It seemed like such a small step, but it represented new relationships with many of the clinic's regular partners. Sara would be busy in the coming months, but today's priorities were the moms, children, and noisy infants.

INTRODUCTION

Public health clinics (PHCs) serve as one of the most important "safety net" institutions. These facilities are available to all Americans, regardless of their health insurance status or health condition. As part of the public health system, the clinics are the only health agency to focus on local populations to emphasize preventing disease and disability rather than simply treating individual health conditions.[1] PHCs can best be described as those clinics operated and sponsored by local-level public health agencies as part of a municipal (city or county) government. Such a clinic may have a permanent physical location or be offered intermittently at different geographic locations throughout a community. PHCs are designed for easy public access, and they serve a neighborhood population, whether it be in a rural location, an inner-city high-rise building, or a suburban municipal office. PHCs are not necessarily autonomous units, and they differ from locally sponsored community health centers (CHCs), which originated in the late 1960s through a federal government program.

The distribution of public health clinics in the United States varies by state and type of municipal governance. In 2002, there were an estimated 3,300 delivery sites for community, migrant, public housing, and homeless centers, but no official data were available regarding the number of public health clinics across the country.[2] Currently, neither the National Association of County and City Health Officials (NACCHO) nor the Health Resources and Services Administration (HRSA; Bureau of Primary Health Care) collects data on the national scope of public health clinics. Unlike CHCs, which are often members of the state and/or national Primary Care Association, most aggregate data available on PHCs

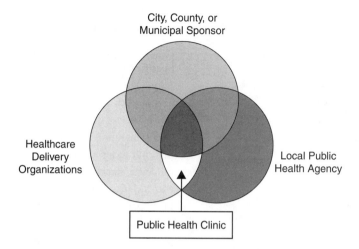

City, County, or
Municipal Sponsor

Healthcare
Delivery
Organizations

Local Public
Health Agency

Public Health Clinic

After providing an overview of the public health clinic setting, this chapter discusses critical human resources issues facing public health clinics including strategic planning, recruitment and selection, retention, compensation, performance evaluation, legal and regulatory issues, and human resources opportunities and challenges.

FIGURE 12-1 Organizations Influencing the Role of a Public Health Clinic

are gathered at the state level and monitored by the state department of health and/or local boards of health. Although PHCs can be sponsored by a city, county, or municipality (town, township, borough), they may receive federal, state, and/or local government support and financing.

Local public health departments serve community populations and are mandated to provide many diverse clinic services. Because of their primary relationship with local government, PHCs offer a unique blend of public services, healthcare services, and population-focused initiatives based on the public health model. Figure 12-1 illustrates the unique position of a public health clinic.

OVERVIEW OF THE SETTING

Role and Characteristics

The most impressive characteristic of public health clinics is the potential range of services provided. Table 12-1 summarizes the scope of health services offered, the diverse priority populations, and the broad range of health conditions covered by a typical public health clinic. This list includes examples ranging from disease-specific clinics, such as clinics for

---

Table 12-1 Types of Clinics Offered by Public Health Organizations

Group 1: Health Promotion/ Disease Prevention	Group 3: Age- and/or Gender- Specific Clinics
Blood pressure screening	Adolescent weight control
Cancer checkups	Child health
Chronic disease checkups	Child vision
Complementary and Alternative Medicine	Family planning
	Immunizations for children
Depression	Influenza/senior clinics
Domestic violence	Men's clinics
Mental health	Orthopedic clinics for children
Osteoporosis screening	Pediatric dental/oral care
Prenatal care	Sudden infant death syndrome
Safety-net clinics	Teen parenthood
Stress reduction	WIC (women, infants, and children)
Substance misuse and abuse	**Group 4: Environmentally Related Clinics**
Vaccinations	
Well-baby days	Environmental exposures (lead poisoning)
Worksite smoking clinic	
Group 2: Disease-Specific Clinics	Lyme disease screening
Asthma	Rabies
Down syndrome	**Group 5: Priority Population Clinics**
HIV/AIDS	American Indian/tribal clinics
Sexually transmitted diseases	Homeless clinics
Tuberculosis	Medicaid recipients
Wound/abscess	Migrant worker's health care
	Screenings for bisexuals and lesbians

---

adults with Down syndrome, to the more typical child immunization clinics. Recently, public health departments have expanded their offerings even further by holding single-event, bioterrorism-related clinics, such as providing smallpox inoculations for first responders. Although HRSA categorizes clinic types into seven service areas for CHCs, the variety of health promotion and disease prevention services offered by PHCs remain essentially focused on primary care. (*Note:* HRSA categorizes clinic services as dental, enabling, mental health/substance abuse services, obstetrics/gynecology, other professional services, primary medical care services, and specialty medical services.) Given this extensive set of operations, obtaining diverse, qualified personnel presents many challenges for health managers.[3]

Some public health clinics may not be available on a 24-hour, workday, or even weekly basis. Many smaller clinics that are staffed with part-time healthcare personnel will have limited operations and may rotate availability by days and county sites. Other, larger PHCs may have weekly schedules that include standard safety-net activities (vaccinations, well-baby days, screenings) interspersed with special hours for disease-specific conditions, such as tuberculosis and HIV/AIDS. Clinic schedules may also reflect the time of year, with immunizations and child vision days occurring in late summer, senior influenza clinic days available in the fall, and Lyme disease screenings in late spring and early summer.

To be most effective, clinic directors often seek to reach specific, underserved populations, and clinics are scheduled for selected locations that will enable workers to better interact with various priority groups, such as adolescents, seniors, working adults (worksites), and elementary-school-aged children (school-based clinics). Although men's clinics appear to be more prevalent than in past years, recent research suggests that PHCs are seldom used by men, especially minority men.[4] PHCs are often scheduled at local cultural centers and community religious institutions to reach diverse populations, although Hispanics and African Americans typically see clinics as the least preferred option for health care.[5]

Each clinic type brings with it accompanying human resources issues for the local health department, the administrative staff, and the clinic healthcare providers. Depending on the size of the clinic and its organizational relationship with the primary sponsor, typical human resources issues can be handled through the local government agency's human resources department, or they can be part of the role and responsibilities of the clinic director. If the clinic director is given specific human resources duties, such as hiring and promotion of personnel, the policies followed by the clinic parallel the sponsoring organization's policies.

Along with the types of clinic services provided, other important characteristics the human resources manager or clinic director will need to consider are clinic size, geographic location, service delivery site location, priority populations being served, and clinic sponsor arrangements (see Figure 12-2). PHCs range in size from a single room and one public health nurse with open appointments to a completely staffed primary care site with 25 clinic support workers serving a large population (more than

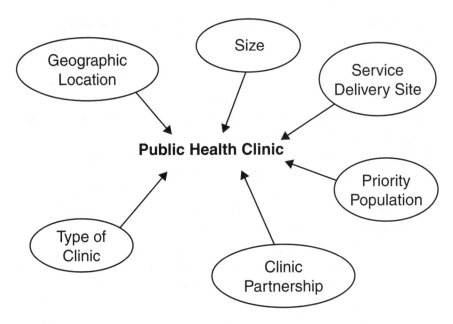

FIGURE 12-2 Characteristics of Public Health Clinics That Affect Human Resources

500 visits) by appointment only. The size range for public health clinics is most often influenced by two other factors: the geographic location of the clinic and the service delivery site location. Public health departments also vary immensely in size and situation, and can be located in urban, suburban, rural, mixed, or frontier areas. The geographic location and population density in turn affect the site location for the clinic. Densely populated areas generally support PHCs at municipal locations, whereas rural PHCs are sometimes transportable and located at schools, local fire departments, and shopping malls. Frontier areas may require the use of mobile clinics to provide services to the entire community.

PHCs operating in a federally designated medically underserved area (MUA) can expect to find a shortage of qualified healthcare providers—especially primary care physicians.[6] In fact, in the last 20 years, the general public health workforce may have diminished by as much as 20%.[7] The emergence of numerous options for other types of employment has greatly hindered recruitment of qualified employees for PHCs.

Public health clinics may partner with a wide variety of other health organizations and develop both informal and formal partnership arrangements. These arrangements can exist with local healthcare delivery organizations (hospitals, ambulatory care facilities), traditional healthcare providers (physicians, dentists, pharmacists), visiting nurse associations, not-for-profit health organizations (American Lung Association, American Cancer Association), or other municipal, city, or state health agencies. Local elected officials or county commissioners are one of the primary constituent groups to exert influence over PHC partnerships. These elected public officials react to public concerns and focus on activities that are important to their constituents. PHCs are directly affected by their decisions, as local match funding is critical to maintaining operations.[8] The Partnerships Project's *Making Strategic Decisions about Service Delivery* is a document that helps PHCs identify appropriate services, develop guidelines for relationships with other community partners, and facilitate strategic HR planning.[9]

Emerging Trends: Internal and External Influences on Public Health Clinics

The three core functions of public health—assessment, assurance, and policy development—serve as the framework for the 10 essential public health services to be provided for every community.[10] Table 12-2 shows the relationship between these three core functions and the role of the public health clinic.

Public health clinics must compete for funding with other primary municipal core services, such as fire, emergency, and police protection; sanitation services; library and recreation services; and schools. Unfortunately, most health departments operate without sufficient funds or staff and remain unable to carry out their stated mission of community protection.[4] Insufficient funds affect public health services negatively by limiting access to qualified personnel and decreasing the number of activities offered, thus requiring the PHC to prioritize the services it will provide and the availability of current services. To maintain their current service delivery levels in the face of inadequate funding, PHCs may begin charging for services, using a sliding fee scale. This type of organizational retrenchment results in longer waits for public access and lessens the opportunities for health promotion and disease prevention among a population that depends on the PHC for primary health care. A recent study of a restructured large urban healthcare system (including clinics and involving primary care services) found that 33% of at-risk clients delayed

Table 12-2 Relationships Between Public Health Functions and Essential Services and the Public Health Clinic

Core Function	10 Essential Public Health Services	Role of Public Health Clinic
Assessment of community need	1. Monitor health status to identify health problems	✓
	2. Diagnose and investigate health problems and health hazards in the community	✓
	3. Inform, educate, and empower people about health issues	✓
	4. Mobilize community partnerships to identify and solve health problems	✓
Policy development	5. Develop policies and plans that support individual and community health efforts	✓
	6. Enforce laws and regulations that protect health and ensure safety	✓
	7. Link people to needed personal health services and assure the provision of health care when otherwise unavailable	✓
Assurance of services	8. Ensure a competent public health and personal healthcare workforce	✓
	9. Evaluate effectiveness, accessibility, and quality of personal and population-based health services	✓
	10. Conduct research for new insights and innovative solutions to health problems	✓

seeking out needed medical care.[11] Clearly, the potential for underserved and at-risk individuals to receive priority health care is undermined when the PHC's funding is cut.

Due to pervasive municipal budget constraints and as a direct result of trying to provide an increasing number of mandated services, some local health departments have opted to privatize clinical services previously offered at their public health clinics.[12] This shift away from providing primary clinical services for the individual has moved the PHC into a newer role, using a population-based approach to health promotion and disease prevention.[13, 14] Community healthcare providers have recognized that fragmented healthcare delivery undermines comprehensive and coordinated care, and the role of the PHC needs to evolve away from providing these kinds of stop-gap measures.[15, 16] Ideally, the outsourcing of primary care services will save money and help to maintain programs at risk for abandonment due to limited budgets.[17]

Another issue that has altered the role of public health clinics is the advent of bioterrorism preparedness and homeland security concerns, especially for urban areas. Establishing the infrastructure necessary to protect the public in the event of a biological or chemical attack requires immense capital and personnel resources. It is estimated that more than $1 billion has been spent in preparing the public health system to prevent bioterrorism.[18] At a local level, the PHC is responsible for providing emergency health screening or care in case of a catastrophic community event. Although funds have been provided to the states, demands related to bioterrorism preparedness at the local level compete with existing demands of the traditional public health clinics, and staffing shortages are continually reported.[19]

The increase in immigrant populations in specific states and certain core urban areas is yet another trend that is affecting the delivery of health care in the PHC setting. Although migrant workers' health has been addressed on a national level in the past, the increase in public health clinic usage by the newly arrived and non-English-speaking immigrant constitutes an additional challenge for PHCs. As states implement special programs for currently underserved or unserved populations, such as Medicaid recipients (family care) and State Children's Health Insurance Program (SCHIP), PHCs will begin to serve individuals and families who are temporarily in transition and become less of a full-time, permanent, primary care provider for these populations.

Labor force issues are key factors feeding many of the challenges facing public health clinics. The drive to attract qualified health professionals to serve in PHCs continues to demand additional resources, but many clinics (both rural and urban) are concentrated in health professional shortage areas (HPSAs). This tension between supply and demand, especially for physicians, has resulted in the continued use of international medical graduates.[20] However, the primary staffing need now appears to be for nurses. Currently, there is a national shortage of nurses, especially those interested in public and community health, which generally pays 10% to 20% less than traditional hospital compensation. The increase in job specialization within the PHC workplace mirrors the trend seen in the general health sector workforce and also contributes to a challenging HR environment.[21] All of these factors have led to increased privatization of local public health department services, including the management and operations of public health clinics.[22] It is estimated that almost three-fourths of all local public health departments in the United States are now involved with some type of privatization efforts.[23]

These twenty-first-century trends will continue to influence the prioritization of services for the PHC. Future HR planning will need to balance the PHC's mandated responsibilities to serve as the safety net for the community and the trend toward partnering with other community health agencies and organizations to provide primary care and service delivery. This transformation will not be easy, and the safety-net focus of PHCs will require them to continue to be the usual source of care for underinsured and uninsured populations.

Understanding and Managing Human Resources for Public Health Clinics

The primary consideration in managing human resources practices for public health clinics continues to be the interrelationship between the municipal or county government with its citizen/voter oversight focus, the public health mandate championed by the local board of health and/or local public health department, and the regulated provision of primary clinical healthcare services through the public health clinic setting. Balancing the policies and regulations surrounding these three foci and the various stakeholders requires familiarity with all of the following:

- State and county public employee policies and procedures
- Public health minimum standards of performance
- Healthcare certifications, licensure issues, and regulations

The rest of this chapter examines these three constraints and applies them to typical human resources functions relevant to public health clinics.

STRATEGIC PLANNING

Developing a successful human resources plan for any public health clinic requires integrating the human resources functions seamlessly with the clinic's mission. The clinic director will generally follow either a leadership or team model approach, the choice of which determines the organizational chart of the clinic as well as the role and relationships of the

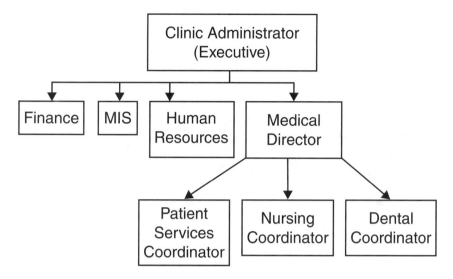

FIGURE 12-3 Leadership/Administrative PHC Staffing Model

various employees. Figure 12-3 portrays an executive chain of command model, and Figure 12-4 illustrates a more typical health team approach. This pivotal management choice will also determine the employee skill sets needed to staff the PHC.

Regardless of the model selected, the PHC clinic director or medical director must be able to provide leadership, work as part of the management and clinical team, and facilitate relationships with primary stakeholders. Like management of other healthcare organizations, PHC management may face thorny issues in balancing administrative roles and responsibilities and the clinical provider role, which has the consumer's health as its primary goal. Unless the PHC is very large, with a budget sufficient for separate administration, this type of organizational dilemma may pose quite a challenge. The range of skills needed can be enormous, depending on the size of the PHC.[15] Filling the clinic director or medical director position with the right person is, therefore, key to the clinic's performance.

Specific workforce data on local public health agencies are limited.[18] Results from current surveys using specific occupational classifications (SOCs) have been inconclusive, as health directors found it difficult to appropriately categorize their staff, who often carry out many multifunctional tasks. Although staffing for PHCs is not separated from general

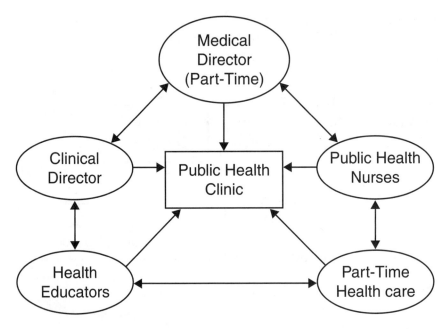

FIGURE 12-4 PHC Team Staffing Model

public health data, the median staff size of a local public health agency is estimated at 13 full-time equivalents (FTEs).[24] Two issues of primary concern to HR management are workforce quantity (staffing levels and mix) and quality (professional education/credentialing).[1]

A pivotal factor for today's HR needs is the national agenda of moving away from individual clinic services and toward a more population-based approach for providing health promotion and disease prevention services.[13] Making this transition requires a workforce that is trained in different skill sets and able to interact with all community populations. To facilitate achieving this PHC goal, clinic management candidates must have experience in developing coalitions and creating partnerships with diverse partners.[25] For all PHC employees, essential knowledge and skills include diversity training, accommodation of community cultural practices, familiarity with other languages, and the accompanying impact on health literacy.[11]

Many states have also adopted public health approaches that require local health departments to complete community needs assessments to ensure that PHCs are providing adequate services. This planning process requires human resources managers to operate within the clinic's budget so that sufficient funds are available to recruit appropriately qualified personnel to meet the identified community needs. This alignment process may also be duplicated at the municipal or county level, as administrators seek to develop balanced budgets and bring standardization to positions and job descriptions. As clinics transition away from their role as primary service providers, the director's role continues to support the local health department agency—but through new activities, such as quality assessment and assurance initiatives, contract development and monitoring, and expanded financial analysis and accountability.[26]

RECRUITMENT AND SELECTION

Past history suggests that many PHCs follow an internal recruitment process and/or promotion protocol, as this practice encourages agency and cultural loyalty, with accompanying low turnover rates. Although not required to hire local or community residents (as are CHCs), PHCs often appeal to local residents as attractive locations for employment. As PHCs assume more of a health promotion and disease prevention focus, new efforts will be needed to attract qualified candidates from an external labor market outside the geographic area if appropriately trained internal or local applicants are not available. However, the standard practice of using part-time healthcare providers (e.g., physicians, dentists, physician assistants) to staff PHCs can still be a legitimate component of the HR strategic plan.

Recruitment strategies for PHCs differ significantly for clinical and management positions. For clinically trained employees, such as infectious disease specialists, orthopedists, and pediatric dentists, recruiters may need to advertise in professional association journals as well as local and regional media. Many times, local health departments will model their job descriptions following state examples. Table 12-3 provides an abbreviated clinic nurse job specification.[27] Table 12-4 presents a recent job advertisement for a public health nurse with clinic duties.[28]

When recruiting for nonclinical positions (administrative and general/clerical), a standard municipal search protocol can be followed. Because of the PHC's relationship to the municipal or county organization, all recruiting strategies will need to adhere to publicly mandated policies and procedures. These steps often include internal job postings

---

Table 12-3 Abbreviated Clinic Nurse Job Specification by State Department of Personnel (For Local Government Use Only)

Clinic Nurse

Definition: Under supervision in a clinic, first-aid unit, or other setting; provides nursing services on a regular or emergency basis; does other related work.

Examples of work: Listed.

Requirements: License—Current and valid registration as a professional nurse in the State of New Jersey. License—Appointees will be required to possess a driver's license valid in New Jersey only if the operation of a vehicle, rather than employee mobility, is necessary to perform essential duties of the position.

Knowledge and abilities: Listed.

Persons with mental or physical disabilities are eligible as long as they can perform essential functions of the job after reasonable accommodation is made to their known limitations. If the accommodation cannot be made because it would cause the employer undue hardship, such persons may not be eligible.

---

and may involve preferences based on union guidelines, seniority, and/or veteran status. Also, candidates for all positions usually are required to pass extensive background checks for criminal or traffic violations. Other common recruitment strategies include participation in job fairs, Internet postings, internships, and employee referrals.

The current health professional shortage phenomenon constrains PHC recruiting efforts significantly. Although physician recruitment is extremely difficult, the demand for nurses is a critical factor, as clinical nurse

---

Table 12-4 Job Advertisement for a Public Health Nurse

Public Health Nurse

We have a full-time position available with excellent benefits for professionals with a BSN degree, current RN license in the State of New Jersey, one year's prior experience in public health, and a valid N.J. driver's license. The position is in Essex County, New Jersey. The successful applicant will assume significant responsibilities with regard to public health emergency preparedness, develop plans for clinic operations, and have responsibilities with communicable disease infection and follow-up in addition to other duties within the specific county. Knowledge specific to clinic operations and communicable disease are preferable. Effective verbal and written communication skills are required. The individual should have the ability to work independently as well as in a team environment and to organize and prioritize work. Bilingual in Spanish is a plus. Salary in the $50,000 range and is based on education and public health experience with excellent full benefits package (paid holidays, vacation, personal and sick days).

specialists are being used as a cost-effective strategy for healthcare delivery.[29] As noted earlier, PHC nursing salaries average 10% to 15% less than other health institutions' compensation levels. The aging of nurses already employed in the public health system places another constraint on the recruiter's ability to find and retain qualified nurses. Some PHC managers estimate the average age of their nurses to be over 45, with many scheduled to retire in the next five years, as baby boomers begin to leave the workforce. The use of part-time allied health professionals is one strategy to supplement clinic staff with older employees. Other recruitment strategies include recruiting retired school nurses and others who live within the geographic location served by the PHC.

To further highlight the PHC's scope and level of HR staffing requirements, Table 12-5 provides an example of the diversity and numbers of PHC staff required for a hypothetical HIV clinic.

The importance of adequate staffing for achieving desired health outcomes is supported by research showing that same-day scheduling at public health clinics results in greater client satisfaction, shorter waiting times, and increased provider productivity. To reach these goals, adequate staff must be available on a daily basis.[30]

Another constraint on the recruiting process is the need for the PHC to adhere to the state's public health minimum standards of performance. These standards often include position requirements for specific degrees, certifications, and specialized training and competencies. One example from New Jersey is presented in Table 12-6.[31] Although outsourcing through the use of visiting nurse associations or proprietary staffing agencies provides an alternative, the additional expense associated with this strategy is usually not a feasible alternative on a permanent basis.

Table 12-5 Example Staffing Needs for an HIV Clinic

Staffing Requirements	Availability	Role
2 infectious disease physicians	Part-time	Weekly appointments
1 internist	Part-time	Weekly appointments
1 nurse practitioner	Full-time	Clinic manager
3 staff nurses (RN/BSN)	Full-time	Clinic care providers
Administrative staff	Full-time	Appointments/clerical

Table 12-6 State Example of Public Health Staffing Qualifications

New Jersey Department of Health: Standards of Performance—Chapter 52

8:52-4.2 Public health staffing qualifications

a. Each health officer shall be licensed by the Department pursuant to the provisions of Licensure of Persons for Public Health Positions, N.J.A.C. 8:7.

b. Each public health nurse shall have the following qualifications:

  1. Hold a baccalaureate degree in nursing from an accredited college or university

  2. Hold a current license to practice as a registered professional nurse by the New Jersey State Board of Nursing

  3. Have a minimum of one year's experience in public health or working with a preceptor or local resource person

  4. Complete a course in population-based health nursing within one year of employment

---

As the designated health provider for the local public health department, the PHC may be invited to participate in many community grants. Federal grants often include specific restrictions on personnel and mandate their degrees, training, and certifications. The Ryan White Act is one example of this regulatory practice; it would influence any hiring strategies used to staff HIV/AIDS clinics. Participation in partnership grants places an additional burden on the PHC recruiter, who must comply with all grant mandates.

The HR recruiting strategy for PHCs requires targeted searches, flexibility in job descriptions, and creative partnering to successfully staff a local public health clinic. The recent Institute of Medicine report, *Who Will Keep the Public Healthy? Educating Public Health Professionals in the 21st Century,* underscores the need for strategic HR initiatives to meet future staffing needs.[32]

RETENTION

Turnover rates for public health clinics vary by clinic size and location. Urban clinics typically compete with other health organizations that usually can provide higher salaries. In contrast, suburban and rural health clinics tend to have less of a retention problem, as employees remain committed to the organization and enjoy the accompanying security. Retention issues are classified into three broad categories:

- *Licensure and certification issues.* Clinical guidelines and regulations require yearly updates of clinical staff eligibility and renewal of licensure and certification. Personnel must maintain these qualifications to be retained through primary and secondary verification.
- *Practitioner impairment issues.* Clinical employees must be able to physically and mentally complete all required tasks without impairment. PHCs, like all other healthcare provider organizations, are required to monitor and report incidents that suggest clinician impairment. Documentation of employee impairment that leads to poor clinical performance would automatically trigger a formal review process.
- *Grant funding issues.* Grant-funded positions may be time delimited, usually for durations of three to five years. Opportunities may be available to retain staff in other full-time positions, transfer them to other grant-funded positions, or seek sustaining monies from the county or original grant funder.

To enhance PHC employee retention rates, human resources directors are encouraged to establish effective employment development strategies.[33] To fully implement an employment development plan, resources and time need to be committed to recognizing quality performance, planning career paths, and providing opportunities for personal and organizational growth. PHCs will need to continually upgrade and upskill their current employees to meet future staffing requirements.

TRAINING AND EDUCATION

Ensuring that the public health workforce as a whole has the appropriate skills and knowledge is an immense task,[34] but opportunities for educational support are plentiful for PHC employees. Many public health managerial and administrative forums and programs are offered by the following organizations:

- CDC/HRSA Public Health Traineeships and Public Health Training Centers[35]
- Public Health Leadership Forum and Public Health Foundation's training initiative: TRAIN[36]
- Management Academy for Public Health[37]

A recent Washington state survey of all public health professionals indicated that the four training topics most highly rated by respondents were (1) interpersonal communication, (2) cross-cultural and cross-age communication, (3) electronic communication, and (4) participatory teaching/training skills. Participants also selected on-site training as the most desirable, although more than 90% of respondents indicated they preferred training with an instructor/trainer. On-site training is often not cost-effective at the local level[38] and for smaller clinics.

In recent years, as PHC's diminished staffing levels have made it difficult for employees to spend time away from the clinic, satellite conferences and Web-based continuing education programs have become preferred options for training. The ready on-site access and ease of participation using this type of educational technology allow workers to invest in the continuing education hours required for licensure or certification. Tracking of educational support activities and certification-related training participation may require the development of a specific database component that ideally would be integrated with the standard HR database (which generally includes personnel, job-related benefits, and miscellaneous information for the individual). Nursing continuing education hours requirements vary according to the certification requirements for each nursing and allied health specialty. PHCs that receive grant funding may also be required to permit staff to attend designated conferences so that these personnel remain up-to-date on treatment protocols.

Training and development efforts can serve as the foundation for any quality improvement initiatives.[39] Local municipal initiatives for quality improvement may also be integrated into the PHC's training efforts. As the role of public health clinics changes, with direct patient care being deemphasized and community health status assessment being highlighted,[39] training needs will, in turn, reflect the new areas of emphasis. PHCs must have a workforce skilled in epidemiology, planning, partnership development, and oversight of contract-service providers.[24]

COMPENSATION

Two significant factors influence compensation plans for PHC workers. First, clinic personnel who are considered public employees receive salaries and benefits based on the municipal or county guidelines and standards. If they are unionized, the elements that make up the union members' compensation will be included in contract negotiations and are not directly part of the clinic manager's responsibility. Second, if union membership does not apply to the PHC staff, additional considerations become important in developing an appropriate salary scale.

The use of part-time employees for staffing PHCs appears to be an established strategy. Unless the PHC is unusually large and operates on a full-time basis, part-time employees offer the flexibility in time and expertise needed to optimally staff a PHC. Compensation guidelines in such a case can be based on professional qualifications, time spent working, and services performed. Because municipal governments often provide significantly less generous benefits for part-time (versus full-time) employees,[40] overall clinic staffing costs will be lower when part-time employees are used.

A local or regional salary survey conducted by PHC management or the state public health officer organization can provide a benchmark for establishing a competitive salary scale. A recent survey of community health center CEOs found a wide salary range—from $40,000 to $100,000.[16] State salary guidelines are often available for comparisons.[41] See Table 12-7.

The issue of physician compensation and market pricing deserves scrutiny, as ranges for full-time and part-time employment may vary by geographic location and by size of clinic. Salaries for consulting physicians often vary depending on whether they provide primary and specialist care and on how many clinic visits they make per week (two times per week

Table 12-7 Example Salary Scale for a State Clinic Nurse, 2003

Increment	$1,424.58
Level 1	$31,509.17
Level 2	$32,933.75
Level 3	$34,358.33
Level 4	$35,782.90
Level 5	$37,207.49
Level 6	$38,632.07
Level 7	$40,056.65
Level 8	$41,481.23
Level 9	$42,905.81

versus three times per week), with physician specialists receiving higher compensation. The Bureau of Health Professions and the National Health Service Corporation can be of assistance in establishing physician salary ranges. Also, the National Center for Health Workforce Analysis produces state health workforce profiles that may assist HR planners in reviewing general supply and demand issues for healthcare workers.

In some cases, PHC specialty clinics may be partially staffed by volunteer physicians who complete a mandated number of clinic hours to satisfy the eligibility requirements at local hospitals. In this case, compensation is not an issue, but legal liability and malpractice insurance should be covered by the partnering hospital facility.

Although equity, incentives, and cost control are all components of any compensation management strategy,[42] cost management emerges as the most critical factor for PHCs.

PERFORMANCE EVALUATION

Within a public health clinic, performance evaluation responsibilities may be delegated to one of three positions: (1) the clinic director (administrative); (2) the medical director (clinical); or (3) the sponsoring human resources department located within the municipal or county agency. A primary concern when engaging in performance assessment activities is to follow any protocols mandated by local union agreements. Staff and clinical employees may be covered by different labor–management agreements, and special efforts should be made to comply with all policies and procedures. Many times, the medical director will be asked to evaluate clinical personnel as well as all clinic administrative staff. If the medical director is inexperienced in evaluating nonhealth personnel, scheduled performance review policy meetings with the primary municipal or county human resources director can help facilitate best practices in this area. Occasionally, PHCs operate fully under the control of the local board of health. In this case, clinic staff may or may not be considered public employees, and performance assessment procedures will vary accordingly.

The PHC's goals for performance evaluation are similar to those of other healthcare organizations and focus on two areas: (1) enhancing the clinic employees' performance through appropriate and systematic feedback and (2) collecting information and documentation for personnel decisions, such as promotions, demotions, or even termination.[43] If the public health clinic requires accreditation from the Joint Commission on Accreditation of Healthcare Organizations (JCAHO), then performance appraisals are required and reviewed as part of the accreditation process.

In general, clinic supervisors or directors complete performance ratings for clinic employees, but in some instances team-peer ratings may be integrated into the process. Performance appraisal methods may involve the use of written standards for the individual or the use of a checklist approach based on attainment of defined task-related goals. This strategy should not be confused with the much more formal approach of "management by objectives." Newer practices applicable to performance evaluation, such as results-oriented performance appraisals and the use of performance-based compensation, are rarely found in PHCs.

LEGAL AND REGULATORY ISSUES

A series of basic human resources laws, policies, and regulations provide a foundation for managing most HR issues of a public health clinic:

- *Basic rights:* Title VII of the Civil Rights Act (1964), Civil Rights Act (1991), Age Discrimination Act (1967), Rehabilitation Act (1973), Equal Pay Act (1963), Pregnancy Discrimination Act (1978)
- *Individual rights:* Worker's compensation (state) laws, Equal Pay Act (1963), workplace incident laws (e.g., hostile environment, harassment), Family and Medical Leave Act (1993)
- *Human resources policy and regulations:* Fair Labor Standards Act, Occupational Safety and Health Act (1970), Employee Retirement Income Security Act (1974), Consolidated Omnibus Reconciliation Act (COBRA), Drug Free Workplace Act (1988), Immigration Reform and Control Act (1986, 1990, 1996)

Clinic managers and directors should also review any state, municipal, or local HR regulations that apply to the public health clinic as part of a larger government entity.

Protocols for Contracts and Agreements

As PHCs transition away from providing actual healthcare services to more prevention-focused activities, they must increase their participation in partnerships and both informal and formal relationships. These more structured agreements between partners create the need to detail and document specialized services and relationships, especially as privatization of direct medical care is increasing.[44] This collaborative type of contract arrangement differs considerably from standard service delivery contracts, such as those negotiated for simple laboratory services. The partnership continuum can range from an informal structure characterized by ad hoc arrangements between the clinic and its partners, to a formal structure with established guidelines and frameworks for all phases of the relationship, to a legal entity status arrangement in which memoranda of agreement or understanding are written as formal contracts.

Indirect consequences of this transition include an increase in outsourcing arrangements and an intensified risk to the PHC as the primary accountable agency. Recent research suggests that contracts are an underutilized but effective alternative for achieving public health outcomes.[45] To manage this risk, the PHC administration will need to be familiar with the principles of contract development, management, and contract monitoring. Basic contract components include price and coverage, with specifications focusing on client services (access, information, provider network), service implementation (quality assurance, reporting requirements), and a detailed performance evaluation plan. Because the potential exists for the PHC to collaborate with many different partners, all agreements and contracts should avoid establishing exclusive relationships with a single agency wherever possible.[45]

Contracts between the PHC and other healthcare organizations will be subject to approval from the municipal or county officer responsible. The PHC manager ultimately has accountability for monitoring compliance with contract agreements, regardless of the category of contract partner. The types of potential PHC contract partners vary greatly, from individuals to large institutions.

- *Healthcare provider organizations:* hospitals, primary care facilities, ambulatory care, visiting nurse associations
- *Healthcare providers:* independent contractors, such as physicians, dentists, and nurse practitioners
- *Health-related organizations:* laboratories, pharmaceutical and medical suppliers
- *Labor organizations:* union organizations representing health workers, as well as municipal or county union organizations

Due to the large number of part-time, contract employees and independent contractors found in PHCs, HR managers should carefully monitor all state and federal antidiscrimination and individual employment rights laws applicable to these groups.[46]

Legal/Regulatory Issues and Compliance

The legal and regulatory issues of interest to HR managers of public health clinics reflect a triad of responsibilities: demonstrating public accountability, meeting health provider standards and compliance, and satisfying public health mandates from the federal and state levels.

Legal issues associated with managing public employees encompass activities that ensure the right to due process in all personnel practices, as well as adherence to union negotiation protocols and contract monitoring. Strategies for promoting labor–management cooperation will also need to include the input of local municipal or county human resources directors and other primary stakeholders. Joint labor–management committees can function proactively in achieving strategic human resources goals if agendas and timing are approached in a collaborative manner.[47] For example, PHC employees may benefit from participation in employee assistance programs (EAPs) that focus on stress management, sexual or workplace harassment, and dealing successfully with co-workers. This perspective may also encourage the formation of other EAPs for risk prevention and management. All employee relationships can be enhanced by taking three basic steps: (1) facilitating reciprocal communication between workers and management, (2) establishing and adhering to a formal grievance protocol, and (3) enhancing effective first-line supervision.[48]

Special regulatory concerns involving the provision and delivery of health services by the PHC include accreditation by JCAHO and achievement of standards where applicable, adherence to the Health Information Portability and Accountability Act (HIPAA), and development and review of clinical treatment documents, including "permission to be treated" and standard "release of information" forms. All PHCs generally follow a standard protocol for reporting any screening abnormalities to the patient and to the identified primary care physician. Under the risk management protocol, consumers are generally not allowed to register for clinic screenings without providing the name and address of their primary care provider. Another prominent concern is the risk of malpractice litigation, which requires PHC managers to follow established best practices and guidelines in all clinical areas. Test results are always accompanied by a letter from the clinic, and abnormal test results should be followed up by a phone call. If results are outside of normal limits, consultation with a physician is recommended. Screenings should not be considered diagnostic and are not a substitute for regular medical care provided by a private physician.

HUMAN RESOURCES OPPORTUNITIES AND CHALLENGES

Integrating diversity into the workforce and the workplace will be the greatest challenge that human resources managers face while working with public health clinics. "Diversity" within the public arena is often broadly defined as differences in ethnicity, race, gender, age, educational level, socioeconomic status, culture, language, religion, physical or mental disabilities, or sexual orientation. Diversity awareness education and training is quickly becoming an essential competency, as the PHC requires employees to interact with members of the public. Newer employees will benefit from cultural competencies, as many health professional degree programs already include learning modules for cultural and diversity sensitivity training. Standard diversity education programs should be enhanced with in-service opportunities or continuing education credits that focus specifically on the local community's culture and preferences. Beliefs about the role of health care and attitudes of clinic providers toward minorities and other diverse populations can either enhance or detract from the quality of services provided. Managing diversity also requires human resources directors to ask themselves if their PHC personnel are reflective of the local community and, if not, why not.

CONCLUSION

The outlook for public health clinics ultimately depends on the ability of the local board of health and the county or municipal department of health to transition from being a provider of direct primary health services to being a facilitator of community health improvements, using a population-based approach that focuses on health promotion and disease prevention. Making this transition successfully will require the human resources manager to develop a strategic plan that replaces retiring and exit-

Table 12-8 Future Challenges and Potential HR Strategies for Public Health Clinics

Challenge	Strategic Options
Reduced funding	• Hire or outsource a grant writer as a part-time position
	• Partner with community health organizations for additional funding
Diversity of population served	• Require multilingual skills for all new personnel
	• Offer cultural sensitivity training
	• Complete an organizational cultural audit
Recruiting constraints	• Partner with other health agencies for part-time or shared clinical workers
	• Develop incentives based on flex time, career path options, and training opportunities for health providers
Mission tensions	• Align municipal administrators' agendas with public health mandates through the strategic planning process
	• Complete quality improvement initiatives to identify service gaps and unmet mandated needs

ing workers with qualified employees who meet the demands of this new public health clinic focus.

The following external and internal environmental challenges will directly impact the major HR functions for maintaining local public health clinics:

- The phenomenon of reduced funding can be expected to occur at all government levels and may directly affect reimbursements from Medicaid and Medicare. Other financial limitations will come from a reduction in state matching funds and municipal government efforts to control budget growth.

- The diversity of populations served will require hiring of additional multilingual staff and clinical health providers who are appropriately culturally trained. These populations will also include more uninsured, immigrants, and elderly patients, all of whom will require additional resources for support services.

- Recruiting constraints will continue to escalate, as fewer physicians are available for primary care and the attractiveness of public health clinics for nurses is negatively affected by lower wages in comparison to other worksites.

• Mission tension—that is, between the role of the public health clinic as the municipal provider of primary care and safety-net services and the emerging health promotion model—will require a strategic plan that blends flexibility and a proactive stance toward recruitment.

These challenges can be met with an emphasis on the role of human resources as a facilitator for change as the public health clinic evolves. Table 12-8 lists specific strategies to counter each of the major trends. Several of these suggested action steps will require additional funding and resources. Other recommended HR activities, such as partnering, offering incentives, and aligning agendas, should be integrated into the overall strategic human resources management plan. The complexity of current and future challenges for the management of human resources in the PHC setting will require a skilled professional who is competent in the standard human resources functions and knowledgeable about the transforming role of public health clinics.

REFERENCES

1. Cioffi JP, Lichtveld MY, Tilson H. A research agenda for public health workforce development. *Journal of Public Health Management and Practice.* 2004; 10:187–192.
2. National Health Center Week. 2002. A Proclamation by the President of the United States. Available at: http://www.whitehouse.gov/news/releases/2002/08/20020816-7.html. Accessed June 17, 2005.
3. Health Resource and Service Administration. Clinic Categories. 2004. Available at: http://ask.hrsa.gov/pc/servicetypedef.htm. Accessed July 27, 2005.
4. Smith AL. Health policy and the coloring of an American male crisis: a perspective on community-based health services. *American Journal of Public Health.* 2003; 93:749–752.
5. Ryan J. Health officials lament minorities' use of clinics as a last resort. *The Star-Ledger.* June 13, 2003; 19.
6. Wells A. San Bernardino, Calif. clinic provides free care, aids poor. *Knight Ridder Tribune Business News.* May 25, 2004; 1.
7. Gebbie K, Merrill J, Hwang I, Gebbie EN, Gupta M. The public health workforce in the year 2000. *Journal of Public Health Management and Practice.* 2003; 9:79–86.
8. Lind P, Finley D. County commissioners as a key constituency for public health. *Journal of Public Health Management and Practice.* 2000; 6:30–38.
9. National Association of County and City Health Officials (NACCHO). Workforce Development. In *Making Strategic Decisions about Service Delivery: An Action Tool for Assessment and Transitioning.* Washington, DC: NACCHO; 2002.

10. American Public Health Association. The Essential Services of Public Health. Available at: http://www.apha.org/ppp/science/10ES.htm. Accessed July 20, 2005.
11. Diamant AL, Hays RD, Morales LS, Ford W, et al. Delays and unmet need for healthcare among adult primary care patients in a restructured urban public health system. *American Journal of Public Health.* 2004; 94:783–789.
12. Halverson PK, Kaluzny AD, Mays GP, Richard TB. Privatizing health services: alternative models and emerging issues for public health and quality management. *Quality Management in Healthcare.* 1997; 5:1–18.
13. Keller LO, Schaffer MA, Lia-Hoagberg B, Strohschein S. Assessment, program planning, and evaluation in population-based public health practice. *Journal of Public Health Management and Practice.* 2002; 8:30–44.
14. Stover GN, Bassett MT. Practice is the purpose of public health. *American Journal of Public Health.* 2003; 93:1799–1801.
15. Kempe A, Beaty BL, Steiner JF, Pearson KA, et al. The regional immunization registry as a public health tool for improving clinical practice and guiding immunization delivery policy. *American Journal of Public Health.* 2004; 94:967–972.
16. Fields T, Welborn RB. Executive directors and community health centers—facing the healthcare transition. *Journal of Health Administration Education.* 1999; 17:211–226.
17. Halverson PK, Haley DR, Mays GP. Current practice and evolving roles in public health. In: Halverson PK, Kaluzny AD, McLaughlin CP, Eds. *Managed Care and Public Health.* Gaithersburg, MD: Aspen; 1998:11–41.
18. Fraser MR. The local public health agency workforce: research needs and practice realities. *Journal of Public Health Management and Practice.* 2003; 9:496–499.
19. McHugh M, Staiti AB, Felland LE. Trends: how prepared are Americans for public health emergencies? Twelve communities weigh in. *Health Affairs.* 2004; 23:201–209.
20. Hagopian A, Thompson MJ, Kaltenbach E, Hart LG. Health departments' use of international medical graduates in physician shortage areas. *Health Affairs.* 2003; 22:241–249.
21. Hernandez SR, Fottler MD, Joiner CL. Integrating management and human resources. In: Fotter MD, Hernandez SR, Joiner CL, Eds. *Essentials of Human Resources Management in Health Services Organizations.* Albany, NY: Delmar; 1998:1–20.
22. Bibeau DL, Lovelace KA, Stephenson J. Privatization of local health department services: effects on the practice of health education. *Health Education and Behavior.* 2001; 28:217–230.
23. Keane C, Marx J, Ricci E. Privatization and the scope of public health: a national survey of local health department directors. *American Journal of Public Health.* 2001; 91:611–617.
24. National Association of County and City Health Officials (NACCHO). *Local Public Health Agency Infrastructure: A Chartbook.* Washington, DC: NACCHO; 2001.

25. Butterfoss FD, Webster JD, Morrow AL, Rosenthal J. Immunization coalitions that work: training for public health professionals. *Journal of Public Health Management and Practice.* 1998; 4:79–87.

26. Brown M. Privatization of public hospitals: trends and strategies. In: Halverson PK, Kaluzny AD, McLaughlin CP, Eds. *Managed Care and Public Health.* Gaithersburg, MD: Aspen; 1998:73–82

27. New Jersey State Department of Personnel. Clinic Nurse Job Specification by State Department of Personnel. Available at: http://www.state.nj.us/jobspec/01277.htm. Accessed July 27, 2005.

28. Essex Regional Health Commission. Public Health Nurse Advertisement. Available at: http://www.essexregional.org. Accessed July 26, 2005.

29. Graveley EA, Littlefield JH. A cost effectiveness analysis for 3 staffing models for the delivery of low risk prenatal care. *American Journal of Public Health.* 1992; 82:180–184.

30. Mallard SD, Leakeas T, Duncan WJ, Fleenor ME, Sinsky RJ. Same day scheduling in public health clinics: a pilot study. *Journal of Public Health Management and Practice.* 2004; 10:148–155.

31. Practice Standards of Performance for Local Boards of Health in New Jersey. Available at: http://www.state.nj.us/health/lh/chapter-52.pdf. Accessed September 7, 2004.

32. Institute of Medicine. *Who Will Keep the Public Healthy? Educating Public Health Professionals for the 21st Century.* Washington, DC: National Academy Press; 2003.

33. Fottler MD. Strategic human resources management. In: Fried BJ, Johnson JA, Eds. *Human Resources in Healthcare: Managing for Success.* Washington, DC: AUPHA, Health Administration Press, Chicago; 2001:1–18.

34. Gebbie K, Merrill J, Tilson H. The public health workforce. *Health Affairs.* 2002; 21:57–67.

35. Kennedy VC, Moore FI. A systems approach to public health workforce development. *Journal of Public Health Management and Practice.* 2001; 7:17–22.

36. TrainingFinder Real-Time Affiliate Integrated Network (TRAIN). Available at: http://www.train.org. Accessed July 27, 2005.

37. Porter J, Johnson J, Upshaw VM, Orton S, Deal KM, Umble K. The Management Academy for Public Health: a new paradigm for public health management development. *Journal of Public Health Management and Practice.* 2002; 8:66–78.

38. Reder S, Gale JL, Taylor J. Using a dual needs assessment to evaluate the training needs of public health professionals. *Journal of Public Health Management and Practice.* 1999; 5:62–69.

39. Johnson JA. Training and development. In: Fried BJ, Johnson JA, Eds. *Human Resources in Healthcare: Managing for Success.* Washington, DC: AUPHA, Health Administration Press, Chicago; 2001:171–184.

40. Roberts GE. Municipal government part-time employee benefits practices. *Public Personnel Management.* 2003; 32:435–453.

41. New Jersey Department of Personnel. Compensation Compendium: State Clinic Nurse 2003 Salary Range. Available at: http://webapps.dop.nj.us/ Comp.Pendium.pdf. Accessed September 15, 2004.

42. Joiner CL, Jones KN, Dye CF. Compensation management. In: Fottler MD, Hernandez SR, Joiner CL, Eds. *Essentials of Human Resources Management in Health Services Organizations.* Albany, NY: Delmar; 1999:248–270.

43. McConnell CR. Performance appraisal: the never-ending task. In: *The Healthcare Manager's Human Resources Handbook. Management Concepts.* Sudbury, MA: Jones & Bartlett; 2003:187–222.

44. Lazzarini A, Elman D. Legal options for achieving public health outcomes. *Journal of Public Health Management and Practice.* 2002; 8:65–75.

45. Halverson PK, Mays GP, Kaluzny AD. Introduction. In: Halverson PK, Kaluzny AD, McLaughlin CP, Eds. *Managed Care and Public Health.* Gaithersburg, MD: Aspen; 1998:3–10.

46. Lehr RI, McLean RA, Smith GL. The legal and economic environment. In: Fottler MD, Hernandez SR, Joiner CL, Eds. *Essentials of Human Resources Management in Health Services Organizations.* Albany, NY: Delmar; 1998: 21–43.

47. American Federation of State, County, and Municipal Employees (AFSCME). Avenues for worker participation. In: *Redesigning Government: The AFSCME Approach to Workplace Change.* AFSCME; 1995. Available at: http://www. afscme.org/wrkplace/redgo.htm. Accessed July 27, 2005.

48. Rakich JS, Longest BB, Darr K. *Managing Health Services Organizations.* Third Edition. Baltimore: Health Professions Press; 1992.

13

The Future Is Now: A Call for Action

Charles F. Wainright III

OVERVIEW OF THE SETTING

In the healthcare industry, just as in other industries, change is inevitable. It is also very difficult to predict the exact direction and type of change that will occur in the future. However, if managers take the position that the future is already here and being experienced by other organizations in other locations, then it may be possible to use this information to plan for similar events or situations that may occur in their geographic community and in their industry. To further this notion, this chapter seeks to provide the reader with an understanding of the future issues and trends in health services human resources management. The material here is presented as a futuristic examination of the issues and information that will affect the health services delivery system. Health services managers can apply the information in the preceding chapters and in this chapter to attain a useful perspective of the future relative to human resources management.

This chapter reviews current and future trends in health care relative to economic, political, social, technological, and regulatory factors in the healthcare environment. Additionally, workforce trends, competencies, education and training needs, recruitment, retention, selection, placement, compensation, quality improvement, productivity, and strategic planning regarding health services management of human resources assets are discussed. Lastly, trends in human resources leadership and

373

mentorship of employees are discussed, and their possible effects on the future highlighted.

ECONOMIC TRENDS

Economic trends in health care include the continued rise in costs and expenditure rates for the United States, which spends more of its GDP on health services than any other country in the world. Health expenditures constitute approximately 15% of the U.S. GDP—more than $5,000 per capita in 2004 (Table 13-1). If this trend continues, the United States will spend approximately 18.4% of its GDP on health expenditures by 2013.[1] Furthermore, medical inflation has continued to accelerate, growing approximately 2.5% faster than the GDP. At the current sustained rate of medical expenditures, it could reach nearly 40% of the GDP by 2050.[2]

This alarming rate of expenditure has significant implications for employment of healthcare personnel. One impact may be the employment of an increasingly large number of individuals in the various healthcare occupations (see Table 13-2).

While healthcare expenditures are increasing, the rest of the U.S. economy appears to be slowing. This may seem contradictory, but Americans are spending increasingly more of their limited funds in the healthcare sector of the economy. Additionally, this trend may be a primary reason why individuals are seeking careers in the healthcare sector—both to improve their personal economic situations and to work in an area that appears to receive the greatest economic support in terms of the GDP.

The stock market has seen several sharp declines over the past three years, indicating that the U.S. economy has slowed. In July 2004, the Federal Open Market Committee (FOMC) of the Federal Reserve raised the prime interest rate for the first time since May 2000.[3] Other factors that have contributed to the slowing of the remaining areas of the U.S. economy include the September 11, 2001, attacks; fears of new terrorism activities, both at home and abroad; the wars in Iraq and Afghanistan; restructuring of various businesses; rising oil prices; and the investigation of corporate fraud. However, the slowdown in the economy has appeared to level off, with the possibility of an upturn in the near future. Indeed, many financial analysts are cautiously optimistic about the future of the U.S. economy over the next few years.

Table 13-1 National Health Expenditures (NHE), Aggregate and Per Capita Amounts, and Share of Gross Domestic Product (GDP), 1993–2014

Spending Category	1993	1998	2002	2003	2004	2005	2006	2014
NHE (billions)	$888.1	$1,150.9	$1,559.0	$1,678.9	$1,804.7	$1,936.5	$2,077.5	$3,585.7
Health services and supplies	856.3	1,112.6	1,499.8	1,614.2	1,735.5	1,862.5	1,997.8	3,451.3
Personal health care	775.8	1,009.8	1,342.9	1,440.8	1,549.0	1,663.6	1,781.3	3,067.0
Hospital care	320.0	378.5	484.2	515.9	551.8	588.6	623.5	1,007.2
Professional services	280.7	375.7	503.0	542.0	581.2	623.6	667.4	1,161.3
Physician and clinical services	201.2	256.8	340.8	369.7	397.2	425.7	453.8	782.5
Other professional services	24.5	35.5	46.1	48.5	52.2	55.6	59.6	102.3
Dental services	38.9	53.2	70.9	74.3	79.1	84.1	90.0	146.9
Other personal health care	16.1	30.2	45.3	49.5	52.8	58.2	63.9	129.7
Nursing home and home health	87.6	123.1	143.1	150.8	160.6	170.9	181.9	290.5
Home health care	21.9	33.6	36.5	40.0	45.2	50.0	54.8	95.9
Nursing home care	65.7	89.5	106.6	110.8	115.4	121.0	127.1	194.6
Retail outlet sales of medical products	87.5	132.5	212.6	232.1	255.4	280.5	308.5	608.0
Prescription drugs	51.3	87.3	161.8	179.2	200.5	223.5	249.3	521.3
Durable medical equipment	12.8	16.9	19.6	20.4	21.2	21.7	22.4	31.6
Nondurable medical products	23.4	28.4	31.1	32.5	33.7	35.3	36.8	55.1

Table 13-1 Continued

Spending Category	1993	1998	2002	2003	2004	2005	2006	2014
Government administration and net cost of private health insurance	53.3	64.9	105.7	119.7	128.2	135.4	147.3	252.9
Government public health activities	27.2	37.9	51.2	53.8	58.3	63.6	69.2	131.4
Investment	31.8	38.3	59.2	64.6	69.2	74.0	79.7	134.4
Research	15.6	20.5	36.5	40.2	43.1	46.4	50.5	90.7
Construction	16.2	17.7	22.7	24.5	26.1	27.6	29.1	43.6
NHE per capita	$3,353.9	$4,097.9	$5,317.4	$5,670.5	$6,039.8	$6,423.1	$6,830.2	$11,045.8
Population (millions)	264.8	280.8	293.2	396.1	298.8	301.5	304.2	324.6
GDP ($billions)	$6,642.3	$8,747.0	$10,487.0	$11,004.0	$11,719.3	$12,375.5	$13,019.1	$19,179.9
Real NHE	$1,009.4	$1,192.9	$1,497.6	$1,583.8	$1,665.8	$1,752.5	$1,843.2	$2,623.8
Chain-weighted GDP index	0.88	0.96	1.04	1.06	1.08	1.11	1.13	1.37
Personal healthcare deflator	0.82	0.94	1.08	1.12	1.16	1.20	1.25	1.68
NHE as percentage of GDP	13.4%	13.2%	14.9%	15.3%	15.4%	15.6%	16.0%	18.7%

Sources: Center for Medicare and Medicaid Services, Office of the Actuary; and U.S. Department of Commerce, Bureau of Economic Analysis, and Bureau of the Census.

Table 13-2 U.S. Healthcare Employment: People Employed in Health Services Sites, 1970–2002 (thousands)

	1970	1980	1990	1995	1997	1998	1999	2000	2001	2002
All employed civilians	76,805	99,303	117,914	124,900	129,558	131,463	133,488	136,891	136,933	136,485
All health service sites	4,426	7,339	9,447	10,928	11,525	11,504	11,646	11,742	12,110	12,653
Physician offices and clinics	477	777	1,098	1,512	1,559	1,581	1,624	1,697	1,799	1,907
Dentist offices and clinics	222	415	580	644	662	666	694	676	699	740
Chiropractic offices and clinics	19	40	90	99	118	127	142	124	117	138
Hospitals	2,690	4,036	4,690	4,961	5,130	5,116	5,117	5,092	5,270	5,340
Nursing and personal care facilities	509	1,119	1,543	1,718	1,755	1,801	1,786	1,737	1,771	1,942
Other health services facilities	330	872	1,446	1,995	2,301	2,213	2,283	2,414	2,454	2,585
Total numbers in all services sites	85,478	113,901	136,808	146,757	152,608	154,471	156,780	160,373	161,153	161,790

Source: U.S. Labor Department, Bureau of Labor Statistics, www.bls.gov.

At the same time, the U.S. population is graying at an alarming rate, and the birth rate is decreasing, indicating that a smaller workforce will be available in the upcoming years. These two factors—the possible upturn in the economy and the graying population—coupled with competition from other industries attracting the best workers, emphasize the importance of appropriately managing and retaining current and future healthcare employees. These economic trends provide a strong basis for healthcare managers to act immediately in preparation for not only costly healthcare expenditures, but also a severe shortage of talented healthcare workers. Because of the economic trends noted, many talented individuals will have numerous avenues through which to choose from a variety of career opportunities that are both health and non-health related. Therefore, it is imperative for healthcare leaders to discover effective ways to attract and retain the best and brightest individuals in the healthcare professions. The economic trends also indicate that salaries and other traditional forms of compensation may not be the only mechanisms that should be used to attract and retain this group of highly skilled workers. Healthcare leaders will need to explore other intangible benefits packages to maintain and sustain the workforce of the future.

POLITICAL TRENDS

The current and future political environment will also create new challenges for the health services manager. The prevailing winds in the political environment have pushed healthcare issues to a top-level priority for most political candidates. The latest trend is for candidates to call for sweeping changes to improve patient privacy, patient access, and increased services. At the same time, Congress has been pressured to cut payment rates, and insurance companies have made their own cuts. This has created a situation in which traditional healthcare facilities experience very narrow profit margins compared to health insurance companies, and free-standing specialty facilities have experienced tremendous gains over the past decade. This situation may also impel hospitals to use more part-time personnel, especially in the area of clinical nursing personnel (see Table 13-3[4]).

Another implication of these events is that not-for-profit hospitals and other tertiary healthcare facilities that have very slim margins will find it increasingly difficult to attract and retain good employees because of their

Table 13-3 Hospital Employment Trends, 1997–2002

	1997	1998	1999	2000	2001	2002
Total U.S. hospitals	5,057	5,015	4,956	4,915	4,908	4,827
Total full-time employees	3,248,861	3,294,274	3,297,689	3,332,232	3,428,159	3,489,000
Total part-time employees	1,246,592	1,242,121	1,246,661	1,320,696	1,285,207	1,329,000
Full-time registered nurses	708,245	733,365	739,086	745,113	751,095	772,000
Full-time licensed practical nurses	112,517	109,882	106,739	101,683	104,534	104,000
Part-time registered nurses	385,909	392,622	397,950	424,801	413,832	431,000
Part-time licensed practical nurses	49,489	47,191	45,561	45,011	43,446	44,000

Source: AHA Hospital Statistics. 1999–2004 editions. Chicago: Health Forum.

reduced ability to enhance pay and other benefits. By contrast, organizations such as insurance companies, free-standing specialty clinics, and assisted living units that have profitable services will enjoy a tremendous advantage and will have more funds available to invest in attracting and retaining high-performing employees.

SOCIAL TRENDS

Social factors will also play a key role in the future management of healthcare employees. As the baby boomers begin to retire, they will have more wealth than generations of the past. Many new millionaires will have high demands for specialized products and services. Their increased level of spending, along with the decrease in the number of offspring per household, will have a spillover effect for the health services industry. The new generation of wealthy retirees will demand higher-quality services and more individualized services, because they will have sufficient assets to pay for their increased demands. At the same time, the population will be living longer and will require greater levels of geriatric services.

At the other end of the spectrum, many aging Americans will not be able to afford their healthcare services. These poor and middle-class retirees will greatly add to the burden on Medicare and Medicaid. This will further strain state and federal programs and subsequently lead to reduced payment levels to public facilities.

These social trends will further divide the classes and promote additional "cherry-picking" of wealthy patients and high-profit services while increasing the public debt. Community, state, and federal programs and facilities that rely on these payment sources will have limited resources available to modify or improve their human resources benefits as a direct result of inadequate reimbursement by governmental authorities (e.g., Medicare and Medicaid programs). This lack of funding, whether as a result of inadequate taxation or allocation of governmental appropriations, will create a deficit in funding new facilities, employee compensation, and equipment. Even more diligent management efforts will be needed to identify new sources of funding employee salaries and benefits.

TECHNOLOGICAL TRENDS

The increased need for technology breakthroughs and improved medical equipment has placed additional burdens on organizations with limited resources that rely on public programs for funding sources. Complex microsurgeries, diagnostic equipment, advanced drug therapies, and increased tests for acute and chronic illnesses have elevated the standards of care and the requirements for healthcare organizations to acquire and assimilate these innovative technologies into their facilities. At the same time, employees who have greater specialization in technological skills are required to deal with these technological advances. Because of the lack of available personnel in the workforce, more employees will be asked to cross-train on various technologies and equipment.

Employers that are able to attract and retain these employees, and employees who are adept at multitasking and learn quickly, will have tremendous advantages over other employers and employees in the health services industry. Many organizations will invest intensely in training programs that improve employees' skills and increase their rate of learning. Moreover, with the advent of electronic medical records, more efficient use of clinical staff personnel will become possible.[5] Successful healthcare organizations will need to recruit and retain employees who are extremely proficient in these technological skills and have the willingness and motivation to adapt quickly to the technologically dynamic environment. Additionally, these employees will need to be able to multitask and handle a variety of software and hardware systems. HR managers will need to devise mechanisms that can identify potential candidates with these exceptional technological skills and abilities.

REGULATORY TRENDS

Over the past few decades, the number and complexity of regulations and legislative amendments affecting healthcare providers and facilities have steadily increased. The trend is highly likely to continue, given the litigious nature of U.S. society, the implementation of the 1996 HIPAA l egislation, and the Institute of Medicine's 2000 report on medical errors. Congress and governmental healthcare agencies have joined forces in attempting to reduce errors in healthcare facilities. Unfortunately, the increased legislation and regulations have further burdened the healthcare system, by forcing providers to incorporate new software and documentation processes within their healthcare operations. While extremely costly and time-consuming, these changes have yet to make a significant difference in error rates. However, the human resources management implication is that many more specialized personnel will be required to implement these new regulations. Compliance officers, Medicare/ Medicaid claims adjusters, software managers, and documentation specialists are just a few of the new employee positions resulting from regulatory changes.

If health services managers desire to successfully and effectively manage the human resources assets within an organization, they must reconcile the organization's operations with these future trends in the economic, political, social, technological, and regulatory environments. Successful health services managers will devise unique and specific strategies to take advantage of opportunities that favorably affect their organizational mission, while simultaneously creating other tactics and strategies to minimize the environmental factors that threaten the successful positioning of their organizations. Organizations that have a distinct competitive advantage in the human resources assets that can accommodate the aging population and have strong learning skills will realize tremendous benefits in the future. Community organizations that rely on federal, state, and local public assistance programs (e.g., Medicare, Medicaid, and local governmental taxes) must be creative in developing human resources benefits under austere conditions. They must react even more rapidly than their for-profit counterparts to attract and retain qualified employees who have the skills necessary to thrive in the technologically complex and highly regulated future environment.

To provide some insight into these future strategies, the various activities of human resources management must be explored relative to the future environment. The major human resources management activities are an excellent starting point when discussing forward-thinking strategies.

IMPLICATIONS FOR HUMAN RESOURCES MANAGERS

First and foremost is the requirement to perform a human resources management needs assessment or gap analysis related to the organization's critical requirements, such as positions, skills, competencies, and operating structures needed for the next three to five years. A review of healthcare organizations often indicates a severe lack of planning and gap analysis concerning their human assets. Many of these organizations place human resources in a personnel services category, where employee benefits, pay, and grievance issues are handled. This department rarely receives recognition, connection, or attention from the executive level—but such strategic integration into the organizational mission and values is required in today's complex healthcare environment.

The needs assessment or critical gap analysis could be performed as a part of the organization's strategic planning process. An external and internal environmental assessment using a TOWS (threats, opportunities, strengths, and weaknesses) grid that matches the future threats and opportunities to the organization's current strengths and weaknesses relative to its human resources assets would be a valuable approach. The organization's executive team and members of the organization's strategic planning committee could use specific brainstorming, the nominal group technique, a Delphi survey, or other tools to develop a list of essential requirements for the future. Additional external sources (research publications, consultants, and forecasting techniques) could be used to further extend this assessment plan.[6] The organization must also use the best available information on economic, political, social, technological, and regulatory trends to honestly assess its strengths and weaknesses.

Past assessments of organizations within the healthcare industry as a whole have shown that many organizations do not have the appropriate human resources necessary to meet future needs. An AHA survey in 2003 revealed that hospitals are struggling to fill certain positions. These include registered nurses (84%), radiology/nuclear imaging workers (71%), pharmacists (46%), laboratory/medical technicians (27%), nurses/clinical aides (20%), physical therapists/occupational therapists/speech therapists (11%), housekeeping/maintenance workers (10%), respiratory therapists (10%), billing/coding workers (8%), and information systems specialists (7%).[7]

There is also a tremendous deficit of employees with high learning skill potential and flexibility in skills. Specific shortages include pharmaco-economic analysts; pharmacists (especially pharmacists knowledgeable in genetic drug advancements); nurses with dual backgrounds (including those with cross-training in at least two or more clinical specialties or administration and clinical specialties); interventional radiologists; documentation specialists to review regulations and records to ensure corporate and organizational compliance with federal, state, and local regulations; computer software experts who can integrate health services software; administrators with regulatory knowledge; physicians with administrative skills; and hospitalists and intensivists who have the ability to monitor critical patients across multiple shifts within the healthcare facility. In addition, there is an immense need for bilingual employees and professional translators to help hospitals treat the 47 million people in the United States who speak a language other than English.[8–10]

Critical shortages will also occur in the near future in the public health workforce. Trends shown in Figures 13-1, 13-2, 13-3, 13-4, and 13-5 indicate that the public health workforce throughout the United States is changing dramatically.

Figure 13-1 reveals the significant aging of public health workers compared to federal and state government workers. The average age of public health workers is approximately 46.6 years, and this average is increasing each year. This average age compares unfavorably to the average age of the

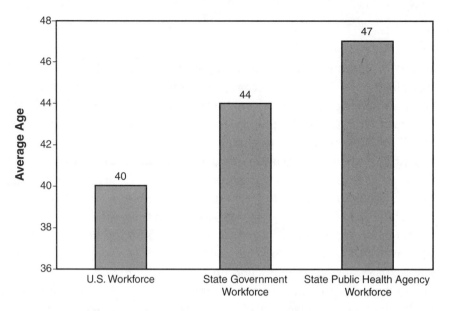

Source: Association of State and Territorial Health Officials (ASTHO). *State Public Health Employee Worker Shortage Report: A Civil Service Recruitment and Retention Crisis.* Available at: http://www.astho.org/pubs/Workforce-Survey-Report-2.pdf. Accessed April 11, 2006.

FIGURE 13-1 Average Age of PH Workers, by Region

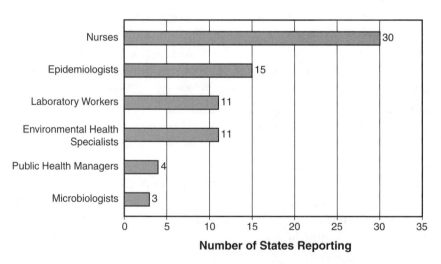

Source: Association of State and Territorial Health Officials (ASTHO). *State Public Health Employee Worker Shortage Report: A Civil Service Recruitment and Retention Crisis.* Available at: http://www.astho.org/pubs/Workforce-Survey-Report-2.pdf. Accessed April 11, 2006.

FIGURE 13-2 State Public Health Occupational Classes Most Affected by Worker Shortage

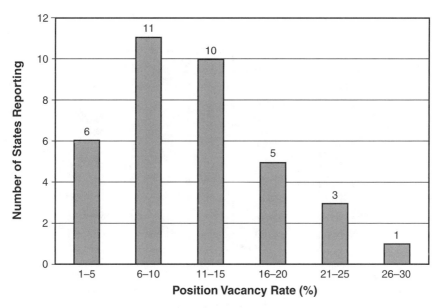

Source: Association of State and Territorial Health Officials (ASTHO). *State Public Health Employee Worker Shortage Report: A Civil Service Recruitment and Retention Crisis.* Available at: http://www.astho.org/pubs/Workforce-Survey-Report-2.pdf. Accessed April 11, 2006.

FIGURE 13-3 Position Vacancy Rates in the State Public Health Agencies

U.S. worker, which is 15% lower, or approximately 40 years. There are also higher percentages of public health employees who are eligible for retirement. This development can be seen as a positive trend, in that more job opportunities will be available to new graduates in health care and public health fields. However, the concern is that state and federal funding will not keep pace with the increase in both the numbers of employees needed and the higher salaries required to attract new employees.

Figure 13-2 indicates the critical shortages by occupational class in the United States. These shortages will persist in the form of unfilled positions in state public health agencies, as shown in Figure 13-3. Like other areas in health care, public health will experience critical shortages in many professional areas, such as epidemiologists, environmental health specialists, data analysts, public health nurses, and other occupations. In the face of the need for increased infrastructure, public health will also experience a significant shortage of professionals to manage the additional requirements and resources. These and other factors will ultimately create a situation characterized by high turnover of current employees due to the

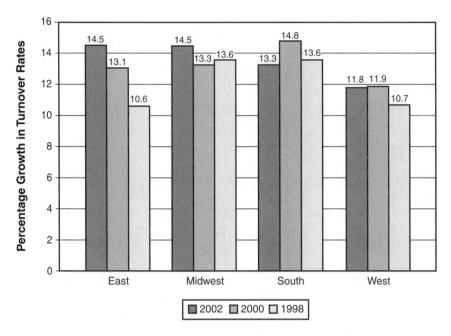

Source: Association of State and Territorial Health Officials (ASTHO). *State Public Health Employee Worker Shortage Report: A Civil Service Recruitment and Retention Crisis.* Available at: http://www.astho.org/pubs/Workforce-Survey-Report-2.pdf. Accessed April 11, 2006.

FIGURE 13-4 Turnover Rates for State Public Health Personnel, by Region and Year

additional workload and pressures created by public and governmental agencies to expand services, provide additional primary care to under-served populations, and improve public health infrastructure. The turnover rate appears to be steadily increasing or remaining high in many regions of the United States, as indicated in Figure 13-4. The increased demand for public health professionals will create even greater levels of competition within a shrinking healthcare workforce.[11] Ultimately, public health leaders will need to make salaries more competitive, improve educational opportunities, and increase outreach opportunities, if they hope to resolve the shortage of trained professionals in this field. See Figure 13-5.

Today's healthcare facilities often lack administrators with the skills needed to manage their human capital needs as well as match organizational strategic objectives with the future skill sets developing in a changing labor market. To correct these deficiencies, health services organizations must develop the competencies needed to assess the strate-

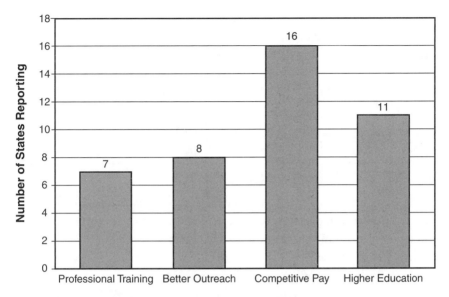

Source: Association of State and Territorial Health Officials (ASTHO). *State Public Health Employee Worker Shortage Report: A Civil Service Recruitment and Retention Crisis.* Available at: http://www.astho.org/pubs/Workforce-Survey-Report-2.pdf. Accessed April 11, 2006.

FIGURE 13-5 Keys to Solving the Public Health Workforce Challenges

gic needs of their organizations. Part of the solution lies in improving the other human resources management functions within their facilities.

A critical step in the process of preparing for the future will be to perform job analysis assessments for current positions within the organization—a review of current employee skills, and a determination of which are and are not needed. Can some skills be eliminated or shifted to other positions? Can positions be combined, eliminated, or transformed into more useful activities that mirror future requirements? Which employment skills/competencies will be needed in the next three to five years, based on the environmental assessment, and what gaps does the organization currently have? Can current skilled employees fill the identified gaps, or do these employees need additional training? Does the organization need to hire new employees who are better equipped to handle the future needs of the organization? Are employees required to think critically about their job tasks and be rewarded for improving their current position requirements? Unfortunately, few health services organizations take the time to analyze their current employee positions unless a critical problem occurs or downsizing becomes necessary. This scenario can be a recipe for disaster, in that it allows an organization to ignore its problems until the organization's back is against a wall. In the future, health services organizations will need to do a better job of proactively analyzing and reviewing all current employee positions by skills and tasks so as to integrate future job requirements into current workforce positions.

RECRUITMENT, SELECTION, AND RETENTION

Recruitment and retention issues of the future and employers' need to be sensitive to traditional family needs—such as two working parents, job security, travel, and family leave—must be carefully examined. How to attract and retain good employees is a critical concern that must be thoroughly addressed. HR managers will need to create more sophisticated tools for determining the fit of each individual worker with the entire organization. Instruments such as surveys, applications, and interviews must be developed that provide a more accurate picture of the motives and desires of potential job candidates to blend with the organization's culture and workforce. At the same time, emphasis should be on family recruitment and recruitment for longer periods (preferably for life). The employees of today and the future will place a high value on their families and family relationships. It is imperative for healthcare organizations to recognize this concern and to create family-friendly environments within their facilities. Providing benefits that attract families and friends will be very advantageous in the future. Providing education and promotion benefits to both employees and their families can also improve the organization's recruitment success and retention rate. In addition, healthcare managers must examine new forms of benefits for employees, such as job sharing and part-time employment opportunities.

Other recruitment issues revolve around the use of the Internet and other direct marketing efforts to attract employees. With an abundance of job search Web sites, efforts must be focused on using the right media to attract employees.

An examination of the hiring process should reflect the type of individuals recruited, the selection tools used, and the corporate culture.[6] Identifying and attracting new candidates at an early age—for example, in high school—and providing undergraduate and graduate scholarships to individuals in early career development stages to lock in future employees are both excellent recruiting tools. Use of new forms of attracting students and future employees through recruitment actions near recreational activities (high school, college, and professional sporting events) is a futuristic method of recruitment. Marketing to parents of potential employees is another way to attract professional workers. Advertising published awards, such as "Best Hospitals to Work For" or making the "Best Hospitals in the United States" list could also help attract employees. Recent studies have projected a shortage of 85,000–96,000 physicians by 2020. Some recruiting incentives offered especially to physicians include reimbursement of moving expenses, income guarantee, signing bonuses, salary guarantee, reimbursement of the recruitment fee, medical education repayment, and low-interest loans.[12]

Retention methods include adding benefits, such as daycare services, on-site primary care services, and travel benefits, to retain highly productive workers. Culture is a key ingredient to making the organization a great place to work.[13] Creating and leveraging the organization's image by branding, establishing high-achievement and recognition programs, partnering with universities and other instructional organizations, and providing family-friendly benefits are among the recruitment strategies that hold promise for the future.[14] Additionally, many organizations are getting employees more involved in their work design and giving them greater decision-making authority. Allowing employees to have more power and responsibility over their work environment makes them more satisfied and increases retention rates.[15]

Approximately 13% of nursing positions in the United States are currently vacant, and this percentage is projected to increase to 20% by 2015. RN positions topped the U.S. Bureau of Labor Statistics' 2003 list of occupations with the largest projected 10-year job growth. In addition, U.S. nursing schools had to turn down 15,994 qualified applicants for entry-level baccalaureate nursing programs in 2003–2004 because of the shortage of nursing teachers.[16] This has led to increased workloads for currently employed nurses, which directly relates to medical errors, quality of care, and job satisfaction. Hence, it is important to retain current nurses by creating better floor plans; offering flexible scheduling; giving nurses the autonomy and authority to delegate tasks that can be performed by workers at less skilled levels; reducing nursing workload and the amount of administrative paperwork by various technologies, such as electronic medication administration records (E-MARs); and creating a culture of nurse appreciation.[17, 18]

Contract Employees and Outsourcing

Contracts/agreements with employees and with service agencies, as opposed to direct-hire employees, should also be considered, along with their advantages and disadvantages relative to benefits, costs, and control issues. Many organizations are currently exploring contracting for employees and worker services rather than hiring full-time employees. Advantages of this practice include reduced requirements to pay large retirement benefits and other fringe benefits, including health, dental, vacation, and other benefits; the ability to eliminate workers on an at-will basis; and reduced burdens of recruitment, selection, training, and evaluation, which are transferred to the contractor or vendor. Disadvantages include concern for the morale of contracted employees; their isolation or a feeling of disconnectedness from other employees; their lack of loyalty to the organization; possible failure to meet exact requirements and skills; and failure to integrate with other employee groups. The use of contractual employees must be carefully evaluated, and all aspects considered prior to committing specific services to contract workers.

Outsourcing may provide opportunities for the healthcare organization to shift HR functions, such as payroll and taxes, to other entities, thus enabling the organization to focus more sharply on its core functions and operations. It will also help the organization in exploiting the skills and expertise of other, more capable organizations for rudimentary or routine tasks.[19] Outsourcing can facilitate the acquisition of the best technology, which in turn can improve performance. On the downside, outsourcing can reduce the organization's workforce knowledge and abilities, which can affect its ability to innovate in the future. Moreover, issues of dependency and loss of control need to be considered when entering the contract arena.[20] Organizations must consider both the advantages and disadvantages of outsourcing and then make the appropriate choices, based on their individual workforce and vision.

EDUCATION AND TRAINING

Training, education, and support priorities and unique opportunities must also be reevaluated for the future. New avenues of training and education should be considered, including use of distance learning, Internet connections, Web-based programs, teleconferencing, partnerships with universities, group learning activities, corporate training programs, in-house seminars by consultants, tuition assistance for employees, structured in-house training programs, tailoring specific training packages for the organization, and splitting of training fees with employees. Training programs offered to current employees and executives should be tailored to the new responsibilities these individuals are expected to take on following completion of the program.

Unfortunately, many organizations lack the ability to properly evaluate various training and education programs to ensure that they are getting quality programs for their money. For example, employers often fail to survey employees three to six months after a training seminar to examine whether the employees gained any skills or knowledge from the training program. Also, it is desirable to evaluate how effectively the knowledge gained has been applied. Failure to capture vital information on usefulness and quality ensures that employers will continue to waste precious resources on low-value education and training programs.

The practice of sending employees to expensive seminars and conferences in distant locations needs to be closely examined, as it becomes more difficult to fund these expensive endeavors. Healthcare leaders will need to weigh carefully the advantages and disadvantages of particular educational venues for training their employees. Less expensive alternatives may include targeted training sessions, either on the Internet or at the worksite, where expert facilitators can train groups of individuals in skills and competencies specifically needed by the organization. Facilitators and educators can assess the training and education needs of the various employees within an organization and then tailor specific education modules that will enhance learning and skill attainment for individual employees. This training method will not just save time and travel costs, but will prove infinitely more useful in terms of providing direct knowledge for specific tasks and overcoming organizational deficiencies.

Employees of the future will be required to master specific competencies in various clinical and nonclinical areas, rather than simply maintaining the routine skills and tasks for the position. Past methods of training an employee, which focused on how to maintain an existing database or perform a current clinical task, will be replaced by general competencies that require learning the latest information surrounding this functional expertise. Competency-based educational requirements are a more suitable way to ensure that an employee maintains the latest knowledge and abilities concerning a functional area, such as information systems management, financial accounting systems, or current records management procedures. Employees may be required to master many of these competencies on their own time to keep pace with their co-workers and remain competitive in their professions. Balancing training, education, work, interpersonal relations, and leisure time will be a difficult challenge for future employees.

Lastly, recent changes, modifications, and innovations relative to performance evaluation methodologies will be reviewed, along with group evaluations and reward opportunities. Modifications to evaluation systems include 360-degree evaluations; group evaluation systems; employee-developed evaluation systems; taking turns when assuming roles and duties, including provision of on-the-spot evaluations; blind review evaluations of supervisors from anonymous employees; and tying pay to performance, based on specific evaluations at the individual and group levels.

COMPENSATION AND BENEFITS

Future changes in compensation packages and innovative techniques to reward employees must be explored, including pay for performance, group evaluation and pay, and promoting employee ownership. These changes can lead to members of the workforce assuming greater responsibility and accountability for the performance of the entire organization. Employees who are rewarded not only for individual performance, but also for team and organizational performance, can significantly enhance the success of the entire organization.[21]

Hospitals that align salaries and bonuses with their operational goals (a combination of financial and human goals) have been found to be successful in promoting employee motivation and involvement within the organization.[22] However, a survey conducted to assess practices to promote employee recognition revealed that the top 10 measures involved praise and appreciation rather than gifts or other tangible rewards. Indeed, the top three measures were support and involvement, personal praise, and autonomy and authority. A variety of simple measures—recognizing employee birthdays via cards, celebrating employee appreciation week, public recognition for high performers, allowing employees to select their colleagues for spot awards, and earning points for annual recognition awards—could prove to be very useful compensation tools to promote employee commitment and satisfaction. To make it interesting for employees, recognition awards or entertaining activities can be planned.[23]

While monetary rewards can be extremely valuable in compensating highly productive employees, nonmonetary reward systems can also serve as powerful motivators. Some companies are using incentives to help employees stay healthy and use fewer of their benefits. For example, Logan Aluminum, a Kentucky-based aluminum plant, uses innovative compensation and benefit mechanisms. Logan Aluminum's consumer-based healthcare insurance and incentives program is extremely effective in changing employee lifestyles and behaviors. The company provides incentive payments to employees if improvements in employee health, plant safety, and utilization of fitness programs are realized during the previous quarter. As a result of these innovative health promotion and consumer-driven health insurance programs, Logan Aluminum has experienced reductions in smoking, alcohol consumption, obesity, cholesterol indicators, accidents, and overall improvements in health indicators (blood pressure and pulse), diet, exercise, and seatbelt use. With these and similar lifestyle improvement mechanisms, other organizations can realize improvements in retention, morale, and healthy employee lifestyles.[24] Such innovative incentives will ultimately lead to increased paid incentives to workers, improved health outcomes, and reduced healthcare costs for the organization.

Another area of possible improvement in benefits is associated with recent legal mandates that have affected the criteria for employee leave and other benefits. Recent changes in the legal and regulatory environment include labor agreement changes, employee assistance programs and benefits, Americans with Disabilities Act requirements, and the Family and Medical Leave Act (FMLA). Ethical ramifications regarding how employers should plan to accommodate and meet employee needs, regardless of the regulatory requirements, should be examined closely. For example, employers will need to plan for accommodations in medical leave for new fathers and other family medical requirements for both male and female employees. Managers will also need to closely monitor supervisory and other working relationships of employees to ensure that sexual harassment, discrimination, and other Equal Employment Opportunity (EEO) policies are not violated. As more employees are changed to independent contractors or current employees are asked to work with external vendors, managers will assume greater responsibility for ensuring the welfare and safety of their employees. The responsibility for monitoring inappropriate behavior of independent contractors working in an organization, for example, will create new managerial challenges. Managers will need to develop, implement, and continuously monitor the activities of external workers inside their facilities. Likewise, managers will need to heighten their awareness of their employees' behavior outside the physical facility for possible EEO violations. In the future, employee behavior outside the workplace will be considered as important as behavior in the workplace. Employee behavior, both on and off duty, will be seen as a reflection of the organization's culture and image.

STRATEGIC PLANNING

Human resources management has a critical role in organizational planning. It must focus on the strategic positioning of the human resources management office, its functions, and the changes needed to support quality initiatives in the healthcare organization. Some of the key topics to be addressed by the HR team include succession planning, job sculpting, and quality improvement initiatives.

Planning for human resources in the context of strategic planning for the entire organization is a critical activity for any healthcare organization. Human resources issues that must be considered include assessments of both the internal and external environments. The organization must determine how future needs in the external environment, in terms of both opportunities and threats, will affect human resources assets. Will health care be delivered in a different setting or using different methods? Will healthcare organizations drastically change their mission, vision, and goals, thus requiring reengineering of human performance systems and job redesign for most employees? Will advances in technology demand new career paths for healthcare workers? Will worker shortages occur in critical clinical and nonclinical areas of the future? Will pay-for-performance and other compensation mechanisms change? Will employees perform their duties via the Internet in a home-based setting? Will retirement systems become so expensive that contracting and temporary employment agencies come to dominate the healthcare workforce?

To answer these questions, one needs merely to look at changes that have occurred in the last five years. Outsourcing of personnel and services has become the norm for many healthcare institutions. Retirement systems, unionization issues, critical personnel shortages, employee health and other benefits, Internet applications, advanced technologies, and changing organizational missions have all created opportunities (or threats) that have prompted healthcare organizations to modify their current work practices. These challenges have squeezed margins in such a manner that healthcare organizations must examine new avenues of delivering healthcare services with fewer full-time personnel. Leasing turnkey operations or outsourcing specific services and activities to contactors who guarantee a level of performance and service to healthcare organizations for a specific price can be attractive alternatives to large employee operations that ensure employees a lifetime of retirement salary and health benefits.

Another critical area of human resources management that must be pondered is the emotional intelligence of the health services workforce. The term "emotional intelligence" was introduced by John Mayer and Peter Salovey in 1990 and further developed by Dan Goleman in his book *Emotional Intelligence.* Emotional intelligence and competencies are the skills that prepare individuals to interact in a professional and mature manner within the work setting. Goleman identifies four components of emotional intelligence: self-awareness, self-management, social awareness, and social skills.[25, 26] An assessment of the emotional intelligence of each employee should be performed, as well as the need to build leadership skills in the organization, such as coaching and mentoring employees, orientation of new employees, and employee empowerment. Numerous examples can be cited of facilities and organizations that are implementing human resources management activities—such as excellence in coaching and mentoring programs—to enhance their future success, as well as handling the difficult problems that are currently developing in health care relative to employee workforce issues.

In the future, it will be absolutely necessary to develop, maintain, and evaluate an employee's emotional intelligence. Employers will insist on hiring and retaining health services employees who have not only the emotional intelligence skills defined by Goleman, but also the skills to detect and nurture the emotional intelligence of teams and co-workers. These skills will empower employees to be both valuable leaders and effective team players within their organizations. The employee's ability to maintain his or her own emotional intelligence, and his or her skill to develop the emotional intelligence of others, will dramatically improve an organization's culture and, ultimately, its competitive advantage. Organizations must strive to retain employees who can work together and make adjustments in working relationships and personal dynamics as needed to satisfy employees at both tangible and intangible levels.

HR managers will need to move beyond traditional thinking and the use of traditional reward systems to improve workforce performance. Healthcare leaders will need to instill a sense of pride in the culture of the organization. High-performing employees and organizations are not motivated solely by traditional perks and reward systems. Instead, they have a sense of pride and ownership in the organization, and they work hard to maintain that image. They are proud of their organization and introduce themselves by using the organization's name rather than their own particular area or specialized skill area. Organizations such as Mayo Clinic, Cleveland Clinic, St. Jude's Hospital, Mount Sinai Hospital, and Sloan-Kettering Hospital are just a few of the outstanding healthcare facilities whose reputations for quality and excellence precede them. At these and similar institutions, employees are proud of where they work and align their interests and priorities with their organizations. They have a strong sense of loyalty to the organization and dedicate themselves to preserving its reputation for excellence. The healthcare leaders of tomorrow must work to instill this same sense of pride into their own organizational culture if they want to transform their facilities into the elite organizations of the future, setting an example as caring and concerned leaders who support their employees and provide an atmosphere of trust, compassion, and quality effort in every aspect of care. These organizations have a much greater chance of achieving this "brand" level of excellence if they are able to instill these attributes in their employees and in their corporate cultures.

Another key issue for human resources management in the future is the generation gap in the workforce. In the next decade, many organizations will experience the obvious differences between various generations within the workforce. There will be groups of individuals who will fall into traditional generational groups: baby boomers, generation X, and generation Y. Each generational group will have its own value sets, priorities, strengths, weaknesses, motivational drivers, and communication skills. Numerous disconnects will inevitably occur between traditional human resources management mechanisms and novel approaches implemented to obtain desired outcomes related to improving employee performance. One size or one policy will not fit all in this mixed generational environment. Healthcare managers will need to individually assess the motivational drivers and values of these distinct employee groups in their drive to achieve success throughout the organization. Modification and reengineering of human resources policies, procedures, and reward systems will be needed to achieve buy-in of all employee groups. Additionally, the disparate employee groups will need to be assimilated and accommodated by one another if team efforts are to be successful. Healthcare leaders will need to show tolerance and sympathy toward all generational groups so as to promote harmony in the workplace. The value systems of each group will need to be examined and communicated to all employees with the goal of improving understanding and awareness of the whole organization. Emphasis on intangible benefits and corporate values will need to be merged with individual value sets to garner collective support for future initiatives. Only by integrating the differences among various generational groups and the organization's goals can the future success of the entire organization be realized.

CONCLUSION

This final chapter has attempted to provide insight into future possibilities in the area of human resources management for health services organizations. Numerous economic, political, technological, social, and regulatory trends will significantly affect the management of vital human resources in the future. Outsourcing, recruitment and retention, training and education, compensation, and continuous quality improvement are specific areas that must be carefully examined. Useful strategies may include performing a gap analysis for the organization, evaluating the emotional intelligence of the workforce, bridging the generational diversity gap, and instilling pride in the corporate fabric of the organization; these strategies represent promising ways to improve future success and performance. While no single recommendation can ever ensure a successful future for any organization, to avoid the future by preserving the status quo will most assuredly lead to failure.

REFERENCES

1. Center for Medicare & Medicaid Services. *National Healthcare Expenditures Projections: 2003–2013.* Available at: cms.hhs.gov.
2. Reinhardt U. *Future Trends in American Healthcare: Micro-Economic Misery on a Sea of Macro-Economic Wealth.* A keynote presentation given at the Annual Association of University Programs in Health Administration, San Diego, CA: June 2004.
3. Federal Reserve. *Federal Reserve Release.* May 16, 2000.
4. AHA Hospital Statistics. 1999–2004 editions. Chicago: Health Forum, LLC, an affiliate of the American Hospital Association.
5. Casey A, Drazen E, Metzger J, Patrino K. *Eleven Critical Success Factors for Implementing Electronic Medical Records.* GE Medical Systems. Available at: http://www.medicalogic.com/emr/user experience/eleven_factors.html.
6. Ginter PM, Swayne LE, Duncan WJ. *Strategic Management of Healthcare Organizations.* Fourth Edition. Cambridge: Blackwell Publishers; 2002.
7. American Hospital Association Annual Survey Database, 2002.
8. Conn J. Faculty shortage limiting nursing school growth. *Modern Healthcare.* December 15, 2004.
9. Greenburn M, Flores G. Professional interpreters needed to help hospitals treat immigrant patients. *Modern Healthcare.* 2004; 34(18):21.
10. O'Brien-Pallas L, Baumann A, Donner G, Tomblin Murphy G, Lochhaas-Gerlach J, Luba M. Forecasting models for human resources in healthcare. *Journal of Advanced Nursing.* 2001; 33:120–129.
11. Association of State and Territorial Health Officials (ASTHO). *State Public Health Employee Worker Shortage Report: A Civil Service Recruitment and Retention Crisis.*
12. Romano M. Doc surplus no more. *Modern Healthcare.* 2003; 33(41):16.
13. May EL. Are people your priority? *Healthcare Executive.* 2004; 19(4):8–10, 12–16.
14. Abrams. Employee retention strategies: lessons from the best. *Healthcare Executive.* 2004; 19(4):18–22.
15. Haley F. Mutual benefit. *Fast Company.* October 2004. Issue 87.
16. Becker C. Workforce report 2004: taking initiative on training. *Modern Healthcare.* 2004; 34(24):26, 34.
17. Morrissey J. Out to set the record. *Modern Healthcare.* 2003; 33(42):28–32, 35.
18. Reilly P. Recruiting and retaining nurses. *Modern Healthcare.* November 24, 2003.
19. Rosto L. The outsourcing option. *Advance.* 2003; 51:53–54.
20. Byrne J. Has outsourcing gone too far? *Business Week.* April 1, 1996:26–28.
21. Joint Commission on Accreditation of Healthcare Organizations. Principles for the construct of pay-for-performance programs. *Joint Commission News Release.* November 22, 2004.
22. Reilly P. Perking up. *Modern Healthcare.* 2003; 33(31):24–28, 34.

23. Garvey C. Meaningful tokens of appreciation: cash awards aren't the only way to motivate your workforce. *HR Magazine.* 2004; 49:8.

24. Watkins C, Wainright C, Lovely T. *Logan Aluminum—A Dynamic Approach to Worksite Health Promotion.* Wellness Councils of America. 2005. Available at: http://www.welcoa.org/freesources/pdf/logan_alum_case_study.pdf. Accessed April 7, 2006.

25. Goleman D. *Emotional Intelligence: Why It Can Matter More Than IQ.* New York: Bantam Books; 1995.

26. Goleman D. *Working with Emotional Intelligence.* New York: Bantam Doubleday Dell Publishing Group, Inc; 1998.

Index

Note: Page numbers with *f* indicate figures, *t* indicate tables.

401